HOME

A Technical Manual For The Professional Nurse

CARE

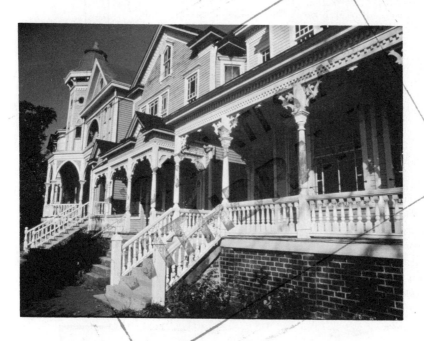

Christine A. Rovinski, RN, MSN
Deborah K. Zastocki, RN, MA, EdM

1989
W. B. SAUNDERS COMPANY
Harcourt Brace Jovanovich, Inc.
Philadelphia · London · Toronto · Montreal · Sydney · Tokyo

W. B. SAUNDERS COMPANY
Harcourt Brace Jovanovich, Inc.

The Curtis Center
Independence Square West
Philadelphia, PA 19106

Library of Congress Cataloging-in-Publication Data

Rovinski, Christine A.

Home care: a technical manual for the professional nurse/Christine A.
Rovinski, Deborah K. Zastocki.

p. cm.

Bibliography: p.

1. Home nursing.   2. Nursing care plans.   I. Zastocki, Deborah K.
II. Title.   [DNLM: 1. Home Care Services—nurses' instruction.
WY 115 R875h]

RT61.R68 1989   649'.8—dc19
DNLM/DLC   88–26319
ISBN 0–7216–2449–9

Editor: Ilze Rader
Developmental Editor: Martha Tanner
Designer: Terri Siegel
Production Manager: Bob Butler
Manuscript Editor: David Indest
Illustration Coordinator: Lisa Lambert
Cover Artist: Michelle Maloney

Home Care: A Technical Manual for the Professional Nurse   ISBN 0–7216–2449–9

Last digit is the print number: 9   8   7   6   5   4   3   2   1

To my parents Frank and Jo Rovinski.

*To my parents Louis and Helen Zastocki
and in memory of my grandmother Harriet Krucker.*

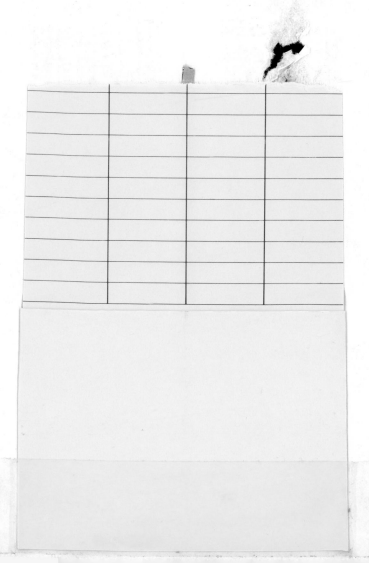

Reviewers

Linda L. Bacon, R.N., M.S.N., O.C.N.
Good Samaritan Medical Center
Zanesville, Ohio

Carolyn Barbier, R.N., B.S.N.
Hospital Home Health Care
Albuquerque, New Mexico

Ann Blues, Ed.D.
Institute for Health Care Education
Portland, Oregon

Barbara Buturusis, M.S.N.
Medical Personnel Pool
Darien, Illinois

Sheron Chisholm, M.S.N.
Michigan Home Health Care, Inc.
Traverse City, Michigan

Davina J. Gosnell, R.N., Ph.D.
Kent State University
School of Nursing
Kent, Ohio

Susan Mullee Herbert, R.N., M.Ed., C.D.E.
Diabetes Education Consultant
Denville, New Jersey

Barbara Husted, Director
Memorial Medical Home Care
Ludington, Michigan

Kathleen Jones, M.S.N.
Valley Home Health Services
Peru, Illinois

Alice D. Maffongelli, M.S.N.
Sheboygan Visiting Nurse Association
Sheboygan, Wisconsin

G. Therese Meyers, M.S.
Visiting Nurse Association
San Antonio, Texas

Madelyn L. Miscally, B.S.N.
Home Health Agency of Chapel Hill
Chapel Hill, North Carolina

Carol M. Patton, R.N., B.S.N., M.S.N.
Wheeling College
Department of Nursing
Wheeling, West Virginia

Debra L. Pinkerton, R.N., B.S.N.
Allied Health Services
Toledo, Ohio

Linda Piper, B.S.N.
Dickinson Iron District Health Department
Iron Mountain, Michigan

Corinne Strandell, Ph.D., R.N.
Independent Practice
Rehabilitation, Home Care and Education
Greenfield, Wisconsin

Libet D. Streiff, R.N.-C., M.S.N., F.N.P.
Yale University
School of Nursing
New Haven, Connecticut

Karen A. Walborn, M.N.
Hospice of Northern Virginia
Arlington, Virginia

Contributors

Susan Havens Lang, R.N., B.S.N., M.S.
Director of Nursing Operations
Community Health Care of North Jersey Incorporated
Orange, New Jersey
Home Care Nursing Documentation

Patricia Partington Murphy, R.N., M.S.N.
Clinical Specialist in Oncology/Nurse Educator
Chemotherapy Care Plan

Suzanne B. Sblendorio, R.N., B.S.N., M.A.
Executive Director
Community Health Care of North Jersey Incorporated
Orange, New Jersey
Productivity and Quality Assurance in Home Care Nursing

Anne S. Shefchik, R.N., B.S.N., E.T.
Program Supervisor
St. Clare's-Riverside Medical Center Division
Tri-Hospital Home Health Care Program
Passaic, New Jersey
Ostomy Care Plan (Colostomy, Ileostomy, Urostomy)
Colostomy Irrigation Procedure

About the Authors

Christine A. Rovinski, R.N., M.S.N. received her B.S. in Nursing from Villanova University, Villanova, Pennsylvania, and her M.S. in Nursing at Seton Hall University, South Orange, New Jersey. She has worked as a staff nurse, oncology clinical specialist, research associate, nursing instructor, and staff development coordinator in a variety of clinical and academic settings. She was administrator of Hospice of Morris County, Morristown, New Jersey, successfully leading the agency to become the state's first Medicare-certified hospice. She is currently Assistant Professor in Nursing at Indian River Community College, Fort Pierce, Florida.

Deborah K. Zastocki, R.N., M.A., Ed.M. received her B.S. in Nursing from the University of Rhode Island, Kingston, Rhode Island, and her M.A. in Nursing Education and Ed.M. in Community Health Nursing from Teachers College, Columbia University, New York. Her previous positions include staff nurse; nursing care coordinator; director of education, training, and research, including community health education; director of specialty nursing, including a skilled-nursing, long-term ventilator unit; and an academic appointment as an adjunct faculty member at Kean College, Union, New Jersey, teaching the well family and community health program. She has served on a professional advisory committee for a home health care agency. She is currently vice president of Nursing at Newton Memorial Hospital, Newton, New Jersey, which is associated with a home care agency.

Preface

Home Care: A Technical Manual for the Professional Nurse is a clinical resource of home health care plans, technical procedures, and documentation guidelines that exemplify skilled nursing care. The manual is a field reference that enhances home health nursing productivity, promotes better patient home care, and guides nurses who need to adapt their acute-care experience to the home.

Home and community health care agencies share the need to document nursing care so that full third-party reimbursement is received. Often it is assumed that greater efficiency and number of visits result in corresponding increases in revenues. Increased productivity, however, does not always add to remuneration. Reimbursement depends largely on the full written description, composed by the professional nurse, of the delivered care. *Home Care* helps the nurse develop skill in documenting care efficiently and accurately and in a reimbursable manner.

In addition to its use in the home care sector, *Home Care* is a reference book for health libraries, colleges of nursing, and intermediate and acute-care facilities. Nurses who are in either external degree or upper division programs, needing to review community oriented procedures and patient education materials, will find the book useful as a clinical resource.

Section I of the book contains three chapters that provide a foundation for the home care nurse. Chapter 1 describes the elements of home care as a nursing specialty. Skilled nursing is presented from the perspective of case management in terms of assessment, nursing diagnoses, planning (with definition of process indicators), intervention (technical skills, teaching, counseling, and coordination) and evaluation/therapeutic achievement. In Chapter 2, nursing activities are further defined as measurable nursing products. Productivity, quality assurance, and standards of practice are also discussed. Chapter 3 is devoted to documentation and the key indicators for successful third-party reimbursement. It features phraseology that concisely conveys skilled nursing, a requirement for favorable intermediary review.

Section II is divided into 14 units containing care plans, procedures, and resources. Although the units in this book are categorized and cross-referenced by medical diagnoses, the home care plan model that is used is closely aligned with the nursing process.

The care plans within each unit promote visualization of care planning as health status alteration. Each care plan includes nursing diagnoses, process indicators, nursing interventions, and therapeutic achievements. The home care nurse can select from these the information required to write a care plan that not only addresses the needs of the patient but also conveys skilled nursing care. The home care nurse's assessment provides the parameters for tailoring each care plan to the unique situation of any patient/family system. The nursing diagnoses, process indicators, and nursing interventions are presented in an open format that is designed to assist the home health care nurse in the creation of individualized patient/family care plans. The importance of individualization is underscored by the absence of designated time frames. The home care nurse must supply the appropriate time frames based on assessment of the particular situation. It is creative thinking that enables the nurse to use the book to translate the actual level of skilled care required by the patient into the language of reimbursement.

In writing a care plan appropriate to a particular individual, the home care nurse may wish to refer to other relevant care plans, procedures, and resources in the book. For this reason, cross-references to related information have been provided in a box at the beginning of each care plan. The alphabetical listing on the inside front and back covers enables the home care nurse to locate the care plans, procedures, and resources easily. In addition, cross-references to related patient instruction sheets are provided in a box at the end of each care plan. These instructions are found in the companion book, *Home Care: Patient and Family Instructions.*

Selected units have care plans composed of generic information from clustered medical diagnoses. Distinctive characteristics from the clustered diagnoses are addressed in separate care plans. Pediatric considerations are also included in some care plans as reminders about the special needs of infants and children.

Procedures most critical to each health status alteration are also in Section II. The procedures enable the professional home care nurse to provide a level of concentrated/ complex patient care that has previously been associated with the acute hospital setting. All of the procedures highlight essential components so that patient/family teaching is complete, consistent, and easily organized. Within each unit of Section II, resources related to the care plans and procedures in the unit are provided.

The appendices at the end of the book include a bibliography, which provides guides for nursing investigation of special interest areas; conversion tables; and a community resource list, in which names and addresses of self-help groups and specialty organizations are included, with space provided for filling in information about local groups.

In summary, *Home Care: A Technical Manual for the Professional Nurse* is an assemblage of home care material in a new, comprehensive format. The features include the following:

1. A process for structuring nursing documentation for favorable intermediary review.
2. Highlighting the prevalent needs of home care clients.
3. Adaptation of high technologic procedures to the home setting.
4. Identification of essential components of procedures to facilitate patient/family teaching that is complete, consistent, and easily organized.
5. A process for transforming generic procedures into agency-specific resources.
6. Facilitating reference by separating nursing procedures from nursing care plans.
7. A format that guides the development of the beginning home care nurse and supplements the knowledge base of the experienced practitioner.

The companion book of patient and family instructions in a format ready for photocopying can be ordered from

W. B. Saunders Company
Order Fulfillment
6277 Sea Harbor Drive
Orlando, FL 32821
1-800-782-4479
1-305-345-2525 (Florida)

Acknowledgments

We would like to acknowledge the following for their support, help, and encouragement: Christopher J. Tighe for his dedication and patience in the preparation and typing of the manuscript; Jeanette Merkl for assistance in gathering resources; friends and colleagues at the Hospital Center at Orange, St. Clare's-Riverside Medical Center and St. Clare's Self-Help Clearinghouse, Denville, and Newton Memorial Hospital, Newton, New Jersey, and the many reviewers who have provided professional expertise.

A special acknowledgment goes to our families and friends for their unflagging confidence in this project and their understanding whenever the book came first.

Contents

Principles of Home Care Nursing

SECTION ONE

1

Home Care Nursing

"Home health service is that component of comprehensive health care whereby services are provided to individuals and families in their places of residence for the purpose of promoting, maintaining or restoring health or minimizing the effects of illness and disability. Services appropriate to the needs of the individual patient and family are planned, coordinated and made available by an agency or institution, organized for the delivery of health care through the use of employed staff, contractual arrangements or a combination of administrative patterns. These services are provided under a plan of care which includes appropriate service components such as, but not limited to, medical care, dental care, nursing, physical therapy, speech therapy, occupational therapy, social work, nutrition, homemaker, home health aide, transportation, laboratory services, medical equipment and supplies."[1]

Using this definition as a common point of reference, both the evolution of and the future trends in home care can be viewed.

EVOLUTION OF HOME CARE

From a historical perspective, nursing's role in caring for patients in their homes has been significant. Under the direction of nurses, agencies in the 1800s provided skilled nursing care to patients of all ages with both acute and chronic needs.[2] Consistent with a nursing model of responding to health care needs throughout the health/illness continuum, agency services focused on illness prevention and health promotion. It was no accident that terms such as public health and community health featured "health" as a theme for services.

Prior to 1965, ". . . it was not seen as necessary or even appropriate for physicians to direct home care."[3] The introduction in 1965 of Medicare and Medicaid legislation impacted upon home health care by shifting the direction and the focus of care to a medical model. Illness prevention and health promotion services became nonreimbursable and were viewed as nonessential; for many nurses, the limitations in the scope of services marked the development of a conflict in values. It became clear that regulation/legislation could change the focus and nature of services dramatically. The 1965 legislation requires that the physician verify the need for services and write orders, including frequency and duration; yet, the physician rarely sees the patient in the home. The services are provided by nurses and other nonphysician professionals and paraprofessionals leading to "split accountability."[4] In essence, the home care professional staff is given a great deal of discretion in the actual care delivery, yet is dependent on the orders of a physician who is not in direct contact with the patient. The nurse is challenged and, at times, frustrated to practice within a framework of medical necessity while attempting to respond to the patient's needs in a wholistic manner.

In many cases, quality of life is a major issue in providing care. In chronic illness, as compared with acute illness, it can be difficult to measure improvement in the disease and in the effectiveness of treatment. Success may be described as the controlled progression of the disease, the patient's expressed satisfaction with the quality of life or both. With the projected increase in the elderly population, the home health care nurse will be confronted with a significant number of elderly patients with chronic illness.

In 1983 a prospective payment system, Diagnostic Related Groups, was introduced for acute care Medicare patients. This system stimulated a shifting of increasing numbers of patients with high acuity levels out of acute care facilities into their homes, extended care/skilled nursing facilities or both. The home health care field responded with additional development of home based (lower cost) high technology for the more acutely ill patient population. Home health care nursing met the challenge of "high tech" while maintaining "high touch."

SCOPE OF SERVICES

It is evident, in reviewing the dynamics of home health care's evolution, that the trend is one of growing diversity and scope of home health care services. For simplicity, most home health care patients can be placed in one of two categories based upon the focus of care as follows: (1) those needing medically oriented service and products and (2) those needing wellness and self-care assistance.[5]

Discharged acute care patients as well as long-term care/disabled patients typically require more medically focused care. Home health care provides the vital linking of services enabling the ill and disabled to live outside of institutions. Medically focused home health care is based upon physician's orders and offers high technology equipment and services, such as nutritional support (oral, enteral, parenteral), intravenous therapy (antibiotics, chemotherapy, blood transfusions), renal dialysis, respiratory support (oxygen, related treatments, ventilators) and rehabilitation. Meeting established criteria and obtaining physician's orders are prerequisites for third party reimbursement.

The demand for wellness and self-care services and products is controlled by people who are health oriented consumers. Many of these services have not been reimbursed by third party payers and a physician's order usually is not needed. Health promotion services and products include health promotion education (nutrition, stress management, smoking cessation), exercise and equipment, self-improvement material and self-testing/screening/diagnostic equipment. Supportive services, such as homemaking, counselling, security homebound communication devices and general assistance with daily living, are needed by both groups. The demand for supportive services is predicted to grow as the population ages and the availability of family members as caretakers diminishes. Restrictive third party reimbursement remains an issue.

With the diversity of needs for services, it is easy to understand the race to enter the home health care field. In addition to the traditional not-for-profit and Medicare certified home health agencies, such as visiting nurse associations and public health nursing, dramatic growth has occurred in hospital-based programs, in private not-for-profit agencies and in proprietary for-profit groups, such as major health care corporations, temporary staffing agencies, private home care services, nursing homes and durable medical equipment/supply companies. This variety in agencies produces considerable lack of uniformity concerning services offered, skills of nurses, types of patients served and focus of care. Home health care, it would seem, has evolved from a homogeneous to a heterogeneous field.

Increasing physician acceptance and utilization of treatments and protocols in the home, along with increasing availability/adaptability of technology, have fostered growth of both products and support services. Agencies are confronted with the need to provide 7 days a week, 24 hours a day admission and visit capabilities. The rapid growth of the industry has created a market for entrepreneurs who desire to provide direct patient services/equipment as well as to offer contractual support services to agencies. Competition among those offering services and products is inevitable. The goal shared by all is to maximize third party reimbursement.

THIRD PARTY REIMBURSEMENT

The third party reimbursement mandates of home health care suggest an emphasis on patient focused treatment, minimizing the family orientation of the nurse: medical model treatment versus prevention and health promotion; cost effectiveness (productivity); increasing documentation, reporting, accountability and quality assurance requirements; and gradually more restrictive interpretation of Medicare home benefits.

Cost containment efforts by the government, third party payers and employers continue to fuel competition. The agency offering the lowest cost may more likely receive special contracts to provide services and products. Internal agency cost constraints will be additionally impacted, if the prospective payment system methodology is applied to home health care reimbursement.[6] The change from a cost based system requires efficiency; it requires delivering only absolutely necessary services and products in order to keep costs to a minimum. If the agency's cost to treat the patient is less than the established reimbursed amount, those monies become profit for the agency. In prospective payment systems, if the agency's cost to treat the patient is higher, the agency is faced with a loss; the patient cannot be billed for the difference. The introduction of the prospective payment system will require agencies and staff to understand the system, to work together and to develop creative strategies in order to survive.

HOME HEALTH CARE AS A NURSING SPECIALTY

Home health care nursing, as a specialty area of professional nursing practice, is in the process of evolving as is the field of home health care. Home health care nurses are developing expertise in clinical specialties and are establishing networks with consultants for periodic referrals in areas such as diabetes, gerontology, hospice, intravenous therapy and high technology products and services. Successful adaptation of acute care technologies to the home setting requires the unique knowledge base of the home health care nurse. The home health care nurse must maintain the patient advocate role and must be able to balance technology, therapeutic interventions and skilled nursing with preservation of the patient's/family's quality of life. By drawing upon multiple theoretical models, such as systems, self-care and adaptation theories, the home health care nurse creates a unique framework to guide his or her practice. The home health care nurse, in conjunction with other members of the health care team, strives to

1. Restore the patient's health and to assist the patient's return to a previous level of functioning as appropriate.

2. Maintain the patient's health and to preserve the patient's functional abilities and independence.

3. Promote the patient's health and to minimize the effects of illness.

4. Improve the patient's health and to help the patient achieve a higher level of functioning than previously existed.[7]

In order to accomplish these nursing goals, the nurse combines case management skills with the application of the professional skills of assessing, diagnosing, planning, intervening and evaluating in the care plan. Effective case management requires the ability to

1. Function autonomously, to make decisions, to solve problems and to manage emergency situations in the home.
2. Consult, collaborate, coordinate and direct other health care providers, contracted equipment/service providers and community resources and to decide when to contact the primary health care provider.
3. Develop a plan of care to assist the patient/family to achieve clearly defined/measurable patient centered outcomes.
   a. The predictive outcomes include an anticipated date of resolution.
   b. Negotiation among the patient, family and nurse is used to determine expectations.
4. Ability to "think interactionally" (to think of family dynamics).[8]
5. Implement appropriate protocols for all procedures and equipment utilized.
6. Communicate verbally (interviewing, teaching, providing feedback) and in writing (documentation of skilled care and patient response to care provided by oneself and other health care providers).
7. Function effectively in regard to cost with an understanding of the economics of legislation and regulatory issues.

The challenge for the nurse as case manager is to maintain coordination of the team's activities so that care procedes in a goal directed manner, in that there is a sequential, purposeful, organized plan of events. Case management skills depend upon the nurse's ability to apply the nursing process so that goals and actions of services are complementary and reflect cooperative care planning.

The Home Care Model translates the nursing process into a framework for home health care nursing. Skilled nursing is made operational as assessment/nursing diagnoses, planning with definition of process indicators, intervention (technical skills, teaching, counselling and coordination) and evaluation/therapeutic achievement (Table 1–1).

Assessment/Nursing Diagnoses

Assessment of the patient and family includes biopsychosocial and environmental status as well as functional abilities as predictors of needs (Table 1–2). During data

Table 1–1
Nursing Process as Applied to the Home Care Model

Nursing Process	Parameters	Home Care Model
Assessment/Nursing Diagnosis	Recognition of biopsychosocial patterns	Assessment/Nursing Diagnosis
	Organization and labeling of patterns in practice domains	
Planning	Statement of outcomes in measurable patient/family behaviors	Planning/Process Indicators
Interventions	Selection of therapeutic nursing actions	Interventions
Evaluation/Resolution	Measurement of clinically significant changes and quantification of patient/family stabilization	Evaluation/Therapeutic Achievement

Table 1–2
Assessment Guidelines

Biopsychosocial
  Physical assessment of body systems
  Ethnicity/culture/language/race/religion
  Socioeconomic status
  Status of support systems/caregiver support
Environmental
  Safety of home/community
  Occupational issues
Functional Abilities/Limitations
PHYSICAL/PSYCHOMOTOR AREAS
  Dexterity
  Senses (impaired)
  Mobility/activities permitted, use of aids
  Body system functioning (impaired) such that it impacts upon activity and homebound status (i.e., dyspnea
    or bowel/bladder incontinence)
MENTAL/COGNITIVE AREAS
  Age/development status
  Functional literacy/learned skills/education level/knowledge level (e.g., of diagnosis and treatment regimen,
    disease progress, time orientation/memory/attention span)
  Conceptualization/discrimination, decision-making
EMOTIONAL/AFFECTIVE AREAS
  Health beliefs/values/practices
  Definition of health illness
  Self-concept/self-value/self-discipline
  Motivation/willingness to engage in care, acceptance of body functioning/ability to work with body and its
    parts

collection, findings are classified into positive and negative categories (Fig. 1–1). Positive findings are the patient's/family's strengths; these are capitalized on during the intervention phase of the process. These strengths can serve to facilitate the resolution of the patient's problem. Negative findings are the patient's/family's limitations, deficits or weaknesses. If the patient and family are coping with these negative findings, no action is warranted. If coping is ineffective, these limitations form the basis for the nursing diagnostic statement and are critical for establishing eligibility for service; negative findings form the basis for favorable reimbursement. By sorting assessment data into positive and negative findings, nursing diagnoses and process indicators become directly related to the negative findings.

Figure 1–1. Classification of findings during data collection. (Courtesy of Suzanne Sblendorio.)

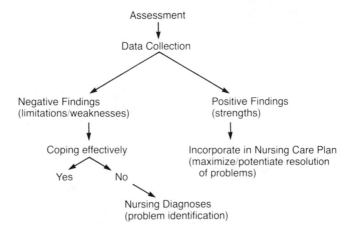

Planning/Process Indicators

As part of the planning process, it is critical to identify whether nursing can effect change (Fig. 1–2). Nursing diagnoses represent patient needs but may not address what is realistic/achievable within each unique patient/family system. The home health care nurse analyzes each patient/family system to develop a plan that focuses resources to areas where changes can be actualized and patient needs can be best met. Definition of the process indicators provides direction for structuring nursing interventions.

Intervention

The positive findings from the assessment are incorporated into the intervention strategies to maximize the resolution of the identified problems. Interventions, prescriptions for care, are viewed in terms of technical skills, teaching, counselling and coordination.

Technical/clinical skills in an environment of increasing "high tech" in the home require continuing education and ongoing documentation of proficiency. Skill requirements vary greatly related to the practice situation and availability of resources. Clinical competence is assumed in the practice setting and is not specifically addressed.

Teaching is directed at achievement of behavior change; therefore, objectives are phrased in terms of patient/family behavior. Successful adult learning is accomplished through mutual goal setting and patient/family contracting. Facilitating a child's participation in goal setting and achievement is equally important. Patient/family progress toward goal achievement should be documented regularly. A few basic principles of learning are

1. Learning is more effective when the learner feels the need to learn. Assess the patient's/family's readiness to learn. Help the patient understand how the learning will benefit him or her based on his or her value system.[9]

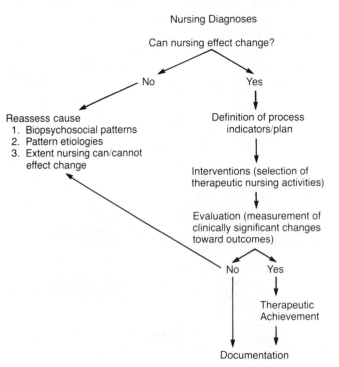

Figure 1–2. Nursing diagnoses. Can nursing effect change?

2. Assess the learner's knowledge level, then relate the information to be learned to what the learner already knows.

3. Actively involve the learner.

4. Arrange to have the learner put the information to use as soon as possible.

5. Give the learner feedback about progress immediately.

6. Provide for periodic reinforcement.

7. Use audiovisual aids/written materials and discussions to convey general information.

8. Build psychomotor skills by demonstration and return demonstrations.

9. Promote the creation of new attitudes through discussion, counselling, role playing and environmental support.

10. Be creative; for example, use photographs (cutouts from magazines are inexpensive but effective) for patients who have literacy, language or visual deficits.

11. Leave some reference material with the patient and family after the teaching session (many organizations supply free literature).

Counselling involves family dynamics as well as one-to-one support. From a systems' perspective, the patient is viewed within the context of the family since illness can change assigned family roles and lead to dysfunctional family dynamics. The nurse strives to maximize the patient's level of independence/control. The home health care nurse is an advocate for patient and family rights and promotes the patient's/family's skills in the decision making process. Responding to the patient's/family's "world view" through counselling requires focusing on the patient and family as people first and on their acquired cultural and behavioral differences second.[10]

Coordination, particularly in relation to high technology, requires organizing, monitoring and evaluating each service and product. The nurse assures that the multitude of agencies, services and products are available and complement each other in the plan of care. She or he prevents the creation of a minihospital in the home, promoting instead an atmosphere of "high tech" with "high touch." The patient's/family's confidentiality and rights are respected and protected.

Evaluation

In the evaluation phase, documentation of the status of process indicators and the patient's/family's therapeutic achievements is essential for reimbursement, quality assurance and liability issues. Clearly describing, throughout each visit, the patient's/family's progress or lack of progress toward the established outcomes is an integral part of structuring nursing documentation for favorable intermediary review. As illustrated in Figure 1–2, lack of goal achievement requires a reassessment of the problem and nursing's ability to effect change. As the last step in the Home Care Model (see Table 1–1), evaluation of therapeutic achievements provides the nurse the opportunity to review the effectiveness of the entire process. Patient/family evaluation of services is more effective if the nurse initially uses contracting and mutual goal setting to establish realistic expectations.

CHALLENGES

In addition to responding to expectations from patients and families, the home health care nurse is faced with expectations and pressures from federal and state regulators and the employing agency. The issues of productivity and qualitative standards that face home health care agencies and staff are depicted in Figure 1–3. The demands continue for

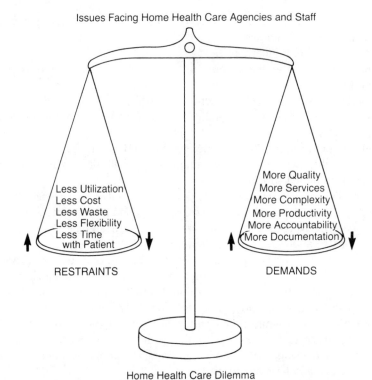

Issues Facing Home Health Care Agencies and Staff

Home Health Care Dilemma

Figure 1–3. Home health care dilemma of restraints and demands weighed against each other. (Courtesy of Suzanne Sblendorio.)

increased volume and more complex services. Growth is restricted, however, owing to decreased number of paid visits, whereas operating costs continue to rise in response to increased regulation.

References

1. McNamara, E. Home Care: Hospitals Rediscover Comprehensive Home Care. Hospitals, November 1, 1982, p. 61.
2. Speigel, A. D. Home Health Care: Home Birthing to Hospice Care. Owings Mills, Maryland: National Health Publishing, 1983.
3. Mundinger, M. Home Care Controversy: Too little, too late, too costly. Rockville, Maryland: Aspen Systems, 1983, p. 40.
4. Mundinger, M. Home Care Controversy: Too little, too late, too costly. Rockville, Maryland: Aspen Systems, 1983, pp. 87–88.
5. Louden, T. Opportunities on the Rise in Home Health Care. Caring, July 1984, pp. 12–14.
6. Simulations of a Medical Prospective Payment System for Home Health Care (GAO/HRD-85-11D). U.S. Government Printing Office Document Handling and Information Service Facility, P.O. Box 6015, Gaithersburg, Maryland 20877. Up to five copies free.
7. Stewart, I. E. Home Health Care. St. Louis, Missouri: C. V. Mosby Co., 1979.
8. Sluzki, C. On Training to Think Interactionally. Social Science and Medicine, 1974, pp. 8, 483–485.
9. Redman, B. K. The Process of Patient Teaching in Nursing, 4th ed. St. Louis, Missouri: C. V. Mosby Co., 1980, pp. 28–32.
10. Lash, M. Community Health Nursing in a Minority Setting. Philadelphia: Nursing Clinics of North America, June 1980, p. 347.

Bibliography

Backscheider, J. Self-Care Requirements, Self-Care Capabilities, and Nursing Systems in the Diabetic Nurse Management Clinic. American Journal of Public Health, vol. 64, no. 12, December 1974, pp. 1141–1145.

Benson, E. R. and McDevitt, J. Q. Community Health and Nursing Practice. Englewood Cliffs, New Jersey: Prentice-Hall, Inc., 1976.

Bille, D. A. Humanizing Patient Education. In Chaska, N. L. (ed.). The Nursing Profession: A Time to Speak. New York: McGraw-Hill, 1983, pp. 479–487.

Coleman, J. and Smith, D. DRGs and the Growth of Home Health Care. Nursing Economics, vol. 2, November-December 1984, pp. 391–395.

Morris, E. and Fonseca, J. Home Care Today—An Interview With E. Griffith. American Journal of Nursing, March 1984, pp. 341–342.

Rogatz, P. Home Health Care: Some Social and Economic Considerations. Home Health Care Nurse, vol. 3, no. 1, 1985, pp. 38–43.

Stuart-Siddall, S. (ed.). Home Health Care Nursing: Administrative and Clinical Perspectives. Rockville, Maryland: Aspen Systems, 1985.

Whitman, N. I., et al. Teaching in Nursing Practice: A Professional Model. Norwalk, Connecticut: Appleton-Century-Crofts, 1986.

Wright, L. M. and Leabey, M. Nurses and Families: A Guide to Family Assessment and Intervention. Philadelphia: F. A. Davis Co., 1984.

2

Productivity and Quality Assurance in Home Care Nursing

The home health care industry is facing new challenges; challenges that have changed the nature of home health care nursing. Some of these challenges can be turned into opportunities while others, if not met, can lead to the collapse of this vital component of the health care delivery system. In the recent past, changes in home health care have included increased competition, more acutely ill patients, reduced coverage by payers, increased regulatory burdens, intensified scrutiny by the consumers and public sector and increased demand for more services. These trends have required the industry to monitor itself in a manner never before required. Indeed, it is the ability of an agency to produce a service of acceptable quality with a high degree of efficiency that will determine its survival. A key factor in home health care survival is the nurse's ability to successfully link productivity, quality and documentation.

Productivity is a measurement often defined in terms of the relationship of input to output. In other words, it is the amount of output (product) that you get for your input (resources). In home health care, output is usually described as "patient visits" and "revenue" whereas input is described as "manpower costs." By defining the home health care product as a unit of service, in this case patient visits, efforts are directed toward assuring that resources are utilized appropriately and efficiently to achieve productivity. In home health care, productivity is a *process* of care delivery (visits) marked by the *efficient* use of manpower.

Quality of care is an end that is achieved when the product (patient visits) is delivered, using standards that are accepted by the profession and industry to achieve an outcome. Quality of health care can mean providing a level of service that is satisfactory to the consumer. Consumers generally rate a service as having quality if it is consistent, reliable and delivered by skilled staff, utilizing available technology. A quality visit in home health care is *effective* when it is marked by the use of the processes and techniques that meet an acceptable standard and produce the desired outcome. These standards can be those required for licensure, certification and accreditation, and are reflective of a profession's body of knowledge. Standards may also be proposed by the payers of third party reimbursement. The successful linking of quality (effectiveness) and productivity (efficiency) is critical to home health care. Figure 2–1 displays this relationship and its relevance to the industry.

12

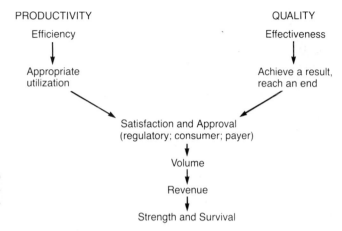

Figure 2–1. The relationship between productivity and quality in the home health care industry.

PRODUCTIVITY

When applying the concepts of productivity to home health care nursing practice, individual productivity is viewed separately from, as well as a part of, organizational productivity. It is important to recognize modifiers/factors that affect productivity. These are the factors an agency takes into consideration when determining staff productivity levels, i.e., number of visits desired per nurse per day. Recognition of these factors will result in more appropriate productivity standards and expectations. The staff nurse who recognizes these modifiers of productivity will be better able to plan and retain control of his or her time.

Significant Modifiers of Productivity

Geography. Rural and urban agencies must deal with different travel situations and different terrains. An agency covering 800 square miles in the Adirondack Mountains will have different travel modifiers than an agency covering 6 square miles within a city's limits. Road systems, traffic and congestion are also travel modifiers.

Climate. Agencies that must deal with inclement weather also have to deal with potential "lost" visits and other travel related modifiers.

Previous Patient Learning and Current Knowledge Level. With much of the home health care nurse's responsibilities centering on teaching, the current patient/family knowledge level and related knowledge deficits are modifiers. Patients with little or no previous health care teaching will require additional home health care interventions.

Acuity Level of Patient. The intensity of the patient's medical problem will also affect productivity. More complex situations demand extended time in assessment and delivery of highly technical care.

Extent of Social Support Available. Patients who are more socially isolated, without significant social support, will often require additional intervention. Without social support, their dependence on the home health care nurse is extended; progress toward self-care management becomes more difficult.

Distribution of Work Among Clerical, Visiting and Supervisory Staff. A significant objective of an efficient home health care operation is to assign visiting staff only those interventions that must be completed by the patient's primary care giver. This objective can be met only if the support of clerical, supervisory and other staff and resources is maximized.

Clear Role Definition and Establishment of Responsibilities. Each component must clearly fit into the whole. Does the organizational structure provide for appropriate levels of supervision without being cumbersome or "top heavy," especially as related to communication and problem resolution?

Availability and Use of Time Saving Techniques. Items such as computers, carbonless documents, tape recorders, nursing care guidelines, policies and procedures can be considered.

Other. Other factors that affect productivity are more controllable by the individual nurse and the agency. These are as follows:

- Attendance at staff conferences, in-services and meetings. Skills in assessment and nursing process.
- Preparation/planning or previsit time. Skills in organization, planning and time management.
- Time spent on telephone and other correspondence. Skill in communication.
- Medical record and other documentation requirements. Ability to use forms and procedures associated with documentation.
- Responsibilities associated with the coordination of multidisciplinary care and other case management responsibilities.
- Distribution of work responsibilities, i.e., delegating tasks better suited for clerical or paraprofessional staff.
- Negotiation within the agency's organization and systems, especially as it relates to problem resolution.
- Clinical skill levels, facility with the nursing process, professional communication and case management.
- Number of patient admissions and discharges.
- Extent of collegial, supervisory and social service support sought and utilized.

Productivity and Tasks Associated with Visit Delivery

Measuring productivity in home health care includes a review of the tasks associated with visit delivery. Some of these tasks are performed during the visit and others are performed at other times in support of the visit. The visit itself comprises the following activities:

1. Data collection
2. Assessment/analysis
3. Direct patient care
   a. patient teaching
   b. observation and monitoring
   c. support, guidance and explanation
4. Evaluation
5. Documentation.

The supportive components include
- Planning and evaluation.
- Telephone, verbal and written communication prior to *and* following the visits.
- Referrals to other services and organizations.
- Coordination of services.
- Consultation with other staff and supervisors.
- Supervision of paraprofessionals.
- Patient care conferences.

- Written documentation including certifications, recertifications, care plans, progress reports and discharge summaries.
- Travel to and from the patient's residence.

A tool that allows the measurement of each of these components is the methodology developed by Janet Bly.[1] This methodology provides specific measurements of productivity and allows for analysis and problem identification. The time associated with visit delivery is broken down sequentially into the basic components identified previously. Each step provides an opportunity to identify the existence of problems. The methodology provides a measurement for the total time associated with a component (across the agency or a subunit or team) *and* for individual full time equivalents (FTE). This analysis leads to the establishment of agency standards. Subsequently, the performance of individuals, groups of individuals and the agency in general can be evaluated against these standards. Problems can be identified and solutions evaluated. In addition, the data can be used to predict staffing needs, to prepare budgets and to develop productivity incentives within the agency. Productivity incentives are a new concept in home health care. Examples of productivity incentives include paying staff per visit for numbers exceeding the standard rather than their hourly rate, compensatory time off and flexibility in work scheduling such as 10-hour days. The effectiveness of these incentives has yet to be proved, however, and it is a basic assumption that the incentives must incorporate quality standards as integral parts of the system.

QUALITY ASSURANCE IN HOME HEALTH CARE

Objectives of quality assurance monitoring in home health care are to prevent unwanted harmful change and to create effective favorable change. A quality assurance program acknowledges the interrelationship of measurement tools to determine the degree to which certain standards are met. These standards relate to three main areas as follows:
1. The structure with which care is provided.
2. The process by which care is provided.
3. The outcome or end result (product) of the care provided.

Monitoring Structure and Process of Care

Historically, most home health care monitoring has occurred in the areas of structure and process. The Medicare certification survey and the state licensure survey are examples of *structure* audits. The main focus is on the organization itself, how services are organized, how personnel are utilized and the framework of the organization as reflected by its policies and procedures. For the most part the *process* of care, as it is delivered, and the end result or *outcome* of care are not closely examined. Current Medicare regulations do not require objective measurement of progress toward or attainment of patient care goals (outcome). In the Medicare conditions of participation for home health care agencies, a clinical record review is mandated. For most agencies this mandated review becomes an assessment of the utilization of services, i.e., appropriations and scope. At least this is a *process* audit that examines the process of meeting patient's needs, including what services were provided and whether all the required elements of the process of care delivery were present. Examples of such elements include consideration of community resources and complete record keeping.

The Joint Commission on Accreditation of Healthcare Organizations (JCAHO) had existing standards for home health care departments of hospitals. The focus was on structure with some process, as evidenced by the mandate for these departments to participate in quality assurance activities as part of the hospital's overall quality assurance program. In an effort to provide more comprehensive standards, new JCAHO standards have been developed for provider based, freestanding home health care agencies as well as for private nursing registries, and equipment and pharmaceutical companies. The standards focus primarily on *process* but also include some outcome criteria.[2]

Other measurement tools for quality assurance in home health care focus on *structure* and *process*. One of the first to be developed exclusively for home health care is the *Phaneuf Public Health Nursing Audit Tool.*[3] This is a *process audit* and reviews care retrospectively. Care is evaluated primarily through a review of the discharged patient's medical record. The application of the nursing process is examined through a review of seven basic functions. This tool is relatively simple to use, has good inter-rater reliability, can be modified for use by other disciplines and provides a basic exposure to general audit techniques. Its value depends on the quality of documentation and focuses on the more technical aspects of nursing.

Another useful audit tool is the *Quality Patient Care Scale* (Qual PACS).[4] This scale was developed to evaluate nursing care while it is being given and, therefore, is a *concurrent process audit*. The scale evaluates for therapeutic, adequate and safe care and is especially useful as a component of performance evaluation. The scale is easy to use but takes 2 hours of observation time and 3.5 hours to score. The measurement criteria are specific and constant with the same rater, but reliability between raters is difficult to achieve. This tool is one of the few quality assurance monitors dealing with care directly observed.

Monitoring Outcomes of Care

As previously noted, a comprehensive quality assurance program for a home health care agency must include monitoring of *outcome* as well as process and structure. Indeed this is often the one component of quality assurance activity that specifically addresses the *effectiveness* of patient care. Significant issues related to determining and monitoring outcomes or end results follow:
- Standard measures of quality used in health care (i.e., the patient completely recovers or is "cured") are not appropriate to home health care. The home health care nurse must respond to measures of quality in relation to the nature of chronic disease, the need to maximize the patient's strengths and the need to educate the patient/family to prevent complications/problems.
- Quality is equated with effectiveness, regardless of the magnitude of change.
- Consumers appear to equate quality with consistency and responsiveness.
- There is an increasing demand placed upon the home health care industry that it be *accountable* for its services and operate in a cost-effective manner, especially regarding utilization of resources.

The use of outcome criteria ("expected outcomes," patient care objectives) provides the mechanisms to measure whether utilization is appropriate and consumption of resources (money, staff time and so forth) is justified. Outcome criteria deal specifically with the patient's behavior at the end of care (e.g., knowledge level, health status, problem resolution, activity tolerance and satisfaction). They are stated in clear, precise measurable terms that are open to little interpretation.

Examples of words with multiple interpretations include
- Know
- Understand

- Value
- Appreciate

Examples of words with restricted interpretations include
- State
- List
- Demonstrate
- Recall

Either the patient does or does not achieve a desired behavioral outcome.

The drafting of outcome criteria can occur in two ways. One way is to use criteria developed by another source. A second way is to develop your own criteria. To develop criteria, first identify a patient population by medical diagnosis, nursing diagnosis, method of treatment and so forth. Greatest success is achieved if nursing diagnoses or treatment methods are used. A group of health professionals then identifies the most common outcomes of care for that group of patients. The number of outcomes should be limited to no more than 20 if possible. After drafting outcomes, critical time periods are addressed. These specify the period of time that is reasonable for achievement of the outcome. Address any acceptable "exceptions" to the achievement of the outcome (Table 2–1). The medical records of a sample group of discharged patients are then audited for evidence that the outcome criteria have been met. Results of the outcome audit are used to identify existence of problems or compliance with standards. Thus, the results are used for problem solving or maintaining appropriate levels of care.

Outcome criteria can be useful in other ways as follows:
- The criteria developed become standards of care that can serve as guidelines in developing and implementing plans of care for the home health care nurse and during orientation of new employees.
- Outcome criteria can be used to monitor the number of visits required to reach specific outcomes in certain patient populations.
- Outcome criteria can be used to monitor service utilization and plan for staffing and budgetary needs.

Promoting and Developing Quality Care

Quality assurance measurement in home health care should include structure, process and outcome monitors. Several existing tools have been presented as well as a method for developing outcome criteria for outcome audits. However, a home health care agency's quality assurance program should include more than a mechanism for measuring quality after care is provided. It must also include methods of promoting and developing quality.

Promotion of quality occurs *before* care is rendered. This is done primarily by staff selection and their functional job descriptions. Development of quality also occurs *during*

Table 2–1
Excerpted Portion of Outcome Criteria for Urinary Catheter for Urinary Retention

Outcome Criteria	Time Frame	Exceptions
Patient /significant other lists signs and symptoms of urinary tract infection.	Two visits	None
Patient /significant other demonstrates appropriate daily catheter care: Soap and water cleansing followed by povidone-iodine (Betadine) ointment daily.	Two visits	None
Patient /significant other reports signs and symptoms of urinary catheter obstruction.	When occurs	None occur

the time care is rendered. This is achieved primarily with staff development programs, availability of policies and procedures and staff assignments.

SUMMARY

As identified in the beginning of this chapter, the home health care nurse's ability to link productivity, quality and documentation is essential for successful home health care. By applying concepts of productivity and quality assurance to home health care, the professional home health nurse can further control and enhance his or her practice.

References

1. Bly, J. Measuring Productivity for Home Health Nurses. Princeton: The Home Health Agency Assembly of New Jersey, Inc. May 1981.
2. Joint Commission on Accreditation of Healthcare Organizations. Chicago, Illinois, 1988.
3. Phaneuf, M. The Nursing Audit: Self-Regulation in Nursing Practice. New York: Appleton-Century-Crofts, 1976.
4. Wandelt, M. and Joel, W. Quality Patient Care Scale. New York: Appleton-Century-Crofts, 1974.

Bibliography

Ballard, S. and McNamara, R. Quantifying Nursing Needs in Home Health Care. Nursing Research, July-August 1983, pp. 236–241.
Blake, R. R. and Mouton, J. S. Productivity: The Human Side. New York: Amacom, 1981.
Bonstein, R. G. and Mueller, J. Improving Agency Productivity. Caring, November 1985, pp. 4–9.
Cabin, W. Home Care Business . . . Productivity Incentives. Home Health Line, February 16, 1987, pp. 62–63.
Crane, V. Quality Assurance as a Problem-Solving Technique. The Health Care Supervisor, October 1984, pp. 58–68.
Decker, F. Using Patient Outcomes to Evaluate Community Health Nursing. Nursing Outlook, April 1979, pp. 278–282.
Foglesong, D. Standards Promote Effective Production. Nursing Management, January 1987, pp. 24–27.
Hamilton, P. Community Nursing Diagnosis. Advances in Nursing Science, April 1983, pp. 21–35.
Harris, M. D. A Patient Classification System in Home Health Care. Nursing Economics, September-October 1985, pp. 276–282.
Holmes, A. Problem-Oriented Medical Records, Nursing Audit and Accountability. Supervisor Nurse, April 1980, vol. 11, pp. 40–44.
Knight, J. Community Health Care: Assuring the Quality of Preventive Care. Quality Review Bulletin, March 1980.
Koerner, B. Selected Correlates of Job Performance of Community Health Nurses. Nursing Research, January-February 1981, pp. 43–48.
Kunkle, V. Accountability Standards Balance Quality and Efficiency. Nursing Management, January 1987, pp. 34–37.
Lackman, V. Increasing Productivity Through Performance Evaluation. Journal of Nursing Administration, December 1984, pp. 19–27.
Mason, E. How to Write Meaningful Nursing Standards. New York: McGraw-Hill, 1979.
Minnesota Department of Health, Section of Public Health Nursing, Outcome Criteria. Minneapolis, Minnesota: Public Health Nursing Services and Home Health Care Services, 1980.
Morano, V. Time Management: From Victim to Victor. The Health Care Supervisor, October 1984, pp. 1–12.
Mundinger, M. Home Care Controversy: Too Little, Too Late, Too Costly. Rockville, Maryland: Aspen Systems, 1983.
Spiegel, A. Home Health Care: Home Birthing to Hospice Care. Owings Mills, Maryland: National Health Publishing, 1985.
Spoelstra, S. Productivity Expectations of Registered Nurses in the Home Health Care Setting. A Michigan Study, Northern Michigan University, August 1986.
Ventura, M. Correlation Between the Quality Patient Care Scale and the Phaneuf Audit. International Journal of Nursing Studies, vol. 17, 1980, pp. 155–162.
Visiting Nurse Association of Omaha. A Classification Scheme for Client Problems in Community Health Nursing. Hyattsville, Maryland: U.S. Department of Health and Human Services, Bureau of Health Professions, Publication no. HRA 80–16, June 1980.
Zander, K. Revising the Production Process: When More Is Not the Solution. The Health Care Supervisor, April 1985, pp. 44–54.

3

Home Care Nursing Documentation

DOCUMENTING FOR CLAIMS REVIEW AND REIMBURSEMENT

Accurate descriptive documentation by the professional nurse is a standard common to all health care settings. The inherent value of the standard's achievement, however, differs in each setting. In home health care the value of nursing documentation relates, in large part, to reimbursement and continuation of patient care services.

Insurance companies demand written accounts, or claim forms, describing the care, service and equipment received by the beneficiaries for whom they are paying. Medical records are not routinely submitted with the claim forms. Depending upon the insurance company, the medical records may be requested routinely or only when absolutely necessary. In particular, a company may request medical records when the agency has been identified as a poor performer based on denial statistics or coverage compliance results.

Company medical auditors review and analyze the documentation on the claim forms in order to determine whether or not an agency should be paid. The documentation should recreate the total picture of service provision and answer the following questions: Who was being served? What was the service? Why was the service performed? When was the service performed? What were the results? The documentation makes the nursing product accessible to the auditors who, of course, cannot be present when home health care services are provided. The process of auditor review is presented in Figure 3–1. Any "Yes" answer supports payment of the claim. Any "No" answer requires supplemental data, if the claim is to be pursued. The auditor may, however, deny the claim based only on the information provided on the claim forms. Typically, there is no requirement for an auditor to request medical records before denying a claim. This factor compounds the subtle reality that the first "No" answer generally causes a change in the auditor's perspective. The analysis of the claim assumes an investigative quality. Requests for supplemental documentation represent a challenge to alter the auditor's concerns whether eligibility requirements have been met.

Therefore, it is essential to complete claim forms carefully and in their entirety. Judicious use of abbreviations, especially "not applicable" ("NA"), is advised. If the item relates to a condition of participation or if it is one the auditor thinks is important to a coverage decision, the claim will likely be denied if information is not provided.

Even when medical records are requested supplemental supporting data can be difficult to obtain. Since home health care claims are often evaluated retrospectively, the

19

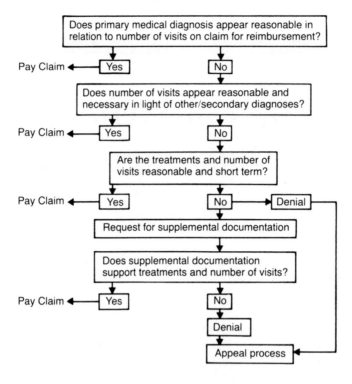

Figure 3–1. Process of auditor review.

patient/beneficiary has usually been discharged by the time the third party review is initiated. As a result, the review process may be further delayed, and the home health care agency's financial viability weakened. Expediting favorable decision making by third party auditors is, therefore, very important.

Documentation Leading to Favorable Reimbursement Decisions

Good documentation eases the medical reviewer's task. Adherence to routine guidelines is essential (Table 3–1). When documentation is free of errors, auditors tend to regard the content as reliable. Correct grammar, syntax and spelling also convey that the nurse's written description is an accurate source of information.

The qualitative, not quantitative, factors in documentation make it a valuable resource for the reviewer. Patient findings can be classified into positive and negative categories

Table 3–1
Routine Documentation Guidelines

1. Write legibly.	9. Record verbal orders from the physician exactly as received.
2. Use blue or black ink.	
3. Label each page with the patient's name.	10. Correct entries by drawing a single line through the error and by adding the date and initials of the person making the correction.
4. Date all entries.	
5. Record events after they occur. Never record before the fact.	
6. Use agency-accepted bbreviations.	11. Do not erase errors or use Liquid Paper for correction of errors.
7. Do not skip lines or leave spaces.	12. Label late entries as such with the dates of both the original situation and the transcription.
8. Use verbatim statements when documenting verbal dialogue.	13. Sign each entry.

Table 3–2
Terminology Associated with Favorable Claims Review

Recommended Terminology When Documenting Skilled Care	Terminology to AVOID When Documenting Skilled Care
Acute	Chronic; stabilized
Assessed; evaluated	Observed; monitored
Instructed	Reviewed; reinforced; retaught; stressed; discussed
Bed confined; chair confined	Stays in bed; sits in chair all day
Requires bodily transfer to move from . . . to . . .; requires assistive device (specify) to move from . . . to . . .	Independent in room with walker; ambulatory in room/house/apartment only; walks with walker/quad cane and so forth
Impaired balance	Falls easily; leans for support; unsteady gait
Unable to . . .	Has problems/difficulty with . . .
Symptoms (specify) exhibited after exertion (specify)	Tires easily; very weak; fatigued after activity
Has functional limitation of (specify)	Generalized weakness; frail
Transported to the physician by (specify)	Went to the doctor's
Homebound	Ambulatory within confines of home
Per the physician's order/request	At the patient's/family's request
Erythematic/inflamed	Appears red; slightly reddened
Beginning to respond to (specify) interventions	Stabilizing
Amount (specify)	Small; minimal; moderate
Frequency (specify)	Often; sometimes; usually
Parameters of response (specify in measurable exact terms, i.e., able to ambulate 10 feet without dizziness)	Monitor response to activity

(see Fig. 1–1). The positive findings or strengths facilitate implementation of the home health care plan. Negative clinical findings are the patient's functional deficits; they establish need. The nurse's documentation of the patient's negative findings, ongoing documentation of the patient's response to the plan of care and documentation of care provided form the bases for favorable reimbursement.

The documentation should be concise but not sparse. If an entry in the clinical record does not make sense or cannot stand alone, it needs amplification. Details should be current and technically descriptive. Use of words and phrases that are associated with payment authorization is helpful (Table 3–2).

The nurse who is documenting must also be attentive to the eligibility criteria for Medicare reimbursement (Table 3–3). Medical auditors review the documentation with these criteria in mind. A patient whose documented needs fall short of the defined parameters is typically not eligible for insurance-paid home health care.

The nurse often holds the key to favorable reimbursement decisions by clearly showing a relationship among the clinical findings, the qualifying parameters and the level of care he or she deems appropriate for the patient. He or she must either respond continually to the eligibility criteria via documentation or terminate the provision of care to that patient. Documentation that successfully responds to the essential criteria answers the following questions:

1. Why are the sophisticated skills of a professional nurse necessary to meet the patient's health care needs?

Table 3–3
Qualifying Parameters for Home Care Reimbursement

1. The individual must be under the care of a physician who medically authorizes home health care services.
2. The individual must be confined to the home.
3. The individual must have an intermittent need for professional skilled intervention.

2. What are the clinical findings and changes that demonstrate that the patient's condition is not stable?

3. Why is the patient unable to manage or coordinate the management of his or her health care needs?

4. Why is the chosen plan of care reasonable and essential in light of the patient's medical diagnosis?

FORMAT OF DOCUMENTATION

The format for the presentation of documentation varies according to agency preference. Agency-selected forms, such as case conference records and assessment forms, delineate the components of an acceptable medical record in that agency. Along with agency-specified documentation forms, additional items may be indicated/required for licensure, certification or both. Sections that respond to the qualifying beneficiary parameters for home health care and the Joint Commission on Accreditation of Healthcare Organizations (JCAHO) criteria for home health care documentation can be found.

While the home health care medical record serves many purposes (Table 3–4), among the most important are to communicate the process of skilled intervention and care rendered and to describe the patient's progress or lack of progress toward therapeutic goal achievement.

The systematic multidisciplinary framework for the documentation process includes the following:

- Collection of data
- Analysis of data
- Identification of significant clinical findings
- Nursing diagnoses or problem identification
- Development of interventions
- Evaluation of outcomes/interventions/responses

Tools developed serve a twofold purpose as follows: (1) to assist the professional care giver through the provision of care and (2) to provide an established model/standard for practice. Selected examples of meaningful documentation tools follow.

Meaningful Documentation

Clinical findings, outcomes and evaluative parameters regarding the appropriateness of medically prescribed interventions can be communicated on well-documented flow sheets/forms. Medication records (Fig. 3–2) effectively document the dose, frequency, route, desired action and probable side effects of the patient's prescription and nonprescription drugs and biologicals. A flow sheet format could include columns to acknowledge instructions to the patient/family and supervision of patient/family return demonstrations. If printed on carbonless paper, the copy can be given to the patient for use as an instruction sheet.

Table 3–4
Purposes of Home Care Documentation

1. To record the services rendered.	4. To forestall unjust legal actions.
2. To describe the patient's condition and response to care/treatment.	5. To validate reimbursement claims.
	6. To provide direction for research.
3. To promote continuity of care.	7. To sustain professional identity.

| PHARMACY: | PATIENT NAME AND ID: |
| TELEPHONE: | |

| DRUG ALLERGIES/SENSITIVITIES: | |

PERSON(S) RESPONSIBLE FOR MEDICATION ADMINISTRATION:

MEDICATION	DESIRED ACTION	SIDE EFFECTS	START DATE	STOP DATE	DOSE	FREQUENCY	ROUTE	TEACHING DONE	RETURN DEMO

Figure 3–2. Sample medication record.

A standardized instruction sheet (Fig. 3–3) provides a framework from which individualized patient/family teaching can derive. Copies of whatever is given to the patient/family can be kept on the medical record and used as a guide to help focus the documentation of all participating disciplines regarding instruction.

In home health care, the members of the caregiving team do not typically visit the patient at the same time. Instead, regularly held case conferences bring together the different team members and their multidisciplinary assessments. Thus, the development of complementary treatment plans and goals is facilitated. The case conferences and their outcomes must be documented and entered into the medical record. A sample of a comprehensive case conference record is illustrated in Figure 3–4.

The ongoing dialogues and collaborations among team members are reflected in the clinical notes and the progress summaries. Clinical notes are written following any contact with the patient, family or persons involved in the patient's care. Progress summaries are done every 30 days and at discharge (unless otherwise regulated by state law). These communication tools address changes in the clinical findings, modifications in the treatment plan, results of and responses to interventions, the identification of interventions that remain essential to continued patient progress and, upon discharge, therapeutic achievement.

CAST CARE

A cast is used to keep a part of the body from moving until the bones can heal. Casts are made of different material. They can be used on almost any part of the body.

FOLLOW THESE STEPS FOR GOOD CAST CARE

For a plaster cast, keep the cast clean and dry.
• White shoe polish can be used for touch-ups (do not paint the cast).
• If your nurse or doctor allows, cover the cast with a waterproof sleeve or a plastic bag to bathe. Tie the bag securely above the cast. Do not wet the cast.

With a fiber glass cast, you may be allowed to wet the cast.
• Dry the cast following your nurse's or doctor's directions.
• Dampness should not be felt under the cast after drying.

Follow your nurse's or doctor's directions for exercise and diet.

Carefully check the skin at the edges of the cast for redness. Cover rough edges on the cast with mole skin. Do not use oils, lotions, or powders on the skin under the cast.

Keep the cast raised (elevated) above the level of your heart.

Minor swelling, discomfort, and change in skin color (blue tinge) are common for the first few days after the cast is put on. This is normal when the casted limb is not raised.

Do not wear rings on the fingers of your casted arm.

Follow your nurse's or doctor's directions for the use of cast aids (crutches or sling).

Do not scratch the skin under the cast. Be careful to keep crumbs and small objects from falling inside the cast.

Using pillows under and around the cast, especially while sleeping, may help to make you feel better.

Use an old hat or a sock to keep your fingers or toes warm.

Figure 3–3. Sample patient instructions.

WHAT YOU SHOULD REPORT TO YOUR NURSE OR DOCTOR IMMEDIATELY

Any break or crack in the cast.

Any softness of the cast.

Any very red skin areas or any break in the skin.

Extreme redness, coldness, or increased swelling of fingers or toes after the casted limb is raised above the level of your heart.

Fingers or toes remaining discolored or blue tinged after the casted limb is raised above the level of your heart.

Numbness, tingling ("pins and needles") or burning of fingers or toes.

Pain that is not relieved by medication or pain that is getting worse.

Unusual or bad odor or drainage from the cast.

Fever over 101°F (39.3°C).

New problems moving fingers or toes.

A child with a cast who is fussy for no reason.

OTHER INSTRUCTIONS

Type of cast _____ Use of cast aids _____
Exercise _____ Diet _____

Figure 3–3 Continued

SAMPLE CASE CONFERENCE RECORD

Date _____   Start of Care Date _____

Patient's Name _____

Diagnoses _____

Disciplines Involved (Initials of Conference Attendees)

   RN _____   OT _____   MSW _____   RD _____

   ST _____   PT _____   HHA _____   MD _____

Services Discontinued Since Last Conference and D/C date

_____

_____

Patient's Current Limitations/Deficits

_____

_____

Professional Interventions and Frequency of Visits

_____

_____

Goals _____

_____

Outcomes _____

_____

Discharge Plans _____

_____

Case Manager's Signature _____

Figure 3–4. Sample for home care nursing documentation.

HEALTH CARE FINANCING ADMINISTRATION (HCFA) DOCUMENTATION REQUIREMENTS

If the clinical record is to meet the objective of maximizing reimbursement, an examination of the Health Care Financing Administration (HCFA) documentation requirements for Medicare claims is essential. Most commercial and private health insurers have adopted the HCFA's definitions of the qualifying beneficiary parameters for home health care (homebound, intermittent, skilled, physician authorized). Most also accept HCFA's standardized claim forms 485, 486 and 487 in lieu of their own.

Claim Form 485

Form 485 (Fig. 3–5) is used to certify the physician's plan of home health care and that the patient meets the eligibility requirements for home health care reimbursement. When reviewing this form, the medical auditor looks for documented answers to the following questions, which are summarized in Table 3–5:

1. Do the primary medical diagnosis and the date of onset justify a predictable need for intermittent home health care intervention?

The primary diagnosis must relate to the services rendered by the home health care agency. Thus, all medical diagnoses that have no bearing on the plan of care are excluded from consideration.

The primary diagnosis may or may not relate to the patient's most recent hospital stay. If the diagnosis and need-for-service are hospital stay–related and appear to have been resolved at the time of discharge, they are not valid reasons for home health care service. If the diagnosis and need-for-service are hospital stay–related and are not resolved at the time of discharge, they may serve as reasonable justification for home health care service.

For example, a stabilized chronic medical diagnosis tends not to justify a current need for skilled home health care. As a case in point, Mr. Smith is recently diagnosed as having multiple sclerosis. He is confined to bed, unless dependently transferred. Mr. Smith would most likely be eligible for reimbursed home health care services as a result of the recent nature of his functional limitation. Alternately, Mr. Jones, who has had multiple sclerosis for 10 years and has been confined to bed for 2 years, would probably not qualify for reimbursement. Although he has the same functional limitation as Mr. Smith, it is of long-term duration.

To meet the requirements for intermittent care, the patient's medical diagnosis must predict and support a short-term need for skilled nursing service. In most instances this qualifying parameter is met if a patient requires a skilled nursing service at least once every 60 days. There are some exceptions (which are thoroughly discussed in the Medicare HM 11 Manual),* with the classic being the patient who has an indwelling urinary catheter that needs changing every 90 days. This qualifies as intermittent care.

2. Do the secondary diagnoses complicate the patient's situation, thus supporting a particular level of care?

The secondary diagnoses must be active conditions that coexist at the time the plan of care is in effect. They may be chronic conditions or conditions that develop during the course of home health care intervention. If the patient will require more extensive skilled intervention as a result of a secondary diagnosis, it is best to describe the secondary diagnosis in terms of functional deficits in order to maximize service eligibility. For example,

---

*U.S. Government Printing Office; Washington, D.C. (A provider number is required.)

Department of Health and Human Services
Health Care Financing Administration

Form Approved
OMB No. 0938-0357

HOME HEALTH CERTIFICATION AND PLAN OF TREATMENT

1. Patient's HI Claim No.	2. SOC Date	3. Certification Period		4. Medical Record No.	5. Provider No.
		From:	To:		

6. Patient's Name and Address

7. Provider's Name and Address.

8. Date of Birth:		9. Sex	M	F	10. Medications: Dose/Frequency/Route (N)ew (C)hanged

11. ICD-9-CM	Principal Diagnosis	Date

12. ICD-9-CM	Surgical Procedure	Date

13. ICD-9-CM	Other Pertinent Diagnoses	Date

14. DME and Supplies

15. Safety Measures:

16. Nutritional Req.

17. Allergies:

18.A. Functional Limitations

1	Amputation	5	Paralysis	9	Legally Blind
2	Bowel/Bladder (Incontinence)	6	Endurance	A	Dyspnea With Minimal Exertion
3	Contracture	7	Ambulation	B	Other (Specify)
4	Hearing	8	Speech		

18.B. Activities Permitted

1	Complete Bedrest	6	Partial Weight Bearing	A	Wheelchair
2	Bedrest BRP	7	Independent At Home	B	Walker
3	Up As Tolerated	8	Crutches	C	No Restrictions
4	Transfer Bed/Chair	9	Cane	D	Other (Specify)
5	Exercises Prescribed				

19. Mental Status:

1	Oriented	3	Forgetful	5	Disoriented	7	Agitated
2	Comatose	4	Depressed	6	Lethargic	8	Other

20. Prognosis:

1	Poor	2	Guarded	3	Fair	4	Good	5	Excellent

21. Orders for Discipline and Treatments (Specify Amount/Frequency/Duration)

22. Goals/Rehabilitation Potential/Discharge Plans

23. Verbal Start of Care and Nurse's Signature and Date Where Applicable:

24. Physician's Name and Address	25 Date HHA Received Signed POT	26. I ☐ certify ☐ recertify that the above home health services are required and are authorized by me with a written plan for treatment which will be periodically reviewed by me. This patient is under my care, is confined to his home, and is in need of intermittent skilled nursing care and/or physical or speech therapy or has been furnished home health services based on such a need and no longer has a need for such care or therapy, but continues to need occupational therapy.
27. Attending Physician's Signature (Required on 485 Kept on File in Medical Records of HHA)	Date Signed	

Form HCFA-485 (C4) (4-87)

Figure 3–5. Health Care Financing Administration (HCFA) Form 485.

Table 3–5
Questions Related to Claim Form 485

1. Do the primary medical diagnosis and the date of onset justify a predictable need for intermittent home care intervention?
2. Do the secondary diagnoses complicate the patient's situation, thus supporting a particular level of care?
3. Do the clinical findings reflect a medical necessity and reasonableness for skilled nursing?
4. Do the specified functional deficits and activity limitations manifested by the patient clearly warrant in home care due to homeboundness?
5. Are the patient's medications and/or treatments newly prescribed or recently changed?
6. Are the goals of the treatment plan realistic and time oriented?

Mrs. Johnson has a primary diagnosis of infected pressure sores (which require cleansing irrigations) and a secondary diagnosis of severe rheumatoid arthritis (which compromises her mobility). The need for home health care service is further supported by Mrs. Johnson's incapacity. If she had no complicating secondary diagnosis, then a reviewer could ask why Mrs. Johnson needed home health care as opposed to health care intervention in an outpatient setting.

3. Do the clinical findings reflect a medical necessity and reasonableness for skilled nursing?

Reimbursable skilled nursing consists of services that are necessary for the treatment of an illness or injury (refer to Medicare HM 11 Manual). Skilled interventions are directed at preventing probable or predictable medical complications as opposed to focusing on the possibility of future problems. Each intervention has as its ultimate goal patient improvement or stabilization at discharge.

Skilled services are performed by or under the direct supervision of a licensed professional nurse, although this alone does not convert any intervention to a skilled level. Additionally, if a service is one that could be done by the average nonmedical person, the unavailability of such a person in the home does not elevate the service to a skilled level.

In determining whether or not a patient requires skilled nursing care, consideration is given to the complexity of the requested service and the condition of the patient. Documentation should identify the service, the patient's inability to otherwise obtain it and the fact that "without (specify) intervention, the patient will experience (specify) symptoms/deficits." Written descriptions of the patient should focus on the unstable, abnormal and dysfunctional signs and symptoms he or she manifests. For example, "The patient experiences shortness of breath during assisted ambulation after distance of 10 feet," or "The patient is unable to bear weight for 2 weeks; lives alone."

The patient's clinical situation must medically support the necessity for skilled intervention. If hypertensive screenings and evaluations are the prescribed treatment modality, then the patient should have an abnormally elevated blood pressure as well as a significantly altered or new medication and dietary regimen.

Only those clinical findings related to the current medical diagnoses will help support payment authorization of skilled nursing care. For instance, when a claim is submitted for nursing visits focused on teaching Mrs. Wilms about insulin administration, a reviewer will ask why the instruction is necessary. Is it because Mrs. Wilms is "new" to insulin and is legally blind? Or perhaps it is because Mrs. Wilms has a recent above-the-knee amputation that confines her to a wheelchair. Any of these findings support the need for skilled intervention. In contrast, if the documentation indicates that Mrs. Wilms has been self-administering insulin for 5 years and has a history of fluctuating blood glucose levels, the reviewer is likely to deny the claim.

4. Do the specified functional deficits and activity limitations manifested by the patient clearly warrant home health care due to homeboundness?

The patient is considered homebound if he or she has a condition that makes leaving the home medically contraindicated, or if he or she has a condition (due to injury or illness) that restricts the ability to leave home except with the aid of supportive devices, special transportation or another person. Unreliable transportation or the taxing effort required for out-of-home travel does not alone satisfy the Medicare requirement for homeboundness.

The normal effects of the aging process are separate from the untoward effects of the current illness or injury. The elderly patient who does not travel from home because of the feebleness and insecurity brought on by advanced age does not qualify under the Medicare program for homebound status. It is essential, if payment for home health care service is desired, that the documented reasons for homeboundness be related to functional deficits induced by the patient's current medical diagnoses.

The functional deficits should be documented in a thoughtful manner. If Mr. Belcastro, for example, was "up as tolerated" during the last home visit, why can't he travel outside his home this week? A functional deficit must be cited to support why this visit is necessary in the home, i.e., "The patient is unable to walk the length of his bedroom without experiencing tachycardia and severe dyspnea."

5. Are the patient's medications and/or treatments newly prescribed or recently changed?

For instance, Mrs. Grant's physician increases her meperidine perscription, necessitating dosage adjustments and a greater awareness of probable side effects. Since the teaching of essential health information is a skilled intervention, authorized payment for Mrs. Grant's home health care is likely. However, if the nurse's teaching efforts are met by Mrs. Grant with recurrent resistance or an inability to learn, the service becomes unreasonable and unnecessary under the Medicare program.

6. Are the goals of the treatment plan realistic and time oriented?

Goals must be identified for each discipline (nursing, social work, physical therapy and so forth) that is part of the patient's care. The goals should be objectively measurable and realistically achievable outcomes with short-term intermittent intervention. For a patient with expressive aphasia, the goal of establishing quality speech patterns for normal communication is unrealistic; whereas, the goal of establishing an alternative communication system is more appropriate.

The goals of treatment are developed as soon as possible after admission. Included in this process are the goals for discharge, or how the patient will be cared for after home health care is no longer needed. Expediency in identifying the goals of treatment and discharge will result in a utilization of skilled services that addresses the patient's need and is cost effective.

Claim Form 486

Form 486 (Fig. 3–6) collects updated medical and patient care information and is used to make coverage determinations on home health care claims. When reviewing form 486, the medical auditor looks for answers to the following questions, which are summarized in Table 3–6:

1. Was the physician consulted regarding changes in the patient's health status?

When the patient's physician is regularly consulted and significant changes in the treatment plan result, the patient is deemed unstable. Continued or expanded home health care service is likely to be approved. Minimal or no medical consultation, however, reflects a stablized patient condition and negates the need for home health care.

2. Do specific services and total visits match the patient's medical diagnoses and current clinical findings?

Department of Health and Human Services
Health Care Financing Administration

Form Approved
OMB No. 0938-0357

MEDICAL UPDATE AND PATIENT INFORMATION

1. Patient's HI Claim No.	2. SOC Date	3. Certification Period		4. Medical Record No.	5. Provider No.
		From:	To:		

6. Patient's Name	7. Provider's Name

8. Medicare Covered: ☐ Y ☐ N | 9. Date Physician Last Saw Patient: | 10. Date Last Contacted Physician:

11. Is the Patient Receiving Care in an 1861 (J)(1) Skilled Nursing Facility or Equivalent? ☐ Y ☐ N ☐ Do Not Know | 12. ☐ Certification ☐ Recertification ☐ Modified

13. Specific Services and Treatments

Discipline	Visits (This Bill) Rel. to Prior Cert.	Frequency and Duration	Treatment Codes	Total Visits Projected This Cert.

14. Dates of Last Inpatient Stay: Admission _____ Discharge _____ | 15. Type of Facility:

16. Updated Information: New Orders/Treatments/Clinical Facts/Summary from Each Discipline

17. Functional Limitations (Expand From 485 and Level of ADL) Reason Homebound/Prior Functional Status

18. Supplementary Plan of Treatment on File from Physician Other than Referring Physician: ☐ Y   ☐ N
(If Yes, Please Specify Giving Goals/Rehab. Potential/Discharge Plan)

19. Unusual Home/Social Environment

20. Indicate Any Time When the Home Health Agency Made a Visit and Patient was Not Home and Reason Why if Ascertainable	21. Specify Any Known Medical and/or Non-Medical Reasons the Patient Regularly Leaves Home and Frequency of Occurrence

22. Nurse or Therapist Completing or Reviewing Form	Date (Mo., Day, Yr.)

Form HCFA-486 (C3) (4-87)   **PROVIDER**

Figure 3–6. Health Care Financing Administration (HCFA) Form 486.

Table 3–6
Questions Related to Claim Form 486

1. Was the physician consulted regarding changes in the patient's health status?	4. Does the updated information section specify new medical diagnoses and new services? Are new diagnoses and services congruent in focus?
2. Do specific services and total visits match the patient's medical diagnoses and current clinical findings?	5. Are clinical findings documented which give evidence that the patient has a changing, deteriorating or unstable health condition?
3. Does the updated information section clearly justify the rationale for the number of home health care visits made?	6. What clinical findings continue to cause the patient to be homebound?
	7. Was the patient ever not home when the home health care professional made a visit?

For example, Mrs. Daniels has had a hypertensive episode. Three years ago she had a cerebral vascular accident resulting in right-sided paralysis. The treatment plan on form 486 would reveal an intensive level of intervention by nursing, physical therapy, occupational therapy and speech therapy directed toward hypertensive screening, medication regulation and a rehabilitation program. The services of multiple disciplines have not been correlated with the current primary medical diagnosis of hypertensive crisis. More than likely this level of home health care service would be denied.

3. Does the updated information section clearly justify the rationale for the number of home health care visits made?

The expectations of the insurance reviewers are that all the significant changes that occurred during the billing period be specified on form 486. For instance, Mr. Dunn, who has a neurogenic bladder, has a Foley catheter to be changed every 4 to 6 weeks. He receives six visits during the billing period specified on form 486. The documentation regarding those six visits must concretely describe why the visits were necessary, e.g., "4/12—Severe bladder spasms, catheter out; reinserted; urine cloudy, c/s with *E. coli* organism; Bactrim therapy begun on 4/15."

4. Does the updated information section specify new medical diagnoses and new services? Are new diagnoses and services congruent in focus?

For example, consider a patient who was admitted for short-term skilled nursing for 3 days of intramuscular injections of gentamicin (Garamycin). On the third day of service, the patient experienced a cerebrovascular accident at home, with no hospital admission. This diagnosis was confirmed by the physician during a home visit. Rehabilitative services were initiated per physician order. To justify the claim, the updated information section needs to reflect the new medical diagnosis and new services required.

5. Are clinical findings documented which give evidence that the patient has a changing, deteriorating or unstable health condition?

For example, the reasons for Mr. Guilbert's home care are medication regulation and instruction. Yet, laboratory values are within normal limits, indicating health status stabilization. Unless there are other complicating factors, home health care services for Mr. Guilbert will be terminated.

6. What clinical findings continue to cause the patient to be homebound?

Again, being specific about homeboundness is important. Documentation should state how the clinical findings relate to the patient's being unable to leave the home. For example, "The patient is confined to bed unless bodily transferred by two people; physician makes home visits due to patient's inability to leave home except by ambulance stretcher."

7. Was the patient ever not home when the home health care professional made a visit?

If a patient can leave the home, it is often interpreted by the reviewer that he or she is not considered homebound. In the event a patient is not at home when the nurse

Department of Health and Human Services
Health Care Financing Administration

Form Approved
OMB No. 0938-0357

ADDENDUM TO: ☐ PLAN OF TREATMENT ☐ MEDICAL UPDATE

1. Patient's HI Claim No.	2. SOC Date	3. Certification Period		4. Medical Record No.	5. Provider No.
		From:	To:		

6. Patient's Name	7. Provider Name

8. Item
No.

9. Signature of Physician	10. Date

11. Optional Name/Signature of Nurse/Therapist	12. Date

Form HCFA-487 (C4) (4-87)

Figure 3–7. Health Care Financing Administration (HCFA) Form 487.

makes a visit, the reason for the patient's absence should be carefully documented. For example, "6/30—RN unsuccessful in making visit; RN confirmed that patient was at General Hospital's emergency room; admitted for 48 hours to stablize acute CHF episode."

Claim Form 487

HCFA form 487 (Fig. 3–7) is used for providing supplemental information to the claim examiners. Form 487 includes updated changes that occur after forms 485 and 486 are completed, thereby expanding upon the transcribed clinical picture. The documentation on form 487 should demonstrate the same attention to detail as on the other forms.

Bibliography

Austin, E. How Your Nursing Notes Can Rob Your Patients of Benefits. RN, September 1978, p. 58.

Barker, L. Progress/Flow Sheets Cut Writing Time, Update Physicians on Patient's Status. Hospital Home Health, September 1985, vol. 2, pp. 120–121.

Bailey-Allen, A. M. and A. McFarland. Avoid Legal Pitfalls in Charting. Orthopaedic Nursing, January/February 1986, vol. 5, no. 1, pp. 21–23.

Baum, R. Guidelines for Referring for Social Work Services for Nurses and Other Members of the Health Care Team. Home Health Agency Assembly. Presentation Materials, September 16, 1986, Princeton, New Jersey.

Bernzweig, E. Avoiding the Legal Pitfalls of Home Care. RN, August 1986, pp. 49–50.

Brown, J. (ed.). Peer Review for Home Health Agencies: HCFA to Implement Only Certain SOBRA Provisions. Washington D.C.: National Association for Home Care, Report no. 215, May 29, 1987, pp. 2–3.

Cabin, W. D. A Primer on the Medicare Claim Review and Denial For Home Care Providers, 3rd ed. September 1987.

Cabin, W. D. Understanding and Reducing Liability Risks in the Delivery of Home Care. Seminar Home Health Agency Assembly, Annual Meeting. Presentation Materials, May 8, 1987, Princeton, New Jersey.

Cell, P., Peters, D. and Gordon, J. Implementing a Nursing Diagnosis System Through Research: The New Jersey Experience. Home Health Care Nurse, January-February 1984, pp. 26–32.

Computerized Nursing Information Systems: An Urgent Need. Research in Nursing and Health, June 1983, pp. 101–105.

Connaway, N. I. Documenting Patient Care in the Home-Legal Issues for Home Health Nurses. Home Health Care Nurse, vol. 3, no. 5, pp. 6–8.

Connaway, N. I. Documenting Patient Care in the Home-Legal Issues for the Home Health Nurse. Part II. Home Healthcare Nurse, vol. 3, no. 6, pp. 44–46.

Creighton, H. Legal Implications of Home Health Care. Nursing Management, February 1987, vol. 18, no. 2, pp. 14–17.

Crownover, K. Shrinking the Demands of Home Care Documentation. Caring, June 1987, vol. 6, no. 6, pp. 20–22.

Deane, D., Mc Elroy, M. and Alden, S. Documentation: Meeting Requirements while Maximizing Productivity. Nursing Economics, July-August 1986, vol. 4, p. 174.

Droste, T. Medicare Denials Threaten the Health of Home Care. Hospitals, June 5, 1987, p. 58.

Engelbrecht, L. Denials Due to Homebound? Ah C'mon. Home Health Journal, March 1987.

Engelbrecht, L. Skilled Observation and Evaluation. Home Health Journal, February 1986.

Fogel, D. Medicare Claims Documentation Tips. National Association for Home Care. (Unpublished Seminar Materials.) March 1987, Washington, D.C.

Gould, J. and Wargo, J. Home Health Nursing Care Plans. Rockville, Maryland: Aspen Systems, 1987.

Greenlaw, J. Documentation of Patient Care: An Often Underestimated Responsibility. Law, Medicine and Healthcare, September 1982, p. 172.

Harris, M., Santoferraro, C. and Silva, S. A Patient Classification System in Home Health Care. Nursing Economics, September-October 1985, vol. 3, pp. 276–282.

Hoffman, J. R. Duplication in Medical Records Is a Problem: How to Avoid It At Your Home Health Agency. Home Health Journal, December 1983, vol. 4, p. 26.

Holmes, A. M. Problem-Oriented Medical Records: Nursing Audit and Accountability. Supervisor Nurse, April 1980, pp. 40–43.

Holloway, V. Documentation: One of the Ultimate Challenges in Home Health Care. Home Healthcare Nurse, January-February 1984, pp. 19–22.

Home Health Coverage Provider Training Manual. Health Care Financing Administration Health Standards and Quality Bureau Office of Medical Review. Washington, D.C., November, 1986.

Joint Commission on Accreditation of Health Care Organizations. Chicago, Illinois: Home Care Standards, 1987.

Lampe, S. S. Focus Charting: Streamlining Documentation, Nursing Management, July 1985, vol. 16, no. 7, pp. 43–45.

Lutz, S. Home Care Agencies Turn to Automation to Reduce Paperwork, Increase Cash Flow. Modern Healthcare, June 19, 1987, pp. 62–64.

Miller, S. Documentation for Home Health Care: A Record Management Handbook. Chicago, Illinois: Foundation of Record Education of the American Medical Record Association, 1986.

New Information—Medicare Update. (Seminar Materials and Presentation.) Cherry Hill, New Jersey: Prudential Insurance Company, Inc., November 13, 1986.

Northrop, C. E. and Kelly, M. Legal Issues in Nursing. St. Louis: C. V. Mosby Co., 1987.

Philpott, M. Rules for Good Charting. Nursing, August 1986, pp. 63.

Rutkowski, B. How DRGs are Changing Your Charting. Nursing '85, October 1985, pp. 49–51.

Schipske, G. Documenting Care for the Patient at Home. The Coordinator, May 1984, pp. 20–21.

Smith, J. Home Care is More Than Medical Regulations. American Journal of Nursing, March 1987, pp. 305–306.

Spath, P. Home Health Services' Expansion Creates Need for Improved Q A Plans. Hospital Peer Review, vol. 11, no. 4, April 1986, pp. 44–46.

Special Task Force Prospective Payment Proposal. Homecare, March 25, 1987, pp. 1–10.

Stewart, P. A Home Health Clinical Documentation System. Computers in Health Care, May 1986, pp. 45–48.

Stuart-Siddall, S. Home Health Care Nursing. Rockville, Maryland: Aspen Systems, 1986.

Stuart-Siddall, S. Home Health Care Nursing: Administrative and Clinical Perspective. Rockville, Maryland: Aspen Systems, 1986.

Tammelleo, A. D. (ed.). Nurses' Notes: Worth Weight in Gold. The Regan Report on Nursing Law, January 1987, vol. 27, no. 8, pp. 1.

Tillman, E. HCFA Holdings on Some of Medicare's Thorniest Home Health Coverage Questions. Home Health Line, December 8–15, 1986, vol. 11, pp. 422–428.

Warling, M. Legal Aspects of the Client's Record: A Guide For Community Health Nurses. Caring, October 1982, pp. 14–17.

Nursing Care Plans, Procedures and Resources

SECTION TWO

Case Management

Procedures
Resources

Procedures

▨▨▨▨▨▨▨▨▨▨▨▨▨▨▨▨▨▨▨▨▨▨▨▨▨▨▨▨▨▨▨▨

Adapting Acute Care Procedures to the Home Care Setting

Adaptation of acute care procedures to home health care requires approaching the procedure with an awareness of acute care biases, such as a sterile orientation (as compared with a clean one), supply/cost intensive materials (high use of prepared solutions/disposables), patient dependent behavior, institution-specific focus (as compared with professional standards' focus) and minimal attention to the patient's/family's home health care management skills. In adapting or developing procedures, professional nursing standards, quality assurance standards and agency standards also can be incorporated as an introduction to each procedure. Some agencies are incorporating the standards into the procedure as a way of satisfying quality assurance requirements. Modify the basic guidelines that follow to be consistent with your agency's protocols.

The basic components of a procedure include the title, purpose, equipment list, content (procedure steps, key points) and documentation. Each component is analyzed for those critical indicators that need to be included in the procedure adaptation/development process.

TITLE

Use of the generic name is preferred. For example, urinary indwelling catheter instead of Foley catheter.

PURPOSE

The rationale for performing the procedure, i.e., what will be accomplished by performing it.

Special Notes. Information that is necessary or useful to review *prior* to performing the procedure is contained in the special notes. This section may include points to clarify with the physician, clarification of indicators for the procedure, helpful hints, safety reminders and options for patients with functional limitations (such as psychomotor, visual or cognitive impairments). For example, "Do not use acetone on the catheter as it will cause the silicone to deteriorate."

EQUIPMENT

- Specify the types (and suppliers if appropriate) of equipment needed. For example, "Intravenous infusion device." (The manufacturer is noted in the documentation section.)
- List the sizes and numbers of items needed. For example, "2 size 25 g 1 inch sterile needles."

- Specify any solutions, medications or ointments that require a prescribed amount and strength. For example, "Heparinized solution (amount/strength prescribed by physician)."
- Specify clean or sterile where appropriate. For example, "4 × 4 sterile gauze." This point is particularly important when adapting acute care procedures; most acute care procedures have a "sterile" bias, whereas in the home certain procedures may safely be done using "clean" technique.
- Assess the cost/benefit ratio for the patient/family when choosing equipment and supplies. A long-term patient may benefit from purchasing a more expensive piece of equipment, which provides longer service and higher reliability. A patient with short-term needs may not require the same caliber of equipment. Most importantly, what is reimbursable remains key.
- Assess the availability/accessibility of equipment. Especially in "high tech" cases, identify who will coordinate equipment/vendor and order/reorder and who will follow up on delivery, trouble shoot and provide backup service. Refer to the manufacturer's user's manual as a reference for the equipment's specific instructions.

UNIT 1

CONTENT

Write the content in two columns.

Steps

1. List in sequential steps.

2. Number all steps.
3. Be thorough/specific (for example, withdraw 6 ml of fluid).
   a. Begin with patient preparation through to the procedure's completion including patient positioning, patient/family teaching and care of equipment.
   b. Be brief but do not assume.
   c. Start each step with an action specific verb (for example, wipe or twist off).
4. Use diagrams/illustrations as needed. Manufacturers frequently can provide illustrations; note the source at the end of the procedure.

Key Points

1. List essential points, scientific rationales, "caution" points to prevent errors, trouble-shooting guides, safety points, special points to reinforce/clarify during patient/family teaching and any points that relate to patient/family functional limitations.
2. Incorporate the nursing process.
3. Match the key points with the appropriate step.

DOCUMENTATION

1. Date, time and result (in measurable terms such as amount and frequency); any difficulties and actions taken.
2. Patient response to the procedure.
3. Type of equipment used (state the manufacturer's name).
4. Date, time and details of communication with the physician and other members of the health care team as appropriate.
5. Patient/family instruction and quality of return demonstration.
   a. Identify content and written material left for reference.
   b. Patient's/family's skill level (if appropriate) at the start and conclusion of the visit. Careful documentation of the patient's/family's progress (psychomotor and cognitive achievement) is critical for reimbursement.
6. Use terms that are technically descriptive and measurable, such as
   a. "instructed" instead of "reviewed/discussed."
   b. "unable to" instead of "has difficulty with."
   c. "state/list/demonstrates" instead of "knows/understands."

Assistive Devices Procedure

PURPOSE

To provide devices that
- aid in the performance of activities of daily living
- facilitate mobility
- increase safety and comfort
- enhance communication.

EQUIPMENT

Assistive devices can be categorized by
- dressing aids: bathroom/toilet/incontinence aids and appliances; hygiene/grooming aids.
- home aids: household aids, kitchen/eating aids, reaching devices.
- mobility accessories: adaptive equipment, splints/braces/straps; ambulatory aids, canes/walkers/crutches/wheelchairs.
- exercise aids: security vests, support/positioning aids, wheelchair accessories, foam.
- recreation/hobby/leisure accessories; books/references/communication aids; sensory, motor stimulation materials.

IMPORTANT POINTS

Selection, fitting and use of certain assistive devices require professional expertise. Resources are as follows:
- your local or state occupational therapy association
- a physical therapist
- American Occupational Therapy Association
  1383 Piccard Drive
  P.O. Box 1725
  Rockville, Maryland 20850-4375
- a physician's order as required for selected devices.

Steps	Key Points
1. Verify the physician's order if appropriate.	1. Review any consultations by the occupational therapist/physical therapist.
2. Wash hands.	
3. Explain the purpose of the device to the patient/family.	
4. Demonstrate the use of the device.	4. Provide for patient privacy as appropriate.
5. Supervise return demonstration by patient/family.	

6. Instruct the patient/family concerning safety measures.

6. Safety measures include care of the skin, care of the device and calling the nurse or physician when indicated.

DOCUMENTATION

1. Type of assistive device used.
2. Consultation with occupational therapist/physical therapist, if appropriate.
3. Instructions to patient/family.
4. Patient/family understanding and return demonstration of device use.
5. Condition of skin or other device-related concerns/safety measures.
6. Report to the primary physician.

Home Health Aide Supervision Procedure

PURPOSE

- To assess the home health aide's performance of personal care and other tasks.
- To assess the patient's/family's relationship with and satisfaction with the home health aide.
- To assess achievement of patient outcomes.

Steps	*Key Points*
1. The registered nurse, as case manager, bases the home health aide's assignment upon the patient's problems/needs and the home health aide's training and skills.	1. Follow the agency's policies/procedures and regulatory guidelines in making assignments. Skilled care must be performed only by the appropriate professional.
2. Provide verbal and/or written instructions.	
3. Assess the home health aide's report to verify that each visit clearly reflects the plan of care and is appropriate for a home health aide visit, i.e., in that the elements of personal care, nutritional support and adherence to the therapeutic/rehabilitative program are supported.	3. Assess pertinent observations and information, adherence to agency policies and procedures, including quality and safe care, use of equipment and supplies and compliance with principles of infection control. Homemaking/housekeeping activities are not an acceptable focus for home health aide visits.
4. Review and/or perform documentation in the clinical record according to agency policy.	4. Documentation must reflect contribution to the plan of care.
5. Perform home health aide supervisory visits. Follow agency policies and procedures for assessment.	5. The frequency of scheduled visits is dependent upon agency and regulatory mandates. The home health aide may or may not be present. Documentation in the clinical record is essential.

Home Safety Procedure

PURPOSE

- To establish/maintain a safe home environment.

EQUIPMENT

- Safety checklist

Steps	Key Points
1. Assess the home environment for safety hazards.	1. A methodical assessment is easily achieved when a safety checklist is used.
2. Alert the patient/family/home health aide to the safety hazards.	
3. Teach the patient/family/home health aide how to correct the safety hazards.	3. Be specific when giving how-to advice. Useful materials/information can be obtained from local health departments/safety engineers.
4. Refer the patient/family to local health department/safety engineers for information/assistance that exceeds the nurse's expertise.	
5. Teach the patient/family/home health aide about accident prevention measures specific to maintaining the patient's safety.	5. Specific measures depend on the patient's medical problem and related nursing diagnoses.
6. Reassess safety hazards for correction/repair during the next visit.	

DOCUMENTATION

1. The assessment according to a safety checklist.
2. The safety hazards discovered.
3. The teaching/referral done pertinent to correction of the safety hazards.
4. The teaching done pertinent to accident prevention measures specific to the patient.
5. The patient's/family's response to the teaching.
6. The reassessment for correction/repair of the safety hazards.

Concern	Precaution/Correction
Bathroom	Handgrips by tub/shower and toilet. Nonskid strips/mat in tub/shower. Seat in tub/shower and/or by sink. High-rise toilet seat.
Electric Outlets/Devices	Unused outlets are covered and appliances are disconnected when not in use. Cords are not frayed/cracked. Cords fit snugly into sockets. Electrical cords run along walls. Electrical devices are not exposed to moisture. Fire safety/drill plan exits are available from all locations in the house. Smoke alarms are installed (hallways, bedrooms, kitchen, basement, attic). Fireplace smoke screen is in place. Fireplace/wood stove maintenance is done on a regular basis. Curtains/flammable items are away from stove/open flames. Adequate number of glass/ceramic ashtrays are available.
Floors	Nonskid wax is used. Scatter rugs are secured by nonskid backing. Large rugs are anchored at the edges. Pathways/hallways are cleared of toys, excess furniture and so forth.
Heating System	Periodic examination/cleaning on a regular basis by utility company.
Lighting	Adequate lights throughout the house and use of night lights.
Stairwells	Nonskid treads on steps with different color edge to indicate change in levels. Securely fastened handrail.
Miscellaneous	Medications, sharp objects and dangerous tools and cleaning substances are in secure areas out of the reach of children/confused adults. Ice/snow removal is efficient and adequate. Sidewalks, curbs and outside stairs are maintained. Hot water heater temperature is no higher than 120°F. Wheeled furniture is secured by caster plates.

UNIT
1

Telephone Contact with Patient/Family Procedure

PURPOSE

- To provide continuity of care.
- To increase patient satisfaction.
- To promote cost effectiveness.
- To check on patient's condition.

EQUIPMENT

- Telephone
- Pen/pencil
- Paper
- Patient home health care record

Steps	Key Points
1. Organize your thoughts and materials prior to making the call.	1. Identification of what you want to accomplish via the call facilitates communication by helping you concentrate on a topic and decreasing your hesitancy.
2. Initiate the telephone call.	
3. Address the patient by name.	3. Frequent use of the patient's name personalizes the interaction.
4. Identify yourself, by name and title, and the agency you are calling from.	
5. State the reason for the phone call.	
6. Assess the patient's current status and level of coping: a. use open-ended and direct questions b. clarify/reflect content c. clarify/reflect feelings.	6. Specific questions vary according to the reason for calling and the responses.
7. Intervene as appropriate: a. give instructions/anticipatory guidance b. schedule an immediate visit c. schedule a future visit d. schedule a future phone call.	7. When giving instructions/anticipatory guidance, clearly identify a. the home management plan b. the signs/symptoms requiring notification of the nurse/physician.
8. Keep the call within a reasonable time frame but do not rush the interaction.	8. Calls should not exceed 10 minutes. If more time is needed, schedule a home visit.

9. Restate the reason for the call and summarize the plan of care.
10. Ask the patient to state his or her understanding of/accord with the plan of care.
11. End the call.

DOCUMENTATION

1. Date of call and time call was initiated.
2. Reason for the call.
3. Name of person spoken with.
4. Assessment with subjective/objective validations.
5. Interventions during the call.
6. Plan of care.
7. Time the call was completed.

Resources

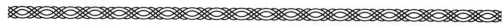

Medication Compliance
Management Guidelines

Prior to designing strategies to promote medication compliance, an assessment of the reasons for noncompliance is a prerequisite.

ASSESSMENT GUIDELINES

1. Sort assessment data into one of two categories.
   a. patient/family strengths
   b. patient/family limitations.
      Strengths are capitalized upon while designing strategies for intervention. Limitations form the basis for problem/need identification.
2. Assess the regimen for factors associated with a higher risk for noncompliance.
   a. recent changes in the regimen
   b. complexity (particularly in patients with chronic diseases)
   c. amount of compliance required (requiring 100% compliance 100% of the time leads to noncompliance in selected patients, such as adolescents with diabetes)
   d. amount of adjustment/decision making required by the patient
   e. age-/disease-related factors (such as chronic illness and progressive disability)
   f. medication side effects (Is the cure worse than the disease?)
   g. overprescribed/polypharmacy (particularly if the patient is managed by more than one physician)
   h. interactions of prescribed and/or over-the-counter medications
   i. all labeled, unlabeled and outdated medications.
3. Assess the patient/family for strengths and limitations in the following areas:
   a. Biopsychosocial. Examples: support systems, financial resources, religion, culture, energy levels, lifestyle and relationship with health care provider.
   b. Environmental. Examples: occupation, safety at home and in the community.
   c. Functional Abilities/Limitations
      • Physical/psychomotor areas. Examples: mobility, dexterity, body system and sense organ functioning.
      • Mental/cognitive areas. Examples: literacy (functional), knowledge level, time orientation and comprehension ability.
      • Emotional/affective areas. Examples: health beliefs (perceived susceptibility, severity, benefits and barriers to the regimen), health/illness practices, self-concept, acceptance of regimen and motivation.

INTERVENTION STRATEGIES

1. After analyzing the patient's/family's needs and perceptions, simplify the regimen to fit the patient's daily life pattern as appropriate.
   a. consult with the physician if prescription changes are necessary

b. attempt to decrease expenses when appropriate. For example, perhaps the patient can take an over-the-counter calcium fortified antacid rather than a more expensive calcium supplement. Refer to financial/community resources as needed.
2. Focus interventions on the patient and family; encourage involvement as much as possible.
3. Telephone visits by the nurse and by volunteers who telephone homebound patients can prove helpful.
4. Encourage the patient/family to call with questions.
5. Identify essential content that needs to be reinforced/taught.
   a. medication, purpose, dosage, side/adverse effects and interactions.
   b. how the medications relate to the disease and the therapeutic regimen.
6. Use principles of patient teaching.
   a. use audiovisual aids (such as photographs, videos, written material, tape recordings)
      • patient education material frequently is available free of charge from national groups (such as the American Cancer Society, American Heart Association, American Lung Association, American Diabetes Association) as well as from drug and medical suppliers
      • use symbols such as the sun, the moon, or a clock face in conjunction with medication names to provide time orientation
      • use a picture of four glasses of water to specify a desired number or a picture with a line drawn through the object to describe something to avoid
      • try to use pictures that convey only one message.
   b. provide for active involvement of the patient/family in the learning process
   c. ask the patient/family for daily routines that can be used as cues for medications, even television shows can help patients with time orientation limitations.
7. Use patient/family contracting when appropriate.
   a. contracts can be formal or informal (written or verbal); the format is not critical.
   b. contracting is based upon mutual goal setting/participative decision making about
      • the problem and the goals; both the process and outcome goals are stated in measurable terms
      • the plan to achieve the goals; the plan can be divided into parts that are prioritized within a time frame
      • roles, responsibilities and expectations of each person in the contract
      • evaluation of progress
      • modifications of contract.
   c. plan the parts/stages of the contract so that the patient/family achieve success as they progress toward the goal
   d. plan a reward at the end of the contract
   e. contracting can work with most age groups.
8. Evaluate interventions and modify strategies as needed.
9. Suggest counselling when appropriate.

UNIT 1

IMPORTANT POINTS

1. Medication management/memory aids include
   a. plastic or cardboard dispenser boxes that can be labeled and taped together as needed
   b. egg cartons can be cut into a group of four for four times a day (QID) medications or grouped together in other ways for other medication time needs.

   c. a posterboard calendar can have small plastic bags or cardboard boxes attached to hold each day's medications

   d. a checkoff list or tally sheet for daily medications can be adequate for the patient who needs minimal assistance

   e. electronic-capped bottles can be programmed for medication times; these represent a more costly alternative.

2. Consider dexterity when designing a medication management/memory aide. Egg cartons, for example, can be easily upset by patients with impaired dexterity.

3. When two or more elderly persons are in the same home, plan for each person's medications to be managed separately. Keep medication management/memory aids labeled and separate.

4. Design the plan so that medications/fluids are accessible.

DOCUMENTATION

1. Date and time of all home and telephone visits.
2. Assessment of reasons for noncompliance.
3. Intervention strategies for compliance management.
4. Use of patient/family contracting as appropriate.
5. Evaluation of progress.
6. All relevant physical findings.
7. Discussions with the physician and other members of the health care team.

Bibliography

American Red Cross. Family Health and Home Nursing. Garden City, New York: Doubleday and Co., Inc., 1979.

Becker, M. and Janz, N. The Health Belief Model Applied to Understanding Diabetes Regimen Compliance. The Diabetes Educator, Spring 1985, pp. 41–47.

Carey, R. Compliance and Related Nursing Actions. Nursing Forum, vol. 21, no. 4, 1984, pp. 157–161.

Creighton, H. Law Every Nurse Should Know, 5th ed. Philadelphia: W. B. Saunders Co., 1986.

Falvo, D. R. Effective Patient Education: A Guide to Increased Compliance. Rockville, Maryland: Aspen Systems, 1985.

Gerber, K. E. and Nehemkis, A. M. (eds.). Compliance: The Dilemma of the Chronically Ill. New York: Springer, 1986.

Gioiella, E. and Bevie, C. Nursing Care of the Aging Client: Promoting Healthy Adaptation. Norwalk, Connecticut: Appleton-Century-Crofts, 1985.

Harnish, Y. and Leeser, I. Patient Care Guidelines: Practical Information for Public Health Nurses, 2nd ed. New York: National League for Nursing (Pub. No. 21-1968), 1984.

Haynes, R. B., Taylor, D. W. and Sackett, D. L. (eds.). Compliance in Health Care. Baltimore, Maryland: Johns Hopkins University Press, 1979.

Helgeson, D. and Berg, C. Contracting: A Method of Health Promotion. Journal of Community Health Nursing, 2(4):1985, pp. 199–207.

Jensen, D. P. Patient Contracting. In Bulechek, G. M. and McCloskey, J. C. (eds.). Nursing Interventions: Treatments for Nursing Diagnoses. Philadelphia: W. B. Saunders Co., 1985, pp. 92–98.

Levitt, D. How to Diagnose, Analyze, and Treat Noncompliance. American Journal of Nursing, January 1985, p. 52.

Loughrey, L. Dealing with the Illiterate Patient. You Can't Read Him Like a Book. Nursing 83. January 1983, pp. 65–67.

Loustau, A. and Blair, B. A Key to Compliance: Systematic Teaching to Help Hypertensive Patients Follow Through on Treatment. Nursing 81. February 1981, pp. 84–87.

Martin, N., et al. (eds.). Comprehensive Rehabilitation Nursing. New York: McGraw-Hill, 1981.

McMillan, J., et al. The Whole Pediatrician Catalog, vol. 2. Philadelphia: W. B. Saunders Co., 1979.

McMillan, J., et al. The Whole Pediatrician Catalog, vol. 3. Philadelphia: W. B. Saunders Co., 1982.

Meichenbaum, D. and Turk, D. C. Facilitating Treatment Adherence: A Practitioner's Guidebook. New York: Plenum Press, 1987.

Providing Early Mobility Nursing Photobook. Nursing 84 Books. Springhouse, Pennsylvania: Springhouse Corporation, 1984.

Rauen, K. The Telephone as Stethoscope. MCH 10(2):1985, pp. 122–124.

Sloan, M. and Schommer, B. Want to Get Your Patient Involved in His Care? Use a Contract. Nursing 80, December 1982, pp. 48–49.

Smith, J. The Patient Who Can't Remember to Take Her Meds. RN, September 1986, pp. 38–41.

Streiff, L. Can Clients Understand Our Instructions? IMAGE: Journal of Nursing Scholarship, vol. 18, no. 2, Summer 1986, pp. 48–52.

Tackett, J. and Hunsberger, M. Family-Centered Care of Children and Adolescents. Philadelphia: W. B. Saunders Co., 1981.

Trekas, J. It Takes Two to Achieve Compliance. Nursing 84. September 1984, pp. 58–59.

Weibert, R. T. and Dee, D. D. Improving Patient Medication Compliance. Oradell, New Jersey: Medical Economics, 1980.

Wesolowski, C. Self-Contracts for Chronically Ill Children. American Journal of Maternal Child Nursing, vol. 13, January/February 1988, pp. 20–33.

UNIT
1

Cardiovascular Alterations

Care Plans

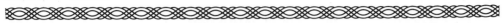

Angina Pectoris Care Plan

This care plan is designed to be used in conjunction with the Generic Cardiac Care Plan. This Angina Pectoris Care Plan supplements angina pectoris–specific information.

CROSS REFERENCES

Depression Care Plan	Oxygen Therapy Procedure
Hypertension Care Plan	Medication Compliance Management Guidelines
Pain Care Plan	

UNIT 2

PROCESS INDICATORS

1. The patient/family/home health aide will verbalize an understanding of how to control angina pectoris.
Indicators
   a. describe situations that may precipitate angina pectoris attacks
   b. describe ways to control the precipitating situations and to decrease cardiac workload
   c. demonstrate how to correctly monitor pulse rate and rhythm
   d. list angina pectoris symptoms
   e. describe step-by-step actions to be taken at the first sign of symptoms
   f. patient carries nitroglycerin at all times (if prescribed)
   g. patient carries emergency medical identification.

NURSING INTERVENTIONS

1. Instruct the patient/family/home health aide about
   a. avoiding situations or activities that result in angina pectoris symptoms such as sudden bursts of activity, straining or lifting, very hot or very cold temperatures
   b. carefully analyzing the living, working and leisure environments to develop a plan to control cardiovascular and emotional stress
   c. using prophylactic nitroglycerin before selected activities (if approved by the physician)
   d. common symptoms of angina
      • pain, tightness, aching or numbness in the chest, arm, neck, shoulder, jaw or throat
      • dyspnea
      • diaphoresis
      • dizziness.
2. Instruct the patient/family/home health aide about an action plan for an angina attack.
   a. stop the activity
   b. sit and look at the time if possible
   c. if nitroglycerin tablets are prescribed
      • take 1 tablet (strength prescribed by the doctor) every 5 minutes up to a total of 3 tablets in 15 minutes

- call physician or emergency services immediately if symptoms continue after 15 to 20 minutes
- begin activity slowly after symptoms are relieved
- have tablets available at all times
- protect tablets from heat, moisture, air and light
- renew tablets every 5 to 6 months (fresh tablets should cause a burning or stinging sensation when placed under the tongue)
- anticipate some of the side effects, such as dizziness, flushing and headache. The side effects should be transient and mild. If they are not, the physician should be contacted. Patients should be instructed to rise slowly from a sitting or supine position.

d. what symptoms to report to the physician or the emergency room personnel
- angina symptoms lasting 20 minutes that are not relieved by nitroglycerin
- symptoms that are becoming more frequent, more intense or occurring at rest
- dyspnea
- syncope
- decreased activity tolerance
- palpitations/tachycardia/bradycardia.

THERAPEUTIC ACHIEVEMENT

- The patient will achieve control of angina pectoris through life style modification and medication.

RELATED PATIENT INSTRUCTIONS

Angina	Restricted Cholesterol Diet
Healthy Heart	Taking a Pulse
Heart Medications	

Congestive Heart Failure Care Plan

This care plan is designed to be used in conjunction with the Generic Cardiac Care Plan. This Congestive Heart Failure Care Plan also supplements specific information in the Congestive Heart Failure.

CROSS REFERENCES

Hypertension Care Plan

Oxygen Therapy Procedure

PROCESS INDICATORS

1. The patient's biopsychosocial integrity is maintained.
Indicators
   a. blood pressure is within the patient's normal range
   b. apical pulse
      • is regular with absence of gallop rhythm
      • is within patient's normal range
   c. respirations are unlabored and within patient's normal range (no adventitious breath sounds)
   d. usual mental status is demonstrated
   e. peripheral pulses are palpable and equal in strength
   f. no evidence of peripheral edema, ascites, neck vein distension, dark amber urine or oliguria
   g. patient/family identifies signs and symptoms of congestive heart failure and strategies to prevent complications.

NURSING INTERVENTION

1. Assess the patient's complaints/symptoms of fatigue, weakness, dyspnea, orthopnea, nocturia, paroxsymal nocturnal dyspnea and activity intolerance. In infants and children assess feeding difficulties, anorexia and failure of growth and development.
2. Assess, monitor and record the patient's
   a. apical and radial pulse rates and rhythm (check for the presence of a third heart sound/gallop rhythm)
   b. blood pressure
   c. peripheral pulses/diminished or alternating pulses
   d. peripheral edema (ankle measurements should be recorded)
   e. ascites
      • measure abdominal girth at the same time of day and in the same place with the patient in the same position
      • percuss abdomen for areas of dullness and shifting dullness
      • look for positive puddle sign and abdominal fluid wave
      • look for unusual tautness of abdominal skin.

3. Instruct the patient/family/home health aide about an activity program (within medically prescribed parameters) that
   a. includes signs of overexertion
      • pulse rate increase of 20 beats/min
      • pulse irregularities
      • marked increase in blood pressure
      • chest pain or increased dyspnea
      • excessive fatigue/weakness
      • diaphoresis
      • dizziness or syncope
   b. includes consultation with an occupational therapist, a physical therapist or a physician for approaches/devices to assist with activities of daily living and diversional activities, such as use of energy-saving techniques like a shower chair or sitting at the sink to bathe
   c. provides for infants and children
      • avoids unnecessary activities (clothing changes or complete baths)
      • suggests diversional activities that require little physical exertion
      • prevents excessive crying (holding child and correcting problems such as wet diapers).
4. Instruct the patient/family/home health aide about a dietary plan that
   a. includes consultations with the dietician or physician when
      • intake and output recording may be needed
      • enteral or parenteral nutrition may be considered (if oral intake is inadequate)
      • a prescription for antiemetics may be needed
   b. provides strategies to minimize vomiting
      • changing positions slowly to avoid dizziness
      • resting before and after meals. After meals the patient should remain in an upright sitting position (if in bed, raise the head of the bed on blocks or with pillows). Infants can be placed in an infant seat.
      • providing good oral hygiene after emesis and before meals
      • eating dry foods without drinking liquids with meals
      • eating small frequent meals with rest periods in between, eating slowly and avoiding large meals and overeating
      • observing for distension and vomiting following meals, especially for infants.
5. Instruct the patient/family/home health aide about
   a. disease processes and complications
      • if dealing with a child use terminology the child and the parents can understand
      • clarify difference between congestive heart failure and myocardial infarction.
   b. measurement and recording of weight as scheduled (probably every day on the same scale)
   c. signs and symptoms that require immediate medical care
      • increased shortness of breath
      • persistent or unusual weight gain
      • edema of extremities/ascites/distended neck veins
      • rapid, labored or irregular respirations
      • increased orthopnea
      • irregular pulse (especially less than 60 beats/min or greater than 100 beats/min)
      • decreased activity tolerance
      • adverse medication reactions
      • cool, pale mottled skin
      • restlessness/confusion/syncope

- signs of pulmonary edema (gurgling respirations; frothy, blood-tinged sputum; diaphoresis; constant coughing and increasing distress)
- in infants and children, report any changes, such as increased temperature, diarrhea, vomiting, upper respiratory infection and changes in cry or mentation.

d. a plan for promoting optimal skin care to prevent irritation and breakdown
  - elevating dependent extremities if edema is present
  - turning and repositioning patient confined to bed at least every 2 hours
  - performing range of motion exercises at least 4 times each day
  - use support devices and correct placement for scrotal edema
  - after consultation with the physician, use elastic wraps or hose for lower extremity edema or pressure minimizing devices/mattresses for patients confined to bed.

e. a plan for promoting adequate air/gas exchange
  - encouraging coughing and deep breathing at least every 2 hours, if patient is confined to bed
  - administering oxygen therapy as ordered
  - performing tracheal suctioning and/or postural drainage as ordered
  - raising the head of the bed on 10-in blocks or achieve a similar position using pillows (sitting in a chair where the legs can be elevated is sometimes preferred, or during difficult periods, some adult patients prefer to rest, sitting forward on a table with good pillow support)
  - being aware that paroxysmal nocturnal dyspnea occurs approximately 2 hours after lying down
  - avoiding exposure to persons with upper respiratory infections
  - providing adequate ventilation and a temperature controlled environment within the home (critical during hot, humid weather)
  - using a humidifier and mucolytic agents as ordered to liquefy secretions.

UNIT 2

THERAPEUTIC ACHIEVEMENT

- The patient/family adapts to the life style changes resulting from congestive heart failure.
- For infants and children, patients will exhibit progression through stages of growth and development within normal limits.

RELATED PATIENT INSTRUCTIONS

Diuretic Medications
Healthy Heart
Heart Medications
Oxygen Therapy

Restricted Cholesterol Diet
Seasonings for Sodium Restricted Diets
Ways to Save Your Energy

Generic Cardiac Care Plan

This care plan is designed to provide a core care plan for patients with cardiovascular disease. Refer to the appropriate cardiovascular supplemental care plans for specific patient conditions.

CROSS REFERENCES

Angina Pectoris Care Plan
Congestive Heart Failure Care Plan
Constipation Care Plan
Cerebrovascular Accident Care Plan

Depression Care Plan
Pain Care Plan

Oxygen Therapy Procedure

Vital Signs: Normal Pediatric Values

NURSING DIAGNOSES

1. Alteration in cardiac output related to
   a. arrythmias
   b. medication side effects
   c. stress/activity intolerance
   d. inadequate medication compliance
   e. exposure to temperature extremes
   f. other.
2. Activity intolerance related to
   a. fatigue/weakness
   b. anxiety/fear
   c. pain (acute or chronic)
   d. impaired gas exchange/dyspnea
   e. abnormal heart rate/rhythm or blood pressure response to activity
   f. exertional discomfort
   g. lack of physical support/mobility assistive devices
   h. dizziness
   i. other.
3. Alteration in comfort related to
   a. abnormal heart rate/rhythm or blood pressure response to activity
   b. imbalance between oxygen supply and demand
   c. other.
4. Anxiety related to
   a. uncertainty of future, disease process, treatment plan, potential surgery
   b. pain/discomfort
   c. fear of disability/death
   d. disturbances in sleep/rest patterns
   e. changes in life style/role functioning/interaction patterns/socioeconomic status
   f. correctly monitoring pulse rate
   g. dependence on others for care
   h. medication side effects (impotence, hypotension, dizziness, headaches)
   i. shortness of breath
   j. activity intolerance
   k. other.

5. Ineffective individual coping such as sleep pattern disturbances, increasing fatigue, trouble concentrating, irritability related to
   a. dysfunctional grieving/depression
   b. multiple life/role changes
   c. inadequate relaxation
   d. inadequate support systems
   e. inadequate activity/exercise levels
   f. inadequate nutrition (lack of appetite or overeating)
   g. inadequate coping skills
   h. inadequate financial resources
   i. impaired interactional patterns
   j. substance abuse
   k. dependence on others for care
   l. other.

6. Alteration in nutrition related to
   a. insufficient financial resources
   b. inadequate support systems (for shopping, cooking)
   c. personal/cultural/religious barriers
   d. not achieving/maintaining range for ideal body weight
   e. noncompliance with prescribed diet
   f. other.

7. Ineffective breathing pattern related to
   a. anxiety/fear
   b. pain (chest)
   c. fatigue/weakness
   d. medication side effects
   e. excessive activity
   f. other.

8. Alteration in bowel elimination (constipation) related to
   a. medications
   b. inadequate physical activity
   c. fear of straining (chest pain/heart attack)
   d. inadequate dietary intake (bulk/fluid)
   e. other.

9. Potential for injury related to
   a. dizziness/weakness
   b. inadequate compliance with the therapeutic regimen
   c. inadequate supervision in the home
   d. excessive activity
   e. lack of mobility assistive devices
   f. impaired skin integrity
   g. denial of severity of condition
   h. other.

10. Noncompliance with therapeutic regimen related to
   a. knowledge deficit
   b. lack of support (family/community/financial)
   c. denial of severity of disease
   d. lack of perceived benefits of compliance
   e. dysfunctional patient/health care provider relationship
   f. medication side effects
   g. difficulty integrating into life style

    h. cultural/religious barriers
    i. dysfunctional grieving
    j. other.

11. Sexual dysfunction (decreased libido/impotence) related to
    a. medication side effects
    b. pain/discomfort
    c. altered self-concept
    d. anxiety about performance/fear of rejection
    e. impaired physical strength/endurance
    f. other.

12. Sleep pattern disturbance related to
    a. pain/discomfort
    b. anxiety/fear of death
    c. paroxysmal nocturnal dyspnea/dyspnea/orthopnea
    d. medication side effects
    e. restlessness/insomnia
    f. other.

13. Ineffective family coping patterns related to
    a. family disorganization/role changes
    b. prolonged disease/disability that exhausts supportive capacity of significant others
    c. sociocultural barriers
    d. inadequate financial resources
    e. impaired parenting
    f. long-term care of elderly family member
    g. difficulty integrating therapeutic regimen into normal childhood growth and development
    h. other.

14. Self-care deficit (feeding, bathing/hygiene, dressing/grooming, toileting, ambulation) related to
    a. fear/anxiety
    b. emotional lability
    c. pain/discomfort
    d. dependence on others for care
    e. dizziness
    f. activity intolerance
    g. other.

15. Knowledge deficit (nature of cardiovascular disease/treatment, therapeutic regimen for medication/diet/activity/follow-up, stress management, signs and symptoms to report to physician, emergency action plan, correctly monitoring pulse rate/blood pressure, community/informational resources) related to
    a. cognitive limitations
    b. misinterpretation of information
    c. lack of readiness to learn
    d. sociocultural barriers
    e. other.

16. Disturbance in self-concept (body image, self-esteem, role performance, personal identity) related to
    a. verbalizations of feelings of hopelessness/powerlessness
    b. sexual dysfunction
    c. dependence on others for care

    d. change in ability to resume role/job/life style

    e. other.

17. Impaired home maintenance management related to

    a. ineffective individual coping

    b. ineffective family coping

    c. excessive environmental demands on the cardiovascular system

    d. inadequate community/financial support

    e. lack of knowledge

    f. weakness/fatigue

    g. other.

UNIT 2

PROCESS INDICATORS

1. The patient/family/home health aide verbalizes an understanding of cardiovascular wellness.

Indicators

    a. demonstrates correct monitoring of pulse rate

    b. describes a cardiovascular risk factor and life style modification plan that minimizes atherosclerosis development and excessive myocardial demands

    c. identifies a diet plan that controls fat, calories, stimulants, alcohol and sodium

    d. describes an activity plan that includes
- planned periods of prescribed graduated activity and rest
- activities that do not induce symptoms

    e. describes a plan for receiving follow-up care

    f. identifies signs and symptoms to report to the physician

    g. describes an appropriate emergency action plan

    h. identifies medication action, dose, administration schedule, side effects and adverse reactions

    i. identifies resources for life style modification/support, such as community groups and the American Heart Association.

2. The patient establishes/maintains a satisfactory level of comfort.

Indicators

    a. reports undisturbed sleep

    b. verbalizes absence of uncontrolled pain/discomfort

    c. verbalizes successful coping with anxiety/stress

    d. demonstrates satisfactory activity levels with ability to perform self-care activities

    e. expresses satisfaction with quality of life

    f. reports decrease in intensity and number of symptoms (fatigue, dizziness, dyspnea, cardiac arrhythmias)

    g. reports satisfactory defecation pattern.

3. The patient/family demonstrates effective coping patterns.

Indicators

    a. reorganizes family roles and activities to incorporate medication, diet, activity and follow-up care as part of the therapeutic regimen

    b. patient and partner express satisfactory level of sexual functioning

    c. demonstrates satisfactory parenting skills

    d. verbalizes decreased anxiety/fear/depression

    e. develops a positive relationship with the health care team

    f. identifies effective and ineffective coping patterns.

NURSING INTERVENTIONS

1. Assess
   a. the patient's/family's understanding of cardiovascular disease, therapeutic regimen and prevention of complications including but not limited to diet, activity and medication compliance
   b. the patient's/family's ability to correctly monitor pulse rate and/or blood pressure
   c. the patient's comfort level/anxiety level/sense of self-esteem
   d. the patient's/family's development of a long-term health care plan
   e. the patient's/family's history of risk factors including dietary pattern, body weight range, smoking behavior, exercise pattern, history of diabetes and/or previous cardiovascular illness
   f. the patient's/family's methods of coping with stress
   g. the patient's reports of pain/discomfort (location, radiation, quality, duration, intensity, circumstances of onset and relief)
   h. the patient's pre-illness and current activity level and complaints of fatigue, weakness and/or dyspnea
   i. the patient's/family's ability to make adjustments within the prescribed regimen as appropriate
   j. the patient's and partner's satisfaction with their sexual relationship.
2. Assess, monitor and record
   a. blood pressure in both arms (take two readings during the visit at least 10 minutes apart, take blood pressure in both arms—supine and standing—and document position and arm selection on subsequent readings)
   b. heart sounds (rate, rhythm, quality, extra sounds) and radial pulse (pulse deficit)
   c. breath sounds (rate, depth, rhythm, adventitious sounds)
   d. skin color
   e. peripheral pulses (palpable, strength)
   f. any evidence of peripheral edema (measure ankles), neck vein distension
   g. intake and output records, if patient is self-monitoring.
3. Instruct the patient/family/home health aide about a dietary plan that
   a. is compatible with the prescribed diet parameters including foods that are
      • high in fiber and bulk (bran, vegetables, fruit, whole grains) to promote satisfactory bowel elimination and maintenance of desirable weight. For example, the patient will eat three food portions with a fiber content of _____% five times per week.
      • high in potassium (bananas, potatoes, raisins, tomatoes) to compensate for potassium depleting medications. For example, the patient will eat half a banana every day.
      • low in caffeine to decrease sympathetic nervous system stimulation (less or no coffee, tea, colas and chocolate)
      • low in sugar to control calories
      • low in cholesterol and saturated fat (decrease intake of whole milk products, eggs, meat; increase intake of fish, poultry, skim milk products) to inhibit progression of atherosclerosis
      • low in sodium (avoid monosodium glutamate, pickled foods, processed meats, salty snacks, added salt) to reduce fluid retention. For infants, low sodium formula is available if prescribed. For example, the patient will maintain a _____ mg sodium diet.
      • nonirritating to the gastrointestinal tract (avoid gas producing foods, spicy foods,

citrus fruit or juice, excessive drinking with meals) if the patient is experiencing discomfort/nausea

b. includes a 3-day diet recall completed by the patient/family. For example, the patient will keep a food log beginning _____ and ending _____.

c. provides written instructions/recipes for reference

d. instructs the patient/family how to read food labels

e. incorporates cultural/religious parameters and personal preferences

f. includes a consultation with the dietician as necessary

g. encourages the patient to eat 3 to 4 meals daily within caloric restrictions (avoid large meals, overeating; plan for a rest period after eating, with head slightly elevated; eat meals slowly; eat portions as specified in the meal plan; use low calorie foods as on the meal plan). For example, divide the day's total calorie allotment into _____ calories for breakfast, _____ calories for lunch, _____ calories for snack, _____ calories for dinner.

h. incorporates weight control strategies (measured portion sizes; decreased use of high calorie sources including butter, sugar, alcohol; increased intake of fiber, bulk, fruit; referral to weight control support groups, as needed).

4. Instruct the patient/family/home health aide about an activity program that
   a. avoids signs and symptoms of overexertion
      - dizziness
      - chest pain
      - shortness of breath
      - marked increase in pulse rate/palpitations
      - marked increase in blood pressure
      - excessive fatigue/weakness.
   b. conditions the cardiovascular system
      - a general isotonic program includes at least a 5-minute stretching and warm up period, approximately 15 to 20 minutes of activity at the currently prescribed target heart rate, and a 10-minute cool down period. For example, a walking program may aim toward a goal of 2 miles in less than 60 minutes.
      - outdoor activity should be avoided in inclement weather with extremes in temperature. For example, stationary bicycling offers an indoor alternative.
      - clarify the difference between isotonic and isometric exercising. (Patients should be cautioned against weightlifting and resistive equipment unless approved by the physician.)
      - the physician should specify the target heart rate as well as the daily/weekly activity targets
      - periods of rest should be planned throughout the day
   c. incorporates pulse taking before and after activity as appropriate
   d. includes signs and symptoms of overexertion and stopping of any activity that results in symptoms or fatigue
   e. avoids Valsalva maneuver (straining to defecate, bending at the waist, lifting above the head, holding breath while lifting, lifting heavy objects)
   f. avoids extremes in temperature (hot or very cold weather/hot or very cold baths)
   g. incorporates diversional activities.
5. Instruct the patient/family/home health aide about
   a. disease process and prevention of complications
   b. cardiovascular risk factor reduction
      - maintain desirable weight
      - maintain a diet low in saturated fats and cholesterol
      - establish a regular pattern of exercise

UNIT 2

- reduce and ultimately stop smoking
- control blood pressure
- develop stress management strategies

  c. medication regimen
- names, actions, dosages, administration schedule, side and adverse effects and drug interactions
- discuss the introduction of any new medications with the physician prior to initiation
- strategies to assist the patient who has an impaired concept of time with adhering to an administration schedule

  d. ways to decrease the demands on the patient's cardiovascular system in the living/working/leisure environments (such as energy saving strategies/devices, planning activities with periods of rest)

  e. a plan for promoting a satisfactory defecation pattern
- including additional high fiber and bulk in the diet as needed
- maintaining an ample fluid intake
- establishing a defecation routine
- avoiding straining at stool
- consulting with the physician for a prescription for stool softeners or laxative

  f. a plan for sleep promotion
- avoiding stimulants 1 to 2 hours before bedtime
- limiting fluid intake 1 to 2 hours before bedtime
- incorporating the patient's previous patterns/strategies to promote sleep

  g. the need for medical identification and an emergency action plan
- posting the emergency service's telephone number
- establishing an emergency action plan.

6. Instruct the patient/family about correctly taking blood pressure and/or pulse rate measurements.
  a. during return demonstration assess for technique and accuracy
  b. provide written instructions for reference.

7. Encourage the patient/family to verbalize fears/anxieties
  a. assist family to identify ways to incorporate life style modifications into a long-term health plan
- foster the patient's/family's sense of control
- identify stressors and possible coping strategies
  b. consult with social worker as needed.

8. Provide the patient and partner with an opportunity to verbalize concerns about their sexual relationship and include sexual activity guidelines
  a. encourage the patient and partner to discuss their feelings about changes (impotence/fatigue) in sexual functioning
  b. discuss with the patient and partner alternative ways of expressing caring/affection
  c. instruct resumption of sexual activity based on the physician's instructions
  d. advise resting before and after sexual activity
  e. encourage avoiding coitus when fatigued or under stress
  f. recommend no eating or drinking alcoholic beverages immediately before engaging in coitus (wait 2 to 3 hours after eating a heavy meal)
  g. advise avoiding anal intercourse (due to vasovagal effect)
  h. recommend taking nitroglycerin before sexual activity, if prescribed
  i. discuss with the physician the patient's need for a consultation with a sex therapist.

9. Identify community resources that can facilitate the patient's/family's adjustment to the effects of cardiovascular disease and life style modification including
  a. cardiovascular wellness and educational materials (American Heart Association)

b. weight loss support groups

c. smoking cessation (American Lung Association)

d. alcohol/drug rehabilitation services

e. stress management/relaxation techniques

f. counselling, psychological therapy or a self-help group for support

g. consulting with the physician and initiating referrals as needed.

10. Coordinate additional members of the health care team such as the social worker, physical therapist, occupational therapist, registered dietician, sex therapist and home health aide.

11. Provide progress reports and a discharge summary to the primary physician.

UNIT 2

THERAPEUTIC ACHIEVEMENT

- The patient/family will adapt to the life style modifications resulting from cardiovascular disease.

RELATED PATIENT INSTRUCTIONS

Healthy Heart	Seasonings for Sodium Restricted Diets
Heart Medications	Taking a Pulse
Restricted Cholesterol Diet	

Hypertension Care Plan

This care plan is designed to be used in conjunction with the Generic Cardiac Care Plan. This Hypertension Care Plan supplements hypertension-specific information.

CROSS REFERENCE

Medication Compliance Management Guidelines

PROCESS INDICATORS

1. The patient/family will verbalize an understanding of how to control blood pressure.
Indicators
   a. the patient will exhibit blood pressure levels within the range established by the physician as reflected in the nurse's/patient's/family's readings
   b. the absence of signs and symptoms of uncontrolled blood pressure levels
   c. the accurate performance by the patient/family of blood pressure readings (if appropriate).

NURSING INTERVENTIONS

1. Monitor and record the patient's blood pressure
   a. take at least two readings during the visit (it takes about 10 minutes for a patient to relax)
   b. establish blood pressure baseline values by taking readings in both the arms, with the patient both supine and standing
   c. document the position and arm selection on subsequent readings.
2. Instruct the patient/family/home health aide about the following strategies for minimizing or coping with side effects of medications (dizziness, nocturia, impotence and gastrointestinal disturbances):
   a. changing from a lying to a sitting, or from a sitting to a standing, position slowly to decrease the dizziness associated with postural hypotension
   b. avoiding prolonged standing in one place or hot baths that lead to peripheral vasodilatation and dizziness
   c. taking diuretics in the morning to avoid nocturia
   d. calling the physician when feeling too ill to eat (if taking a diuretic to avoid dehydration)
   e. avoiding foods with tyramine (if taking a monoamine oxidase (MAO) inhibitor).
3. Instruct the patient/family/home health aide about signs and symptoms that require immediate medical care, including
   a. progressive severe headache, severe dizziness, stupor, convulsions, transient ischemic attacks (TIAs), weakness in arms or legs
   b. changes in vision
   c. stomach pain, nausea, vomiting
   d. increased shortness of breath, persistent cough
   e. chest pain, palpitations
   f. dysphagia

g. diastolic pressure greater than 120 mm Hg (if monitoring blood pressure readings)
h. adverse reactions to medications
i. swelling of ankles, feet, abdomen
j. weight gain of greater than 5 lb in 1 week
k. increased frequency and severity of nosebleeds.

THERAPEUTIC ACHIEVEMENT

- The patient will achieve blood pressure control within a range of _____ by adhering to the therapeutic regimen.

RELATED PATIENT INSTRUCTIONS

Diuretic Medications
Healthy Heart
Heart Medications
High Blood Pressure Medications

Medication Compliance
Restricted Cholesterol Diet
Seasonings for Sodium Restricted Diets
Warning Signs of a Stroke

Myocardial Infarction Care Plan

This care plan is designed to be used in conjunction with the Generic Cardiac Care Plan. This Myocardial Infarction Care Plan supplements myocardial infarction–specific information.

CROSS REFERENCES

Angina Pectoris Care Plan
Constipation Care Plan
Depression Care Plan
Hypertension Care Plan

Oxygen Therapy Procedure

Medication Compliance Management Guidelines

PROCESS INDICATORS

1. The patient achieves biopsychosocial integrity.
Indicators
   a. maintains an apical pulse rate that is within the patient's normal range (regular rhythm or an irregular rhythm that is not life-threatening)
   b. maintains blood pressure within the patient's normal range
   c. maintains unlabored respirations within the patient's normal range with no adventitious breath sounds
   d. verbalizes/demonstrates that symptoms (such as angina, dyspnea, chest/neck/jaw/shoulder pain) are decreasing in number and/or intensity
   e. no evidence of peripheral edema or neck vein distension
   f. maintains weight within optimal range.
2. The patient/family verbalizes an understanding of how to maintain the cardiac rehabilitation plan.
Indicators
   a. patient/family identifies signs and symptoms of myocardial infarction and the appropriate emergency action plan
   b. patient/family describes the phases (progressive nature) of the rehabilitation plan
   c. family is competent in cardiopulmonary resuscitation (CPR)
   d. patient/family is able to accurately monitor pulse rate.

NURSING INTERVENTIONS

1. Assess
   a. the patient's premyocardial infarction parameters of living/work/leisure activity
   b. the patient's/family's understanding of the cardiac rehabilitation plan particularly to clarify preinfarction and postinfarction adjustments in activity, diet and medication.

2. Instruct the patient/family/home health aide about an activity program (within the medically prescribed parameters) that
   a. allows for frequent rest periods during the first 4 to 8 weeks after hospital discharge as described within the phases of the patient's prescribed rehabilitation plan
   b. emphasizes the importance of resting heart rate, target heart rate and myocardial demands
   c. clarifies restrictions on air travel and return to work activity schedule.
3. Instruct the patient/family/home health aide about signs and symptoms that require immediate medical care including
   a. recurrence of previous heart disease signs
   b. chest pain unrelieved by nitroglycerin (if prescribed)
   c. increased shortness of breath
   d. edema of extremities/weight gain
   e. decreased activity tolerance
   f. adverse medication reactions
   g. irregular pulse.

UNIT 2

THERAPEUTIC ACHIEVEMENT

- The patient/family adapts to the life style modifications as a result of cardiac disease.
- The patient will achieve optimal rehabilitation physically, emotionally and functionally within his or her limits.

RELATED PATIENT INSTRUCTIONS

After Your Heart Attack	Heart Medications
Anticoagulant Medications	Seasonings for Sodium Restricted Diets
Aspirin and Aspirin-like Medications	Restricted Cholesterol Diet
Diuretic Medications	Taking a Pulse
Healthy Heart	Ways to Save Your Energy

Pacemaker Care Plan

This care plan is designed to be used in conjunction with the Generic Cardiac Care Plan. The Pacemaker Care Plan supplements pacemaker-specific information.

CROSS REFERENCE

Telephone Contact with Patient/Family
    Procedure

PROCESS INDICATORS

1. The patient/family/home health aide will verbalize an understanding of pacemaker care and safety.
Indicators
    a. describes the function of the pacemaker including any special equipment for testing
    b. identifies situations that may interfere with proper pacemaker functioning/safety
    c. describes an activity plan that incorporates pacemaker safety guidelines (such as contact sport restrictions)
    d. lists pacemaker malfunction symptoms (vary depending upon the type of pacemaker)
    e. identifies emergency actions to be taken at the first sign of symptoms
    f. verbalizes the importance of carrying a medical emergency and pacemaker identification card at all times
    g. describes the importance of and a plan for
        • pacemaker checks
        • routine physician follow-up.
2. The patient/family/home health aide will demonstrate wound care procedure
Indicators
    a. follows principles of infection control
    b. describes signs and symptoms of wound infection
    c. independently performs dressing change within correct procedural guidelines.

NURSING INTERVENTIONS

1. Assess pacemaker functioning
    a. following any manufacturer's instructions for testing as applicable
    b. performing an electrocardiogram (ECG) (if ordered)
        • pacer spikes should appear before QRS complex
        • if a demand pacemaker the spikes will occur only when the pulse rate is less than the present rate
    c. including documentation of patient parameters
        • regular pulse within 2 to 3 beats of present rate
        • stable blood pressure readings
        • absence of symptoms.
2. Instruct the patient/family/home health aide about an activity program (within the medically prescribed parameters) that
    a. incorporates full range of motion exercises at least four times per day for the operative side's arm and shoulder

b. limits vigorous movement, stress, pressure on the operative side's arm for about the first 6 weeks after surgery
c. requires physician's approval prior to engaging in contact sports
d. promotes safety by avoidance of environment/equipment that causes electromagnetic interference
  • sources of high voltage
  • television and radio transmitters
  • industrial arc welders
  • diathermy and some electrocautery in some health care facilities
  • certain older microwave ovens
  • large running motors/engines.
e. incorporates pulse taking before and after physical activity as indicated.
3. Instruct the patient/family/home health aide about
a. function of and type of pacemaker including the prescribed preset rate
b. palpating radial pulse rate for 1 minute and assessing regularity of rhythm every day
  • reconfirming that patient/family understands the significance of a variance between the preset rate and the palpated pulse rate
  • assessing for technique and accuracy during the return demonstration.
4. Instruct the patient/family/home health aide about common symptoms of pacemaker malfunction
a. any pulse rate reductions greater than 4 to 5 beats/min from the preset pacemaker rate
b. any periods of bradycardia or tachycardia
c. dizziness
d. syncope
e. irregular pulse rate
f. prolonged hiccups
g. chest pain
h. dyspnea
i. peripheral edema
j. persistent/unexplained weight gain.
5. Instruct the patient/family home health aide about
a. an emergency action plan for pacemaker malfunction
  • if near electrical equipment or in a high voltage environment when experiencing symptoms move at least 5 ft away from the equipment, take pulse, call the physician or emergency services immediately when symptoms continue after moving out of range
  • if not in range of a high voltage environment or near electrical equipment when experiencing symptoms take pulse, call the physician or emergency services when symptoms first appear.
b. a pacemaker safety plan
  • patient/family will inform other health care providers (nurse, dentist, chiropractor, physical therapist) about the presence and type of pacemaker
  • avoid known environment/equipment that interferes with pacemaker function
  • have another person (who is aware the patient has a pacemaker) nearby when trying new electrical equipment, in case of symptoms in order that the other person can assist the patient to leave the area; most electrical equipment in the home will not cause pacemaker interference.
c. travel precautions
  • notify the physician if travel involves long distances or extended time away from

UNIT
2

home (physician may provide the name of another physician or a pacemaker clinic for emergencies)
- request airplane seating away from the kitchen/galley
- show airport security staff pacemaker identification card since the security alarm will be triggered by the pacemaker; the pacemaker will not be affected by screening devices.

   d. remember not to turn or twiddle with the pacemaker which can lead to pacemaker damage or dislodged wires

   e. plan for routine pacemaker function checks and medical follow-up
- including awareness of eventual battery replacement (perhaps in 6 to 7 years)
- teaching the patient/family about the type of pacemaker function checks they will be using (daily pulse check, in-person checks at the physician's office or pacemaker clinic, by telephone using a special transmitter, by transistor radio and a special magnet)
- assisting the patient/family to rent/purchase any prescribed special equipment for home use
- teaching the patient/family how to use any special equipment (provide written reference material that includes all of the appropriate steps, such as positioning of equipment, application of lubricant, application of electrodes, placement of magnet over pacemaker site, pacemaker recording over telephone).

   f. need for pacemaker identification
- type (include model and serial number)
- rate
- physician's name and telephone number
- hospital where the pacemaker was inserted
- all pertinent medical information.

6. Instruct the patient/family/home health aide about
   a. wound care procedure
   b. wearing loose-fitting clothing around pacemaker area
   c. signs and symptoms of infection
   d. keeping incision clean and dry
- confirm bathing restrictions with physician
- use agency procedure for wound care.

   e. clarify plan for removal of sutures/staples.

7. Incorporate age-specific modifications into interventions
   a. families need specific support for promotion of normal growth and development of children as well as care of the elderly as appropriate
   b. consult with the social worker as needed.

THERAPEUTIC ACHIEVEMENT

- The patient will perform activities of daily living without experiencing symptoms of cardiac dysrhythmias.
- The patient/family adapts to life style modifications as a result of living with a pacemaker.

RELATED PATIENT INSTRUCTIONS

Healthy Heart	Restricted Cholesterol Diet
Heart Medications	Taking a Pulse
Pacemaker	

Bibliography

Andreoli, K. G., Fowkes, V. K., Zipes, D. P. and Wallace, A. G. (eds.). Comprehensive Cardiac Care: A Text for Nurses, Physicians, and Other Health Practitioners, 5th ed. St. Louis: C. V. Mosby, 1983.

Boogaard, M. Rehabilitation of the Female Patient After Myocardial Infarction. Nursing Clinics of North America, Sept. 1983, pp. 433–439.

Brody, M. The Role of the Nurse in Modification of Cardiac Risk Factors. Nursing Clinics of North America, Sept. 1984, pp. 387–396.

Cousins, N. The Healing Heart: Antidotes to Panic and Helplessness. New York: W. W. Norton, 1983.

Douglas, M. K. and Shinn, J. A. (eds.). Advances in Cardiovascular Nursing. Rockville, Maryland: Aspen Systems, 1985.

Guzzetta, C. E. and Dossey, B. M. Cardiovascular Nursing; Bodymind Tapestry. St. Louis: C. V. Mosby, 1984.

Hijeck, T. The Health Belief Model and Cardiac Rehabilitation. Nursing Clinics of North America, Sept. 1984, pp. 449–457.

Kern, L. and Gawlinski, A. Stage-Managing Coronary Artery Disease. Nursing 83, April 1983, pp. 34–40.

Michaelson, C. R. Congestive Heart Failure. St. Louis: C. V. Mosby, 1983.

McCauley, K. and Weaver, T. E. Cardiac and Pulmonary Diseases: Nutritional Implications. Nursing Clinics of North America, March 1983, pp. 81–96.

McGurn, W. C. People with Cardiac Problems: Nursing Concepts. Philadelphia: J. B. Lippincott, 1981.

Pinneo, R. Living with Coronary Artery Disease: The Nurse's Role. Nursing Clinics of North America, Sept. 1984, pp. 459–467.

Purcell, J., Fletcher, B. and White, S. Angina Pectoris. Atlanta: Pritchett and Hull Associates, Inc., 1985.

Sadler, D. Nursing for Cardiovascular Health. Norwalk, Connecticut: Appleton-Century-Crofts, 1984.

Sheps, D. S. The Management of Post-Myocardial Infarction Patients. New York: McGraw-Hill, 1987.

Slvsarczyk, S. and Hicks, F. Helping Your Patient Live With a Permanent Pacemaker. Nursing 83, April 1983, pp. 58–63.

Wenger, N. K. and Hellerstein, H. K. (eds.). Rehabilitation of the Coronary Patient, 2nd ed. New York: John Wiley & Sons, 1984.

Wenger, N. K., Hurst, J. W. and McIntyre, M. C. Cardiology for Nurses. New York: McGraw-Hill, 1980.

UNIT 2

Respiratory Alterations

Care Plans

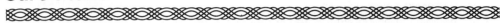

Apnea Care Plan

CROSS REFERENCES

Bereavement Care Plan
Bronchopulmonary Dysplasia (BPD) Care Plan

Home Safety Procedure
Infection Control Procedure

Medication Compliance/Management Procedure
Oxygen Therapy Procedure

Mental Health Assessment/Intervention Guide
Vital Signs: Normal Pediatric Values

UNIT 3

NURSING DIAGNOSES

1. Potential/actual skin impairment related to
   a. inadequate hygiene
   b. electrode placement
   c. inadequate/inappropriate skin care
   d. other.
2. Potential for injury related to
   a. inadequate supervision of the monitor or the patient and siblings
   b. inaudible monitor alarms
   c. environmental hazards
   d. other.
3. Potential for ineffective airway clearance related to gastroesophageal reflux.
4. Alteration in nutrition (less than body requirements) related to gastroesophageal reflux.
5. Potential/actual alteration in parenting related to
   a. lack of support from significant others
   b. unmet social needs of parenting figures
   c. unmet maturational needs of parenting figures
   d. no previous model/experience of parent-child interactions
   e. resentment over forced reallocation of family resources/priorities
   f. financial stress
   g. unrealistic expectations of parenting figure/patient/siblings/partner/others
   h. limited cognitive ability
   i. other.
6. Alteration in family process related to
   a. situational crisis of a chronically ill family member
   b. disruption of usual pattern of family life
   c. diminished parental focus on healthy siblings
   d. other.
7. Social isolation related to
   a. lack of qualified babysitters
   b. anxiety about leaving the patient
   c. other.
8. Familial sleep pattern disturbances related to sensory overload.
9. Familial grieving related to loss of their perfect/healthy child ideal.
10. Familial anxiety/fear related to
    a. perceived threat of patient's death

    b. change in environment
    c. perceived powerlessness
    d. potential of giving birth to another medically fragile child
    e. responsibilities accompanying home apnea monitoring
    f. other.
11. Knowledge deficit (skin care, use of monitor, safety precautions, emergency precautions/plans, alarms and responses, cardiopulmonary resuscitation (CPR), reflux precautions, medications, normal growth and development, when family should contact nurse/physician/rescue squad, reorganization of daily patterns of living, counting pulse rates and respirations, assessment of patient's status/symptomatology) related to
    a. misinterpretation of information
    b. cognitive limitations
    c. lack of motivation
    d. sociocultural differences
    e. low readiness for acceptance of information
    f. other.

PROCESS INDICATORS

1. The patient is at minimal risk for life-threatening apneic episodes.
Indicators
    a. the patient is monitored during all sleep times and when out of visual range
    b. the family expresses an accurate understanding of the monitor and its purpose and their inherent responsibilities
    c. the family describes the appropriate response to each type of monitor alarm
    d. the family identifies emergency precautions/plans
    e. the family is competent in CPR
    f. the family verbalizes the indications for contacting the physician/nurse/emergency squad/durable medical equipment (DME) supplier
    g. the family recalls the purposes, side effects and dosages of prescribed medications.
2. The patient's/family's biopsychosocial integrity is maintained.
Indicators
    a. the patient has no skin irritation/breakdown at electrode placement sites
    b. the family identifies appropriate skin care techniques
    c. family members identify no sleep pattern disturbance or a return to their previous sleep pattern
    d. family members express a feeling that the crises of apnea monitoring (rehospitalization, insurance-related problems, monitor alarms) are manageable.

NURSING INTERVENTIONS

1. Assess the patient
    a. apical rate
    b. respiratory rate
    c. respiratory pattern
    d. skin color
    e. skin integrity
    f. electrode placement/wires come out of lower ends of clothes
    g. serial measurements (weight, length, head circumference)
    h. dentition
    i. behaviors/feeding skills.

2. Inspect the monitor
    a. accuracy of digital readouts (if present)
    b. control settings (if not set internally)
    c. situated on a hard surface at patient's bedside
    d. not situated on other electrical equipment
    e. situated with at least 8 in of ventilation space above and behind
    f. no extension cord
    g. grounded outlet/grounding adaptor in use
    h. situated out of reach of children and child-proof panel in use
    i. presence of extra supplies (optional battery pack, two sets lead wires, four sets disposable patches, manufacturer's manual/troubleshooting guide).
3. Obtain assessment data from the family
    a. patient's color changes during feeding, sleeping, changing air temperature alterations or at stool
    b. occurrences/durations of apnea/bradycardia alarms
    c. status of patient during alarms
    d. symptoms preceding alarms
    e. degree of stimulation needed for arousal after alarms
    f. occurrence of short apneic periods that do not set off alarms
    g. frequency of monitor use
    h. changes in family's daily pattern of living
    i. ways the family is coping with changes
    j. frequency, amount and activities preceding reflux episodes.
4. Contact/alert the attending physician if occurrences of short apneic periods that do not set off the alarm are frequent/persistent.
5. Assess
    a. that the frequency of monitor use is as prescribed
    b. that the monitor can be heard from all locations in the home
    c. the verbal/nonverbal interactions among family members
    d. the completeness/accuracy of the family's knowledge/understanding about the patient's condition/reason for monitoring
    e. the family's capacity to learn.
6. Teach/review with the family
    a. skin care (bathe the patient with soap and water, do not use baby bath products/lotions/oils)
    b. electrode placement/care (place symmetrically on sides of chest, replace as attachment loosens or every 2 days, reposition to prevent skin breakdown, no electrode belt until patient weighs at least 9 lb)
    c. safe use/care of monitor (refer to manufacturer's manual and troubleshooting guide)
    d. safety precautions (remove the leads from the patient unless they are attached to the monitor, unplug the power cord from the wall when it is unplugged from the monitor, use safety covers on electrical outlets, detach the monitor prior to bathing the patient, thread wires out lower end of clothes)
    e. appropriate response to and identification of each type of alarm
        • apnea alarm—observe patient for respiratory movement; if not noted or if lethargic, call loudly and touch, proceeding from gentle to vigorous as needed; if no response, initiate mouth-to-mouth resuscitation and CPR
        • bradycardia alarm—call loudly and touch, proceeding from gentle to vigorous as needed
        • loose-lead alarm—depends on the monitor and refer to the manufacturer's manual and troubleshooting guide.

UNIT
3

    f. emergency procedure for infant CPR

    g. emergency precautions/plans (24-hour phone access; indications for calling nurse/physician/rescue squad/DME supplier; emergency numbers next to telephone; notification of police, telephone company, electric company, fire department, rescue squad)

    h. how to accurately count pulse rates/respirations

    i. reflux precautions (position the patient in an infant seat inclined 35 to 45 degrees or in a prone position with shoulders 30 degrees higher than feet during and for 45 to 60 min after feeding, give small frequent feedings, thicken formula with small amounts of rice cereal)

    j. factors that cause alarms (growth, stretching, feeding, hiccups, flatus, defecation, crying, fever, cold, immunization reactions)

    k. importance of keeping written records of all alarm/nonalarm apnea/bradycardia episodes

    l. purpose, side effects, dosage and administration of prescribed medications

    m. that medication dosages increase as the child grows

    n. age-appropriate developmental stimulation for the patient

    o. normal patterns of growth and development

    p. importance of being able to hear the monitor alarm

    q. importance of providing intervention to the patient within 10 seconds after an alarm

    r. importance of carefully watching the patient when off the monitor (particularly the patient who easily falls asleep).

7. Assist the family to
    a. reorganize daily patterns of living (avoid showering/vacuuming/using hairdryer, other activities that drown out sound of alarm, if only one family member is home with patient)

    b. identify ways of accomplishing tasks/meeting responsibilities (use of an intercom system) without jeopardizing the patient

    c. train babysitters in responsibilities of watching a monitor-dependent infant in CPR technique and emergency action plan

    d. develop safe travel plans.

8. Create opportunities for the family members to express their feelings.
9. Obtain medication prescriptions from the attending physician.
10. Determine criteria for concern with the attending physician, i.e., when the family should contact the nurse/physician/rescue squad.
11. Coordinate referrals, as necessary, to social worker, dietitian, financial counselling service, self-help support groups.
12. Send progress notes and a discharge summary to the attending physician.

THERAPEUTIC ACHIEVEMENT

- The patient is not dependent on the apnea monitor for the management of hypoxic episodes.
- The family relinquishes its emotional dependency on the apnea monitor.

RELATED PATIENT INSTRUCTIONS

Apnea Monitoring
Medication Compliance
Oxygen Therapy

Pediatric Diet
Skin Care

Bronchopulmonary Dysplasia (BPD) Care Plan

CROSS REFERENCES

Apnea Care Plan
Bereavement Care Plan
Generic Cardiac Care Plan
Tracheostomy Care Plan
Ventilator Care Plan

Infection Control Procedure
Oxygen Therapy Procedure

Suctioning (Oronasopharyngeal) Procedure
Suctioning (Tracheostomy) Procedure
Tracheostomy Tube Changing Procedure

Pediatric Injection Sites
Suction Catheter Sizes
Suction Vacuum Settings
Vital Signs: Normal Pediatric Values

UNIT 3

NURSING DIAGNOSES

1. Ineffective airway clearance related to
   a. copious/tenacious secretions
   b. gastroesophageal reflux
   c. respiratory infection
   d. subglottis stenosis
   e. fluid overload
   f. other.
2. Impaired gas exchange related to
   a. inadequate oxygen supply
   b. cystic changes in lungs
   c. respiratory infection
   d. other.
3. Alteration in fluid volume (excess) related to
   a. compromised regulatory system
   b. parental inaccuracy in administering medications
   c. other.
4. Alteration in nutrition (less than body requirements) related to
   a. gastroesophageal reflux
   b. easy fatigability
   c. increased metabolic demands (infection, work of breathing)
   d. disturbed parent-infant interactions
   e. other.
5. Knowledge deficit (pathophysiology and clinical course of BPD, signs and symptoms of respiratory distress/respiratory infection/congestive heart failure/digoxin toxicity, oxygen/inhalation therapy, chest physiotherapy, medications, suctioning, tracheostomy care, assessment of vital signs, reflux precautions, when to call nurse/physician/rescue squad, CPR, emergency plan/precautions, use/maintenance of equipment, normal growth and development) related to
   a. misinterpretation of information
   b. cognitive limitations
   c. lack of readiness to learn

     d. sociocultural differences
     e. lack of confidence
     f. other.

6. Alteration in family process related to
     a. situational crisis of a chronically ill family member
     b. disruption of usual pattern of family life
     c. diminished parental focus on healthy siblings
     d. other.

7. Familial grieving related to loss of their perfect/healthy child ideal.

8. Familial fear/anxiety related to
     a. perceived threat of patient's death
     b. change in environment
     c. perceived powerlessness
     d. potential of giving birth to another medically fragile child
     e. responsibilities of managing the patient at home
     f. threat of frequent hospitalizations
     g. other.

9. Social isolation related to
     a. lack of qualified babysitters
     b. anxiety about leaving the patient
     c. other.

10. Potential/actual alteration in parenting related to
     a. lack of support from significant others
     b. unmet social needs of parenting figures
     c. unmet maturational needs of parenting figures
     d. no previous model/experience of patient-child interactions
     e. resentment over forced reallocation of family resources/priorities
     f. financial stress
     g. unrealistic expectations of parenting figure/patient/siblings/partner/others
     h. limited cognitive ability
     i. other.

PROCESS INDICATORS

1. The patient is at minimal risk for life-threatening respiratory/cardiac decompensation.
Indicators
     a. improved respiratory pattern
     b. no hypoxia during feedings
     c. family recalls signs/symptoms of respiratory distress/infection and cardiac failure
     d. family describes appropriate response to respiratory distress
     e. family identifies adoption of precautions/household modifications to protect the patient
     f. family verbalizes indications for contacting the nurse/physician/emergency squad/ DME supplier
     g. family demonstrates adequate skill in the performance of respiratory procedures, bronchopulmonary toilet, care of equipment
     h. family recalls purposes, side effects and dosages of prescribed medications
     i. family is competent in CPR.

2. The patient's biopsychosocial integrity is maintained.

Indicators
    a. adequate weight gain
    b. health maintenance needs are met (immunizations, dental care, safety)
    c. patient is exposed to experiences that foster normal growth and development
    d. positive/nurturing patient/family relationships (attachment, interaction) are ob-
       served.
  3. The family's psychosocial integrity is maintained.
Indicators
    a. familial feedback reflecting an accurate understanding about the etiology/patho-
       physiology of BPD
    b. each member participates in the patient's care
    c. family meets its social/occupational responsibilities
    d. family expresses a feeling that the crises of BPD (rehospitalization, insurance-
       related problems, respiratory distress) are manageable.

UNIT 3

NURSING INTERVENTIONS

  1. Assess the patient
    a. respiratory rate/pattern
    b. apical rate/pattern
    c. adventitious lung sounds
    d. signs/symptoms of respiratory distress/infection
    e. signs/symptoms of cor pulmonale
    f. signs/symptoms of congestive heart failure
    g. signs/symptoms of fluid retention
    h. skin color
    i. levels of activity/alertness
    j. side/toxic effects of medications
    k. serial measurements (weight, length, height, head circumference)
    l. behaviors/feeding skills
    m. dentition.
  2. Obtain assessment data from the family
    a. the patient's color changes during feeding, sleeping, changing air temperature or
       at stool
    b. frequency, amount and activities preceding reflux episodes
    c. patient's nutritional intake
    d. the medication schedule is as prescribed.
  3. Assess the family
    a. completeness/accuracy of the family's knowledge/understanding of the patient's
       condition
    b. competency in bronchopulmonary toilet, suctioning, administering nebulized med-
       ications
    c. changes in daily pattern of living
    d. ways of coping with changes in patient/parent interactional patterns
    e. verbal/nonverbal interactions among family members and between family mem-
       bers and the patient
    f. capacity to learn.
  4. Assess the equipment
    a. no extension cords
    b. grounded outlets/grounding adaptor in use
    c. specific safety/care precautions visible/demonstrated

    d. oxygen tubing is long enough to enable the patient to move around

    e. does not interfere with the patient's practice of developmental skills

    f. the degree to which patient/family interactions are inhibited

    g. adequate/appropriate extra supplies are stocked

    h. clean and in working order

    i. service/follow-up is regularly scheduled/done by the DME vendor.

5. Determine criteria for concern with the attending physician (when the family should contact the nurse/physician/rescue squad/DME vendor).

6. Request/obtain orders, as necessary, from the attending physician concerning

    a. medications

    b. oxygen flow rate/concentration

    c. theophylline levels

    d. electrolyte levels

    e. digoxin levels

    f. arterial blood gas values

    g. nasogastric feeding

    h. increased caloric intake.

7. Refer to and coordinate nutrition-based interventions with the dietician.

8. Monitor/adjust, in collaboration with the attending physician and dietician, the rate/concentration of tube feedings.

9. Teach/review with the family

    a. bronchopulmonary toilet (percussion/vibration, postural drainage, humidification)

    b. emergency procedure for infant/child CPR

    c. how to accurately count pulse rates/respirations

    d. purpose, side effects, dosages and administration of prescribed medications

    e. that medication dosages increase as the child grows

    f. normal patterns of growth and development

    g. expected responses/reflexes of a premature infant/child

    h. age-appropriate developmental stimulation for the patient

    i. importance of maintaining the patient's immunization schedule

    j. pathophysiology/course of BPD (that frequent rehospitalizations are normal, that symptomatology may continue up to 7 years of age, that symptomatology/prognosis improves as the lungs develop, that the patient is especially vulnerable during winter/early spring)

    k. signs/symptoms of respiratory distress (tachypnea, nasal flaring, cyanosis, tachycardia, retractions, wheezing)

    l. signs/symptoms of respiratory infection (change in respiratory patterns, irritability, change in color/amount/consistency of secretions, fever, change in appetite, change in sleeping pattern)

    m. signs/symptoms of cardiac decompensation (rapid weight gain, diaphoresis, nasal flaring, anorexia, other change in appetite, fatigability)

    n. signs/symptoms of altered fluid balance (rapid weight gain, change in number of wet diapers, change in color/odor/consistency/number of bowel movements, peripheral puffiness, depressed fontanel, decreased skin turgor, increased respiratory rate)

    o. reflux precautions (position the patient in an infant seat inclined 35 to 45 degrees or in a prone position with shoulders 30 degrees higher than feet during and for 45 to 60 minutes after feeding, give small frequent feedings, thicker formula with small amounts of rice cereal)

    p. emergency precautions/plans (24-hour phone access/indications for calling nurse/physician/rescue squad/DME vendor, notification of police/telephone company/

electric company/fire department/rescue squad, emergency numbers next to telephone)
 q. safe use/care of equipment (refer to manufacturer's manual/troubleshooting guide, coordinate with DME vendor/respiratory therapist)
 r. oxygen therapy guidelines/safety precautions
 s. tracheostomy care/safety precautions (if appropriate)
 t. ventilator care/safety precautions (if appropriate)
 u. suctioning technique
 v. ways to encourage nutritional intake and decrease oxygen expenditure during feedings (small frequent feedings, use of oxygen during feedings, schedule feedings to include time for frequent burping/rest periods, have patient eat with the family, use of tube feedings).
10. Teach the family precautions for protecting the patient against respiratory infections
 a. handwashing
 b. good personal hygiene
 c. well-ventilated rooms
 d. avoid exposure to persons with respiratory infections
 e. avoid/minimize exposure to bronchopulmonary irritants
 f. humidified air
 g. cleaning/sterilizing respiratory equipment.
11. Assist the family to
 a. reorganize daily patterns of living
 b. identify ways of accomplishing tasks/meeting responsibilities without jeopardizing the patient
 c. train babysitters in responsibilities of watching a child with BPD in CPR technique and in emergency action plan
 d. develop safe travel plans.
12. Coordinate referrals, as necessary, to social worker, physical therapist, occupational therapist, speech therapist, DME vendor, financial counselling service, mental health service, respite volunteers, self-help support groups.
13. Create opportunities for family members to express their thoughts and feelings.
14. Send progress notes and a discharge summary to the attending physician.

THERAPEUTIC ACHIEVEMENT

- The patient does not exhibit/experience the complications of chronic hypoxia.
- The patient's developmental findings are appropriate for gestational age.
- The family adapts to the life style changes induced as a result of living with a child with chronic respiratory compromise.

RELATED PATIENT INSTRUCTIONS

Antibiotic Medications
Bronchopulmonary Health
Diuretic Medications
Heart Medications
Infection Control for the Home
Measuring Liquid Intake and Output
Nasogastric, Orogastric, Nasointestinal Tube
 Feedings

Oral Suctioning
Oxygen Therapy
Pediatric Diet
Percussion and Postural Drainage
Taking a Pulse
Tracheostomy Care
Tube Feeding—Special Conditions
Ventilator Care

UNIT
3

Chronic Obstructive Pulmonary Disease (COPD) Care Plan

CROSS REFERENCES

Depression Care Plan
Generic Cardiac Care Plan

Home Safety Procedure
Infection Control Procedure
Oxygen Therapy Procedure

NURSING DIAGNOSES

1. Activity intolerance related to
   a. inadequate nutritional status
   b. exhaustion
   c. imbalance between oxygen supply and demand
   d. other.
2. Ineffective airway clearance related to
   a. copious mucus
   b. stasis of secretions
   c. unproductive/minimally productive cough
   d. narrowing of bronchioles
   e. other.
3. Impaired gas exchange related to alveolar/vascular alterations.
4. Ineffective breathing patterns related to
   a. trapped air
   b. anxiety/fear
   c. decreased energy/fatigue
   d. decreased lung expansion
   e. other.
5. Alteration in oral mucous membrane (dryness) related to
   a. oxygen therapy
   b. mouth breathing
   c. other.
6. Alteration in nutrition (less than body requirements) related to
   a. nausea/vomiting
   b. decreased energy/fatigue
   c. depression
   d. other.
7. Sleep pattern disturbance related to
   a. orthopnea
   b. coughing
   c. fear/anxiety
   d. nocturnal diaphoresis
   e. other.

8. Anxiety/fear related to
   a. dyspnea
   b. feeling of suffocation
   c. lack of control over disease progression
   d. financial stress
   e. actual/perceived lack of adequate support system
   f. other.
9. Self-care deficit (feeding, hygiene, grooming, toileting) related to
   a. decreased strength/endurance
   b. dyspnea
   c. depression
   d. inability to relinquish secondary gains of COPD
   e. other.
10. Powerlessness related to chronic fatal illness.
11. Alteration in self-esteem/body image related to
    a. barrel chest
    b. clubbing of fingers/toes
    c. dependence on others/machinery
    d. other.

12. Knowledge deficit (COPD and its progression, breathing patterns, pulmonary toilet, nutritional maintenance, personal energy conservation methods, medications, community resources, bronchopulmonary irritants) related to
    a. cognitive limitation/impairment
    b. misinterpretation of information
    c. lack of motivation for learning
    d. other.
13. Social isolation related to
    a. embarrassment
    b. decreased energy/endurance
    c. discrepant perceptions of illness between patient and others
    d. preoccupation with illness
    e. depression
    f. other.
14. Anticipatory/actual grieving related to
    a. loss of job/income
    b. loss of health/function/life style
    c. other.
15. Alteration in family process related to
    a. role modifications
    b. situational crisis of a chronically ill family member
    c. disruption/change in usual pattern of family life
    d. other.
16. Noncompliance related to
    a. denial
    b. anxiety
    c. depression
    d. decreased strength/endurance
    e. other.
17. Alteration (excess) in fluid volume related to alveolar-capillary membrane changes.

PROCESS INDICATORS

1. The patient's symptoms are controlled.
Indicators
    a. vital signs/laboratory values are within the patient's normal limits
    b. no cyanosis
    c. breath sounds are heard in all lungs fields
    d. no signs of cor pulmonale (dependent edema, distended neck veins, pain in liver region)
    e. weight is maintained
    f. no signs of dehydration/overhydration
    g. decreased amount/loose bronchial secretions
    h. patient demonstrates recommended methods of preventing/relieving breathlessness
    i. patient decreases/stops smoking
    j. patient verbalizes/demonstrates increased tolerance for exercise/activity
    k. patient/family demonstrates measures that improve bronchial hygiene
    l. patient/family verbalizes an understanding of how to minimize/prevent further pulmonary damage/irritation
    m. patient/family validates adherence to the prescribed medical regimen
    n. patient/family recalls signs/symptoms of respiratory infection/deterioration
    o. decreased frequency of hospitalization
    p. decreased use of emergency services
    q. patient/family recalls purposes, side effects and precautions for prescribed medications/treatments.
2. The patient participates in the activities of life to the extent of his or her capabilities.
Indicators
    a. patient realistically identifies physical limitations
    b. patient demonstrates personal energy conservation techniques
    c. patient revises daily pattern of interaction with others to incorporate the limitations imposed by COPD and its treatment
    d. patient maintains social/occupational responsibilities
    e. patient/family realistically identifies the amount/type of activity the patient can undertake
    f. patient/family validates a balance between rest, nutrition and exercise
    g. patient verbalizes acceptance of and comfort with the need to be dependent
    h. patient/family identifies the adoption of household precautions/modifications to protect the patient.
3. The family's psychosocial integrity is maintained.
Indicators
    a. familial feedback reflecting an understanding of COPD and its disabilities
    b. familial feedback reflecting an understanding of the typical behavior patterns of chronically ill respiratory patients
    c. patient/family verbalizes acceptance of and comfort with role modifications
    d. patient's/family's utilization of community resources.

NURSING INTERVENTIONS

  1. Assess the patient's
    a. cardiopulmonary status
    b. coexisting health problems

   c. psychosocial strengths/weaknesses
   d. smoking habits
   e. pattern of physical activity
   f. pattern of oxygen use
   g. cognitive ability
   h. medications (beta-adrenergic blockers aggravate bronchospasm; sedatives depress respirations).
2. Assess the patient's occupational/avocational/home environments for the presence of
   a. bronchopulmonary irritants (dust, fumes, smoke, chemicals with strong odors, powders, paint, smog, particulates, dogs, cats, pigeons, farm animals)
   b. safety hazards.
3. Assess the family's
   a. psychosocial strengths/weaknesses
   b. changes attributed to the disease
   c. availability/reliability of support systems
   d. cognitive abilities.
4. Provide instruction to the patient/family/home health aide
   a. pathophysiology of COPD
   b. identification of bronchopulmonary irritants
   c. how to avoid/reduce bronchopulmonary irritation (seek vocational/avocational environments without irritants; check air pollution levels daily and avoid outdoor activity when levels are high; keep the home temperature above 70° F during the day and 65° F at night; use radiant heat/air conditioning, when feasible; change/clean air filters in forced air conditioning systems; do not use fireplaces or wood and coal burning stoves; use exhaust fan in kitchen and bathroom; keep bathroom door ajar when bathing/showering; do not use substances with ammonia and avoid chlorine bleach; avoid heavy drapes and carpets in the home; frequently dust or damp mop; wear a mask or face scarf in cold weather; avoid individuals with colds; avoid crowds)
   d. the benefits of not smoking (less coughing, reduced sputum production, increased resistance to respiratory infections, renewed sensitivity to taste and smell)
   e. medications (purpose, side effects, administration)
   f. personal energy conservation techniques (slower pacing of activities; sitting instead of standing; wearing of loose/lightweight clothing; using slip-on shoes; putting on a terrycloth robe after bathing instead of towel drying; avoiding straining, bending, and squatting; including "fatigue-time" when scheduling the day's activities; moving more slowly)
   g. measures to improve bronchial hygiene (postural drainage with percussion/vibration; adequate fluid intake; slow, deep breathing with prolonged expiratory phase; pursed-lip breathing)
   h. coughing technique (sit in forward flexed position with feet supported; drop head, sink chest and bend forward while breathing out of pursed lips; sit up and slowly sniff air in; refrain from coughing until repeated six times; when ready to cough, take a deep abdominal breath; bend forward; produce a soft staccato cough using the abdominal muscles)
   i. positions to relieve dyspnea (sit in a firm chair, rest forearms on thighs; sit in a firm chair, lean forward, rest forearms on table)
   j. modifications in diet (avoid gas-producing foods; eat small frequent meals; decrease sodium intake; increase proteins and carbohydrates)
   k. importance of getting weighed daily (on the same scale at the same time of day)

UNIT
3

    l. importance of notifying the nurse/physician of an overnight weight gain of 2 to 3 lb

    m. stress management/relaxation techniques

    n. methods to induce sleep (consistent bedtime; similar ritual each night at bedtime; water, lamp, tissues, aerosol device within easy reach of the bed; use of a wedged pillow, lightweight pillows and blankets; avoid use of alcoholic beverages/over-the-counter sleeping aids at bedtime)

    o. the importance of annual immunizations for influenza

    p. progressive/graded exercises

    q. environmental modifications for home safety

    r. use/cleaning/maintenance of respiratory equipment.

5. Teach the patient/family/home health aide about oxygen therapy.
   a. need for low flow rate
   b. use at mealtimes, when febrile and during exercises
   c. not to use oxygen near an open flame
   d. not to increase the flow rate without a physician/nurse so advising
   e. regarding oxygen as a medication.

6. Teach the patient/family/home health aide the importance of notifying the nurse/physician if the patient experiences
   a. chest tightness/pain
   b. change in color/amount/consistency of sputum
   c. blood/unusual clumps in the sputum
   d. excessive fatigue/weakness
   e. fever
   f. puffy ankles
   g. tightening fit in rings/belts
   h. leg cramps
   i. tingling/numbness of fingers.

7. Teach the patient/partner how to adapt their sexual activities to COPD-induced disabilities.
   a. patient takes a passive sexual role
   b. use a position that is comfortable and doesn't restrict breathing
   c. patient uses pursed-lip breathing
   d. emphasize enjoyment over performance
   e. avoid sexual intercourse during extremely hot or cold environmental temperatures, when strenuous activity is anticipated after sex, and when partners are angry/anxious
   f. select a time for sexual intercourse that provides sufficient rest periods.

8. Assist the patient/family to
   a. reorganize daily patterns of living (reorganize work areas/habits, plan one major chore each day, set priorities for daily activities)
   b. develop safe travel plans.

9. Request/obtain orders, as necessary, for medications, laboratory tests, equipment and so forth from the attending physician.

10. Monitor
    a. arterial blood gas values
    b. white blood cell counts
    c. sputum analyses
    d. pulmonary function tests
    e. electrocardiograms (EKG)

    f. fluid and electrolyte balance

    g. blood levels for prescribed medications.

11. Refer the patient/family to

    a. American Lung Association

    b. Emphysema Anonymous

    c. Meals-on-Wheels

    d. smoking cessation counselling

    e. state division of motor vehicles (for handicapped license plates)

    f. local self-help/support groups.

12. Confer and coordinate interventions with

    a. social worker

    b. occupational therapist

    c. physical therapist

    d. dietician

    e. hospice

    f. respite volunteers

    g. DME suppliers.

13. Provide opportunities that facilitate the patient's independent action/decision-making.

14. Create situations that encourage the patient/family to express their thoughts and feelings.

15. Send progress notes/discharge summary to the attending physician.

THERAPEUTIC ACHIEVEMENT

- The patient experiences a deceleration of degenerative symptomatology.
- The patient/family adapts to life style changes induced as a result of COPD.

RELATED PATIENT INSTRUCTIONS

Antitussive Medications	Making the Home Environment Safe
Diuretic Medications	Measuring Liquid Intake and Output
Healthy Heart	Percussion and Postural Drainage
Heart Medications	Seasonings for Sodium Restricted Diets
Infection Control for the Home	Ways to Save Your Energy

UNIT 3

Cystic Fibrosis Care Plan

CROSS REFERENCES

Bereavement Care Plan
Constipation Care Plan
Pain Care Plan
Spiritual Distress Care Plan

Domestic Violence Procedure

Home Safety Procedure
Infection Control Procedure
Oxygen Therapy Procedure

Mental Health Assessment/Intervention Guide
Pain Perception in School-Age Children

NURSING DIAGNOSES

1. Alteration in nutrition (less than body requirements) related to
   a. deficiency/absence of pancreatic enzyme
   b. obstruction of pancreatic ducts
   c. deficiency/absence of vitamins A, E and K
   d. decreased energy/fatigue
   e. depression
   f. other.
2. Ineffective airway clearance related to
   a. thick/copious mucus
   b. unproductive/minimally productive cough
   c. bronchial obstruction
   d. stasis of obstruction
   e. other.
3. Ineffective breathing pattern related to
   a. trapped air
   b. anxiety/fear
   c. decreased energy/fatigue
   d. pain
   e. chronic inflammatory process
   f. bronchial obstruction
   g. other.
4. Impaired gas exchange related to pulmonary vascular changes.
5. Activity intolerance related to
   a. inadequate nutritional status
   b. decreased energy/fatigue
   c. imbalance between oxygen supply and demand
   d. other.
6. Alteration in comfort (pain) related to
   a. gastrointestinal obstruction
   b. musculoskeletal changes
   c. other.
7. Potential/actual skin impairment related to
   a. inadequate hygiene
   b. inadequate/inappropriate skin care
   c. frequent/prolonged contact with the products of elimination
   d. enzymatic irritation
   e. other.

8. Alteration in bowel elimination (constipation/diarrhea) related to
   a. less than adequate dietary intake
   b. intestinal obstruction
   c. anxiety
   d. bowel malabsorption
   e. other.
9. Alteration in self-esteem/body image related to
   a. barrel chest
   b. clubbing of fingers/toes
   c. small/emaciated body
   d. frequent, productive cough
   e. foul-smelling flatus
   f. other.
10. Powerlessness related to chronic fatal illness.
11. Social isolation related to
    a. embarrassment
    b. decreased energy/endurance
    c. depression
    d. lack of qualified babysitter
    e. parent's anxiety about leaving the patient
    f. other.
12. Sexual dysfunction related to
    a. chronic fatal prognosis of cystic fibrosis
    b. sterility
    c. fear of pregnancy
    d. lack of intimate partner
    e. other.
13. Anticipatory/actual grieving related to
    a. perceived potential loss of a significant other
    b. chronic fatal illness
    c. other.
14. Potential/actual alteration in parenting related to
    a. lack of support from significant others
    b. unmet social needs of parenting figures
    c. resentment over forced reallocation of family resources/priorities
    d. financial stress
    e. unrealistic expectations of self, parents, siblings, partners, others
    f. limited cognitive ability
    g. other.
15. Alteration in family process related to
    a. situational crisis of a chronically ill family member
    b. diminished parental focus on healthy siblings
    c. disruption of usual pattern of family life
    d. other.
16. Knowledge deficit (cystic fibrosis and its progression, percussion, vibration, postural drainage, nutritional maintenance, personal energy conservation methods, medications, normal growth and development, oxygen therapy, assessment of patient's status/symptomatology, reorganization of daily pattern of living, community resources) related to
    a. cognitive limitations
    b. misinterpretation of information

UNIT 3

    c. low readiness for acceptance of information
    d. sociocultural differences
    e. unfamiliarity with information resources
    f. other.

PROCESS INDICATORS

1. The patient's symptoms are controlled.
Indicators
    a. breath sounds are heard in all lung fields
    b. no cyanosis
    c. rib cage is normally mobile
    d. weight gain/maintenance
    e. no signs of cor pulmonale (dependent edema, distended neck veins, pain in liver region)
    f. no skin rash/irritation/breakdown
    g. soft, nonfloating stools
    h. vital signs/laboratory values within the patient's normal limits
    i. decreased amount/loose bronchial secretions
    j. no signs of respiratory infection
    k. patient/family demonstrates percussion and postural drainage
    l. patient/family verbalizes measures to minimize/prevent pulmonary irritation
    m. patient/family validates adherence to the prescribed medical regimen
    n. patient/family recalls side effects, purposes, precautions and guidelines for administration of prescribed medications/treatments.
2. The patient participates in the activities of life to the extent of his or her capabilities.
Indicators
    a. patient demonstrates personal energy conservation
    b. patient maintains a satisfactory level of social/community interaction
    c. patient's independent performance of the activities of daily living is realistically commensurate with his or her capabilities
    d. patient/family validates a balance between rest-nutrition-exercise.
3. The family's psychosocial equilibrium is maintained.
Indicators
    a. family members express a feeling that the crises of cystic fibrosis are manageable
    b. familial feedback reflects an understanding of cystic fibrosis and its accompanying disabilities
    c. patient/family utilization of community resources
    d. each member's participation in the patient's care.

NURSING INTERVENTIONS

1. Assess the patient
    a. rate/pattern of respirations
    b. frequency/pattern of cough (daytime and nighttime)
    c. quantity/consistency/color of sputum
    d. presence/degree of retractions, cyanosis, orthopnea
    e. presence/degree of digital clubbing
    f. lung sounds

    g. presence/degree of abdominal distension/cramps/pain
    h. presence/degree of joint pain or swelling
    i. anterior-posterior diameter of the chest
    j. frequency/appearance of stools
    k. presence/degree of polydipsia, polyuria, polyphagia
    l. skin integrity
    m. pattern of physical activity
    n. pattern of oxygen use
    p. psychosocial strengths/weaknesses.

2. Assess the family
    a. changes in family's daily pattern of living
    b. verbal/nonverbal interactions among family members
    c. psychosocial strengths/weaknesses
    d. cognitive abilities
    e. completeness/accuracy of family's understanding of patient's condition
    f. availability/reliability of support systems.

3. Assess the environment
    a. bronchopulmonary irritants
    b. safety hazards
    c. other.

4. Provide instruction to the patient/family about
    a. pathophysiology of cystic fibrosis
    b. how to identify/avoid/reduce bronchopulmonary irritants
    c. need for extra salt
      • in hot weather
      • during strenous exercise
      • when the patient is febrile.
    d. oral hygiene
    e. personal hygiene
    f. exercises to correct postural deficits
    g. signs/symptoms of respiratory infection
    h. techniques to conserve personal energy
    i. medications (purpose, side effects, administration)
    j. importance of avoiding individuals with colds
    k. diet modifications (high carbohydrates and proteins, moderate amount of fats, restrict fats if persistent abdominal pain is present)
    l. signs/symptoms of heat prostration (muscle cramps, listlessness, abdominal pain, vomiting)
    m. use of moist heat for joint pain
    n. importance of not using aspirin
    o. importance of maintaining an adequate daily fluid intake
    p. enzyme therapy (take enzymes throughout/during meals, mix powdered form with cold food, wipe/clean food containing the medication off the skin as it may cause local irritation/ulceration, avoid inhalation of powder while mixing as it may irritate respiratory tract and/or cause an allergic asthmatic response, titrate amount of medication prescribed individually by number and type of stools).

5. Provide instruction to the patient/family about techniques of bronchopulmonary hygiene
    a. nebulization therapy (inhalations are done before or after postural drainage depending upon physician's prescription and medication used)
    b. importance of daily percussion/postural drainage/vibration

UNIT
3

    c. scheduling of percussion/postural drainage/vibration (at least twice a day upon arising and at bedtime, more frequently when the patient has a cold or accumulated airway secretions; long enough before meals so that the patient doesn't vomit and has sufficient time to rest before eating)

    d. contraindications to postural drainage/percussion (hemoptysis; acute asthma episodes)

    e. positions for postural drainage (no head-down positioning if vertigo, arthritis, or hypertension present)

    f. how to incorporate play into bronchopulmonary hygiene (patient can hang upside down on a Jungle gym; teach patient to stand on head, blow up balloons, blow soap bubbles, blow a pinwheel; use an incentive spirometer with a ball mechanism)

    g. how to protect the patient's skin from irritation (have the patient wear a lightweight cotton shirt; place a thin towel over the area to be percussed/vibrated; do not wear jewelry while percussing/vibrating the patient)

    h. how to percuss (an infant, two or three fingers are tented together; an older child, the whole hand is tightly cupped; use a brisk, relaxed flexion and extension of the wrist; a hollow, not slapping, sound should be produced; use both hands to achieve an alternating, rhythmic percussion; do not percuss over sternum, vertebrae, kidneys, tender areas)

    i. to percuss/drain the areas of greatest involvement first

    j. to limit/rotate positions for postural drainage (children usually cannot tolerate more than four to six different positions during any one session)

    k. effective coughing technique (to cough two to three times after each positioning during postural drainage; importance of not suppressing a cough)

    l. importance of staying with and supervising the patient.

6. Teach/review with the family

    a. how to assess respiratory patterns/characteristics

    b. how to accurately count pulse rates and respirations

    c. importance of monitoring the characteristics (bulk, consistency, frequency, odor) of the patient's stool

    d. skin care

    e. importance of weighing the infant patient daily and the older patient at least twice a week (on the same scale)

    f. importance of notifying the nurse/physician of an unexpected/unexplainable weight gain

    g. importance of having the patient wear clothes that fit properly

    h. environmental modifications for home safety

    i. that medication dosages increase as the patient grows

    j. age-appropriate developmental stimulation for the patient

    k. normal patterns of growth and development

    l. use/cleaning/maintenance of respiratory equipment

    m. oxygen therapy.

7. Assist the family to

    a. reorganize daily patterns of living

    b. identify ways of accomplishing tasks/meeting responsibilities without jeopardizing the patient

    c. train babysitters in the responsibilities of watching a child with cystic fibrosis

    d. develop safe travel plans.

8. Request/obtain orders, as necessary, for medications, laboratory tests, equipment and so forth from the attending physician.

9. Confer and coordinate interventions with
   a. social worker
   b. dietician
   c. respiratory therapist
   d. hospice
   e. respite volunteers
   f. teachers
   g. play therapist
   h. DME suppliers.
10. Refer the patient/family to
    a. Cystic Fibrosis Foundation
    b. American Lung Association
    c. financial counselling service
    d. local self-help/support groups
    e. handicapped children's services.
11. Provide opportunities that facilitate the patient's independent action/decision-making.
12. Create situations that encourage patient/family to express their thoughts and feelings.
13. Send progress notes/discharge summary to the attending physician.

UNIT 3

THERAPEUTIC ACHIEVEMENTS

- The patient experiences a deceleration in the degenerative symptomatology.
- The patient/family adapts to the life-style changes induced as a result of cystic fibrosis.

RELATED PATIENT INSTRUCTIONS

Antibiotic Medications
Bronchopulmonary Health
Care for the Patient Confined to Bed
Clinical Signs of Imminent Death
Comfort Measures for Dehydration
General Comfort Measures
Healthy Heart
Heart Medications
Infection Control for the Home
Medication Compliance

Oral Suctioning
Oxygen Therapy
Pain Medications
Pediatric Diet
Percussion and Postural Drainage
Reading a Thermometer and Taking
  a Temperature
Skin Care
Taking a Pulse
Ways to Save Your Energy

Laryngectomy Care Plan

CROSS REFERENCES

Alcohol Abuse Care Plan
Depression Care Plan

Home Safety Procedure
Infection Control Procedure

Suctioning (Tracheostomy) Procedure

Gum Disease Warning Signs
Suction Catheter Sizes
Suction Vacuum Settings

NURSING DIAGNOSES

1. Ineffective airway clearance related to
   a. copious/tenacious mucus
   b. stasis of secretions
   c. nonproductive/minimally productive cough
   d. other.
2. Alterations in nutrition (less than body requirements) related to
   a. dysphagia
   b. changed olfaction
   c. drooling
   d. inadequate oral/dental hygiene
   e. learning esophageal speech (swallowed air)
   f. other.
3. Potential/actual impairment of skin integrity related to
   a. inadequate skin/stoma care technique
   b. copious mucus production
   c. other.
4. Ineffective breathing pattern related to inadequate humidification of the environment.
5. Potential for injury related to
   a. hazardous environmental conditions
   b. inadequate protection of stoma
   c. other.
6. Impaired verbal communication related to
   a. surgical intervention
   b. fatigue
   c. resistance to voice rehabilitation/speech therapy
   d. other.
7. Anxiety/fear related to
   a. perceived/actual inability to communicate
   b. potential/actual recurrence of cancer
   c. potential/actual metastatic disease
   d. fatalistic misperceptions
   e. financial stress
   f. other.
8. Disturbance in body image/self-esteem related to
   a. facial disfigurement
   b. prosthesis
   c. method of communication
   d. other.

9. Social isolation related to
   a. embarrassment
   b. depression
   c. reactions of others to speech/method of communication/facial disfigurement
   d. frequent coughing episodes
   e. reaction of others to patient's continued smoking/drinking
   f. other.
10. Knowledge deficit (speech therapy, voice rehabilitation, prosthesis/corrective surgery options, pulmonary toilet, community resources, tracheobronchial irritants/hazards, tracheostomy/stoma care, cancer of the larynx and its prognosis, oral/dental hygiene, normalcy of taste/smell changes) related to
    a. cognitive limitation/impairment
    b. misinterpretation of information
    c. low readiness for acceptance of information
    d. unfamiliarity with information resources
    e. patient's/family's request for no information
    f. other.

PROCESS INDICATORS

1. The patient's physical integrity is sustained.
Indicators
   a. patent airway
   b. no signs/symptoms of infection/aspiration
   c. weight maintained
   d. decreased amount/loose tracheobronchial secretions
   e. patient decreases/stops smoking
   f. patient/family verbalizes understanding of how to minimize/prevent tracheobronchial irritation
   g. patient/family demonstrates appropriate care of laryngeal dressings, laryngostomy tube, stoma
   h. patient/family demonstrates adequate facility in the care/application of prosthesis
   i. patient/family verbalizes emergency plans for prosthetic mishaps
   j. patient wears an emergency medical identification tag/bracelet
   k. no skin irritation/breakdown around stoma.
2. The patient/family's psychosocial equilibrium is maintained.
Indicators
   a. the patient can/does communicate
   b. patient's/family's verbalizations reflect satisfaction with communication effort/technique
   c. patient/family maintains social/occupational responsibilities
   d. patient/family appropriately utilizes community supports/resources
   e. each family member verbalizes thoughts and feelings about the laryngectomy.

NURSING INTERVENTIONS

1. Assess the patient
   a. tracheobronchial status
   b. condition of the stoma

     c. method/quality of communication
     d. acceptance/rejection of method of communication
     e. coexisting health problems
     f. signs/symptoms of metastatic disease
     g. smoking habits
     h. patterns of alcohol use
     i. cognitive ability
     j. understanding of and ability to perform physical care techniques
     k. acceptance/rejection of physical appearance
     l. nutritional status
     m. psychosocial strengths/weaknesses
     n. factors that aid/impede intelligible speech.

2. Assess the family
     a. method/quality of communication with the patient
     b. meaning the family attaches to the laryngectomy
     c. each family member's willingness to participate in the patient's care
     d. effects on each family member of the patient's smoking, alcohol use, surgery
     e. cognitive abilities.

3. Teach the family/home health aide guidelines for effective communication with the patient
     a. respond to the patient's speech efforts, no matter how awkward or minimal the effort
     b. avoid pressuring the patient into a conversation
     c. ask the patient questions so that yes or no answers suffice
     d. do not yell when speaking with the patient
     e. do not answer questions or give responses for the patient
     f. encourage the patient's self-expression through any available means (hand signals, magic-erase slates, flash cards, music, writing, lip reading, art).

4. Provide instruction to the patient/family/home health aide about
     a. verbal/nonverbal communication techniques
     b. identification of tracheobronchial irritants (aerosol sprays, powders, smoke, dry heat, air conditioning, loose hair after shaving and haircuts)
     c. how to reduce tracheobronchial irritants (wear a filter and bib of porous material; avoid crowded areas; keep doors and windows closed; use humidifiers and cool mist/steam vaporizers; ensure adequate fluid intake)
     d. benefits of not smoking (less coughing, reduced sputum production, increased resistance to respiratory infections, renewed sensitivity to taste and smell)
     e. stoma care (wash stoma area twice daily with 1:1 hydrogen peroxide/normal saline solution, then apply bland ointment around stoma; do not use cotton applicators/fluffy swabbing; remove crusts/dried secretions with tweezers; clean inner cannula twice a day with hydrogen peroxide, rinse with tap water, dry with noncotton 4 × 4 pad; clean and change outer tube daily; keep stoma area as free of mucus as possible; change bibs when soiled)
     f. suctioning (if appropriate)
     g. prosthesis care (application, examination, cleaning, preparation of the prosthetic site)
     h. safety precautions (wear neck shield when bathing/showering, install gas/smoke detectors, no swimming, use amplifiers on telephone)
     i. importance of annual immunizations for influenza
     j. need for balancing rest, exercise, nutrition
     k. importance of adequate oral/dental hygiene

    l. stress management/relaxation techniques

    m. importance of wearing a medical emergency tag/bracelet

    n. coughing position (forward flexed position; keep stoma below lung level)

    o. clothing (ascots, scarves, high-necked dresses, necklaces to protect the stoma)

    p. importance of having enough supplies on hand

    q. signs/symptoms of infection (fever, chills, shortness of breath, change in color/amount/consistency of sputum, excessive fatigue/weakness).

5. Teach the patient how to burp as a prelude to esophageal speech.
6. Provide opportunities that facilitate the patient's independent action and/or decision-making.
7. Develop, with the patient/family, plans to deal with prosthetic mishaps.
8. Create situations that encourage the patient/family to express their thoughts/feelings about
   a. laryngectomy and resultant changes
   b. esophageal speech/artificial speech devices
   c. cosmetic/corrective surgery
   d. prosthetic devices.
9. Refer patient to the dentist, as necessary.
10. Coordinate referrals, as necessary, to social worker, speech therapist, occupational therapist, DME suppliers, pastoral care and mental health counselor.
11. Determine criteria for concern with the attending physician, e.g., when the patient/family should contact the nurse/physician/rescue squad.
12. Refer to the dietician and coordinate the patient's utilization of the dietician's teaching to promote/maintain the patient's nutritional status.
13. Refer to
    a. International Association of Laryngectomees
    b. American Cancer Society
    c. Lost Chord Club
    d. Alcoholics Anonymous/Alanon
    e. vocational rehabilitation services.
14. Send progress notes and a discharge summary to the attending physician.

UNIT 3

THERAPEUTIC ACHIEVEMENT

- The patient/family adapts to the life style changes induced as a result of the laryngectomy.

RELATED PATIENT INSTRUCTIONS

Antibiotic Medications	Skin Care
Bronchopulmonary Health	Tracheostomy Care
Infection Control for the Home	

Ventilator Care Plan

CROSS REFERENCES

Apnea Care Plan
Bereavement Care Plan
Depression Care Plan
Generic Cardiac Care Plan

Domestic Violence Assessment/Intervention
    Procedure
Home Safety Procedure
Infection Control Procedure

Oxygen Therapy Procedure
Range of Motion Exercises Procedure
Suctioning (Tracheostomy) Procedure
Tracheostomy Tube Changing Procedure

Mental Health Assessment/Intervention Guide
Suction Catheter Sizes
Suction Vacuum Settings

NURSING DIAGNOSES

1. Ineffective breathing pattern related to
    a. neuromuscular impairment
    b. inflammatory process
    c. inappropriate ventilator settings
    d. other.
2. Potential for injury related to
    a. inadequate supervision of patient or ventilator
    b. environmental hazards
    c. inaudible ventilator alarms
    d. inadequate pulmonary ventilation
    e. other.
3. Alteration in family process related to
    a. situational crisis of a ventilator-dependent family member
    b. disruption of the usual pattern of family life
    c. role modifications
    d. other.
4. Patient/family social isolation related to
    a. anxiety about leaving the patient
    b. lack of qualified respite care givers
    c. lack of knowledge about portable equipment
    d. other.
5. Anxiety/fear related to
    a. perceived threat of patient's death
    b. changes in environment
    c. perceived powerlessness
    d. responsibilities accompanying home ventilator care
    e. other.
6. Impaired home maintenance management related to
    a. insufficient planning/organization
    b. insufficient resources
    c. lack of reliable/adequate support systems
    d. knowledge deficit
    e. other.

7. Alteration in nutrition (less than body requirements) related to depression.
8. Knowledge deficit (use/maintenance of the ventilator; emergency precautions/plans; alarms and responses; cardiopulmonary resuscitation (CPR); medications; when to call nurse/physician/rescue squad; reorganization of daily patterns of living; assessment of patient's status and symptomatology; medications; resources) related to
   a. misinterpretation of information
   b. cognitive limitations
   c. sociocultural differences
   d. low readiness for acceptance of information
   e. other.
9. Impaired physical mobility related to
   a. neuromuscular impairment
   b. depression
   c. other.
10. Grief related to loss of physiopsychosocial well being.
11. Sleep pattern disturbance related to
   a. anxiety/fear/depression
   b. sensory overload
   c. other.
12. Ineffective (compromised/disabled) family coping related to
   a. lack of support from significant others
   b. resentment over forced reallocation of resources/priorities
   c. financial stress
   d. unrealistic expectations of care giver/patient/others
   e. prolonged disability of the patient
   f. highly ambivalent relationships
   g. disorganization and role changes
   h. other.

UNIT 3

PROCESS INDICATORS

1. The patient experiences no interruption of ventilatory support.
Indicators
   a. ventilator alarm is plugged into power source
   b. manual ventilation equipment near patient and ready for emergency use
   c. family expresses accurate understanding of ventilator and its purpose and of their inherent responsibilities
   d. family identifies emergency precautions/plans
   e. family is competent in CPR
   f. family verbalizes indications for contacting the nurse/physician/emergency squad/ DME supplier
   g. family recalls purposes, side effects and dosages of prescribed medications.
2. The patient's biopsychosocial integrity is maintained.
Indicators
   a. weight is maintained
   b. arterial blood gas values are within normal limits
   c. breath sounds are heard in all lung fields
   d. decreased amount/loose bronchial secretions
   e. family demonstrates measures that promote the patient's bronchopulmonary hygiene

    f. family recalls signs/symptoms of respiratory infection/distress/failure

    g. patient/family realistically identifies amount/type of activity the patient can undertake

    h. patient maintains a reasonable level of social interaction.

3. The family's psychosocial integrity is maintained.

Indicators

    a. family verbalizes acceptance of/comfort with role modifications

    b. family utilizes community resources

    c. family identifies no sleep pattern disturbance or a return to their previous sleep pattern

    d. family members express a feeling that home ventilator care is manageable

    e. family identifies the adoption of household precautions/modifications to protect the patient

    f. each family member participates in mental health counselling/self-help support group (if needed)

    g. each member participates in the patient's care.

NURSING INTERVENTIONS

1. Assess the patient
   a. vital signs
   b. respiratory pattern/spontaneous respirations
   c. skin color
   d. skin integrity
   e. lung sounds
   f. signs/symptoms of respiratory distress/failure
   g. signs/symptoms of pneumothorax (diminished/absent breath sounds; acute pain on affected side; trachea deviated away from pneumothorax)
   h. signs/symptoms of fluid imbalance
   i. signs/symptoms of respiratory infection
   j. observed respiratory rate against ventilator rate.
2. Obtain assessment data from the family
   a. occurrence of alarms
   b. status of the patient during alarms
   c. changes in the family's pattern of living
   d. ways the family is coping with changes
   e. can ventilator alarms be heard from all locations in the house
   f. verbal/nonverbal interactions among family members
   g. completeness/accuracy of the family's understanding about the patient's condition and the reasons for mechanical ventilation
   h. each family member's ability to perform CPR
   i. family's knowledge of equipment use and maintenance
   j. financial situation
   k. degree of family's acceptance of home ventilator care
   l. availability/reliability of support systems.
3. Assess the ventilator
   a. actual control settings against prescribed settings
   b. alarm lights are on
   c. bellows are rising
   d. humidifier is filled
   e. tubing is not water filled and has no kinks

    f. connections are secure

    g. no extension cord

    h. in a grounded outlet or a grounding adaptor in use

    i. presence of extra supplies (tracheostomy tube with ties attached; a tube one size smaller; manual resuscitator with tracheostomy adaptor attached; oxygen equipment; 12-volt batteries/electrical generator as back-up power source; manufacturer's manual/troubleshooting guide)

    j. childproof panel in use

    k. enough slack in the ventilator lines and tubing so that the patient can move his or her head without disconnecting the lines and tubing

    l. ventilator is positioned close to the patient.

4. Assess the environment

    a. electrical capability of the home (confer with DME supplier)

    b. space for equipment/supplies

    c. telephone availability

    d. safety hazards

    e. supplies are at bedside and wherever else care is provided.

5. Teach/review with the family

    a. signs/symptoms of cardiorespiratory problems (dyspnea, restlessness, pallor, fatigue, periorbital edema)

    b. measures to prevent atelectasis (frequent position changes, regular percussion/postural drainage, periodic hyperinflation/hyperoxygenation, suctioning as needed)

    c. ventilator settings/functions (post the prescribed settings on/near the ventilator, check the settings every 3 to 4 hours when the ventilator is in use, identify the source of humidification, describe the ventilator circuitry)

    d. emergency procedure for CPR

    e. appropriate responses to ventilator alarms (assess the patient; if not a circuitry disconnection, remove the patient from the ventilator and manually ventilate until the reason for the alarm is identified and corrected)

    f. emergency precautions/plans (24-hour phone access and indications for calling nurse/physician/rescue squad/DME supplier; emergency numbers next to telephone; notification of police/telephone company/electric company/fire department/rescue squad of presence of ventilator-dependent individual in the home)

    g. how to accurately count pulse rates/respirations

    h. signs/symptoms of respiratory distress/failure

    i. basic guidelines for intervention in the event of respiratory distress

    j. measures to prevent respiratory infection (handwashing, avoiding exposure to individuals with colds, emptying of accumulated water from ventilator tubing away from cascade, regular cleaning/disinfecting of reusable equipment, sterile technique for tracheostomy care)

    k. tracheostomy care/suctioning

    l. apnea monitoring (if appropriate)

    m. factors that cause ventilator alarms (tubes disconnected, nebulizer hood off, internal ventilator malfunction, tracheostomy tube out, plugged tracheostomy tube, air leaks, inadequate ventilator settings)

    n. purpose, side effects, dosages and administration of prescribed medications

    o. importance of being able to hear the ventilator alarms

    p. importance of providing quick intervention to the patient after an alarm sounds

    q. oxygen therapy

    r. age-appropriate developmental stimulation for the patient

    s. skin care

    t. personal care/hygiene.

UNIT 3

6. Assist the family to
   a. determine optimal locations for equipment/supplies
   b. reorganize daily patterns of living
   c. identify ways to accomplish tasks/meet household responsibilities without jeopardizing the patient
   d. train respite workers in the responsibilities of watching a ventilator-dependent individual, in CPR technique and in emergency action plan
   e. develop safe travel plans
   f. plan a clear daily schedule of patient care
   g. develop an inventory list/schedule for ordering of supplies
   h. maintain a schedule and procedure for cleaning and changing the ventilator circuitry.
7. Determine with the physician
   a. criteria for concern (when the family should contact the nurse/physician/rescue squad)
   b. basic guidelines for intervention in the event of respiratory distress.
8. Request/obtain orders, as necessary, for medications, laboratory tests, equipment and so forth from the attending physician.
9. Coordinate referrals, as necessary, with
   a. social worker
   b. physical therapist
   c. occupational therapist
   d. speech therapist
   e. financial counselling service
   f. educational/vocational teachers/counsellors
   g. respite volunteers
   h. dietician
   i. DME suppliers
   j. respiratory therapist
   k. self-help support groups
   l. mental health counsellors.
10. Provide opportunities that facilitate the patient's independent action/decision-making.
11. Create opportunities for the patient/family to express their feelings.

THERAPEUTIC ACHIEVEMENT

- The patient/family adapts to the life style changes induced by the dependency on mechanical ventilation.

RELATED PATIENT INSTRUCTIONS

Antibiotic Medications	Oxygen Therapy
Comfort Measures for Dehydration	Percussion and Postural Drainage
Healthy Heart	Range of Motion Exercises
Heart Medications	Skin Care
Infection Control for the Home	Taking a Pulse
Making the Home Environment Safe	Tracheostomy Care

Procedures

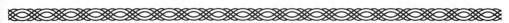

Oxygen Therapy Procedure

PURPOSE

- To prevent hypoxia.

Steps	Key Points

1. Obtain orders from the attending physician
  a. oxygen therapy
  b. flow rate or concentration
  c. arterial blood gas values
  d. respiratory therapy consultation.	

2. Discuss the indications/purposes/anticipated outcomes of oxygen therapy with the patient/family.	2. Knowing what to expect increases patient/family compliance.

3. Evaluate the patient's oxygen needs
  a. prescribed flow rate or concentration
  b. desired portability
  c. humidity requirements
  d. continuous or intermittent use.
	3. These factors influence the choice of oxygen equipment.

4. Select an oxygen delivery system.	4. Consultation with a home health care respiratory therapist can be helpful.
5. Coordinate order and delivery of equipment/supplies with the vendor.	5. Selection of a DME vendor is determined by agency policy.
6. Teach/review with the patient/family oxygen safety precautions a. no smoking	a. Post prominent no smoking signs.
b. do not use oxygen near stove/space heater/heat source	b. Oxygen under pressure explodes if it gets too hot.
c. do not use electric blankets/heating pads	
d. do not use polyester/nylon bed linens/clothing	d and e. Avoid creating static electricity.
e. use all cotton bed linens/clothing	
f. keep oxygen at least 5 ft away from electrical outlets/appliances	f. Oxygen supports combustion.
g. avoid the use of alcohol- and oil-containing skin care products	g. Oil and alcohol are flammable.
h. do not run oxygen tubing under clothes, bed linens, furniture, rugs and so forth	
i. keep the oxygen container upright	
j. turn off the oxygen when it's not in use	j. This step prevents oxygen leaks.

k. alert the local fire department and rescue squad about the use/storage of oxygen in the home.

k. Post the numbers of the fire department and rescue squad plus the oxygen vendor near the telephone.

7. Teach/review with the patient/family
   a. signs/symptoms of hypoxia (anxiety/apprehension, decreased ability to concentrate, decreased level of consciousness, dizziness, pallor, cyanosis, increased pulse rates/respirations, increased fatigue, behavior changes)
   b. how to assess respiratory status

   b. Supervised assessments validate the learner's progress.

   c. to minimize nasal dryness and stuffiness by using a single nasal prong and alternating nostril
   d. techniques for oral hygiene/comfort
   e. cleaning/maintenance of supplies/ equipment

   e and f. Return demonstration may be necessary.

   f. information specific to use of the selected oxygen delivery system
   g. importance of not changing the flow rate/pattern of oxygen use from that prescribed by the physician.
8. Monitor
   a. patient's pattern of oxygen use
   b. patient's respiratory status/response to oxygen therapy
   c. oxygen/humidity settings against prescribed rates
   d. functioning/supply level of oxygen source.

DOCUMENTATION

1. The steps of the procedure.
2. The type of oxygen delivery system used.
3. The prescribed flow rate/concentration.
4. The patient's baseline/ongoing respiratory status.
5. Patient's/family's understanding of and reaction to the need for oxygen therapy.
6. The content of teaching.
7. To whom the content was taught.

OXYGEN DELIVERY SYSTEMS

1. Oxygen concentrator
   a. Cost-effective indication
      • Long-term use of low flow oxygen (extracts oxygen from room air)

b. Humidity
- Some models do not require external humidifier
c. Portability
- Mobile (on wheels) but is bulky; compressed oxygen tank recommended for portability
d. Points to consider
- Home must have available space/access lanes
- Requires direct electrical current/grounded outlet
- Oxygen tank necessary as emergency back-up unit
- Cannot be used with Venturi masks or medication nebulizers
- Occasional release of room air gasses results in mechanical "burps"
e. Special care
- Clean filter at least twice weekly
- Do not use with extension cords
- Turn off, use back-up oxygen and call vendor if alert buzzer doesn't come on when power switch is pushed, if power light goes out and alert buzzer goes on during use and if alert buzzer sounds
- If power failure occurs, turn off and use back-up oxygen until power is restored
- Alert electric company about presence of concentrator in home.

2. Liquid oxygen
   a. Cost effective indication
   - Intermittent or continuous use of low flow or moderate flow rates
   b. Humidity
   - Need to add external humidifier to system
   c. Portability
   - Large stationary units are not mobile; portable liquid oxygen units are available
   d. Points to consider
   - Some units cannot be used with Venturi masks or medication nebulizers
   - Home must have available space
   e. Special care
   - Always keep unit upright in a well-ventilated area
   - Avoid touching the unit's metal parts with bare hands as frostbite may result.

3. Compressed oxygen
   a. Cost effective indication
   - High flow use of oxygen
   - Intermittent use up to 12 h/day
   b. Humidity
   - Need to add external humidifier to system
   c. Portability
   - Rolling tank stands are available; portable cylinders are recommended
   d. Points to consider
   - Can be used with any mask/cannula/nebulizer via an appropriate regulator/connector
   - Tanks must be replaced at frequent intervals (lasts about 50 hours at 2 L/min)
   e. Special care
   - Keep tank away from congested areas in the home
   - Keep at least a 3-day supply on hand
   - Open windows and call the vendor if the tank is emptying too quickly or the tank is hissing.

UNIT 3

Suctioning (Oronasopharyngeal) Procedure

PURPOSE

- To remove accumulated upper airway secretions.

EQUIPMENT

- suction machine
- connecting tubing
- suction catheter with a control device or a y-connector (a Yankauer or a tonsillar tip suction catheter may be used to remove extremely thick/copious oral secretions)
- 2 nonsterile gloves
- clean basin or disposable cup filled with tap water
- 2 clean towels
- clean gauze pad
- rubber band

Special Note. This is a clean procedure since suctioning is confined to the oral, nasal and pharyngeal areas.

Steps	Key Points
1. Assess the patient's lung sounds and respiratory pattern.	
2. Explain/review the procedure with the patient/family.	2. Knowing what to expect increases patient compliance and allays patient/family anxiety.
3. Wash your hands.	3. Good handwashing is an essential component of clean technique.

4. Position the patient
  a. oropharyngeal, semi-Fowler position with neck turned toward you.
  b. nasopharyngeal, semi-Fowler position with neck hyperextended.
	4. If patient is unconscious, place him or her in a lateral position facing you.

5. Place a towel under the patient's chin.	
6. Attach the connecting tubing to the suction machine.	
7. Turn on the suction machine and adjust the regulator so that the desired negative pressure is achieved.	7. Always use the lowest level of suction that will adequately clear secretions.

8. Put on the gloves.

8. Gloves reduce the possibility of microorganism transmission.

9. Attach the catheter to the connecting tubing.

10. Approximate the distance between the patient's ear lobe and nose and hold the catheter at that point.

10. This minimizes the possibility of the catheter being inserted past the pharynx into the trachea.

11. Moisten the catheter tip in tap water; apply suction.

11. This lubricates the catheter, reduces friction, eases insertion and enables you to check the equipment for proper functioning.

12. Instruct the patient to cough and deep breathe.

12. This mobilizes secretions in the pharynx.

13. Release the suction; gently insert and advance the catheter through one side of the patient's mouth/naris. *Do not apply suction during insertion.*

13. If the naris is obstructed, remove the catheter and reinsert it into the other naris. If both are obstructed, stop the procedure and notify the physician.

14. If the patient coughs during insertion, continue to advance the catheter.

15. Apply suction as you withdraw the catheter with a gentle rotating motion.

15. Gentle rotation of the catheter reduces mucosal irritation and maximizes secretion removal.

16. While suctioning, observe the patient for

   a. hypoxia (yawning, cyanosis, increased restlessness, shortness of breath)

   a. If hypoxia occurs, administer oxygen as prescribed.

   b. laryngospasm (crowing respirations)

   b. If laryngospasm occurs, stop suctioning, administer oxygen and notify the attending physician.

   c. bleeding; isoproterenol (Isuprel) and red gelatin may cause secretions to be pink tinged.

   c. If bleeding occurs, the suction pressure is too high or the mucosa has been traumatized.

17. Limit suctioning to 15 seconds.

17. If the patient is elderly or debilitated, limit suctioning to 10 seconds to prevent severe depletion of the patient's oxygen.

18. Flush the catheter with water.

18. Flushing maintains patency of the suction catheter and tubing and provides a rest period for the patient.

19. Repeat steps 12 to 17 until the airway is clear or the patient is able to cough productively.

20. Suction the oral cavity after the oropharyngeal/nasopharyngeal suctioning is completed.

21. Flush the catheter and connecting tubing thoroughly with fresh tap water.

21. Flushing reduces the possibility of microorganism transmission.

UNIT 3

22. Turn off the suction machine and detach the catheter from the connecting tubing.

22. Cover the end of the connecting tubing with a clean gauze pad, secure the pad with a rubber band and hang the tubing with the tip pointing up.

23. Rinse the catheter with running tap water and dry it.
24. Store the catheter in a clean towel until its next use.
25. Remove and discard your gloves.
26. Assist the patient to a comfortable position.
27. Reassess the patient's lung sounds and respiratory pattern.

27. Notify the physician of worsening respiratory distress, need for supplemental oxygen, need for another means to provide a patent airway.

28. Offer to perform or assist with oral hygiene.
29. Wash your hands.
30. Thoroughly clean reusable equipment with warm soapy water. Dry and store equipment in an accessible place until its next use.
31. Teach/review with the patient/family
    a. importance of maintaining adequate hydration
    b. importance of having the patient cough and expectorate secretions
    c. importance of keeping adequate/ appropriate supplies on hand
    d. indications for suctioning (ineffective coughing, restlessness, excess oral/nasal secretions, drooling)
    e. signs/symptoms of respiratory tract infection (fever, increased amount of secretions, change in color of secretions, foul smelling secretions)
    f. when to notify the nurse/physician
    g. need to change the connecting tubing every day
    h. need to empty the collection cannister once a day
    i. importance of disinfecting reusable equipment (collection cannister, connecting tubings, basin, catheters) at least once a week

    a. At least eight 8-oz glasses of water daily are recommended.
    b. Productive coughing is preferable to frequent suctioning.

    d. The patient should be suctioned as necessary.

    h. The Centers for Disease Control suggests that cannisters don't have to be emptied/changed until full.
    i. Boil reusable equipment that has been thoroughly washed for 15 minutes. Let cool. Dry using clean towels. Store in clean plastic bags, fresh jars or freshly laundered towels.

j. need to replace cracked or hard-
ened catheters, tubings and can-
nisters.

32. Have the patient demonstrate the procedure without nursing assistance (if appropriate).

32. Repeat this step on future visits to assess whether the patient has cor-rectly learned and is compliant with the procedure.

33. Teach the procedure to at least one other responsible family member.

33. It is important for another family member to know the procedure in the event the patient is unable to do the suctioning.

DOCUMENTATION

1. The teaching, the procedure, the equipment used, the number of times the patient was suctioned, the quality of the return demonstration and the name and relationship of the person taught, if other than the patient.
2. Assessment of the patient's lung sounds/respiratory pattern before and after the suctioning.
3. The color, consistency, odor and amount of suctioned secretions.
4. The patient's/family's response to the procedure.
5. Date, time and details of consultations with the attending physician.
6. Plans for follow-up.

Suctioning (Tracheostomy) Procedure

PURPOSE

- To remove accumulated tracheobronchial secretions.

EQUIPMENT

- suction machine
- connecting tubing
- sterile or disinfected suction catheter with a control device or a y-connector
- manual resuscitator attached to oxygen source
- 2 clean gloves
- clean basin or disposable cup
- normal saline or boiled tap water
- 3 to 5 cc syringe filled with sterile normal saline (optional)
- clean gauze pad
- rubber band
- mirror (optional)

Special Note. This procedure uses the principles of medical, rather than surgical, asepsis. The decision to teach this procedure as clean or sterile depends upon the nurse's assessment of the patient's needs and the patient's/family's capabilities.

Steps	*Key Points*
1. Assess the patient's lung sounds and respiratory pattern.	
2. Explain/review the procedure with the patient/family.	2. Knowing what to expect increases patient compliance and allays patient/family anxiety.
3. Help the patient to a comfortable semi-Fowler or high Fowler position.	3. Positioning the patient in front of a mirror facilitates his or her understanding of the procedure.
4. Wash your hands.	
5. Attach the resuscitator to the oxygen source and adjust the flow meter to 12 to 14 L/min.	
6. Attach the connecting tubing to the suction machine.	
7. Turn on the suction machine and adjust the regulator so that the desired negative pressure is achieved.	7. If the DME supplier has not preset the negative pressure, use the lowest level of suctioning that will adequately clear secretions.
8. Put on gloves.	
9. Attach the catheter to the connecting tubing.	

10. Moisten the catheter tip in normal saline/water; apply suction.

10. This step enables you to check the equipment for proper functioning, lubricates the catheter, reduces friction and eases insertion.

11. Release the suction; gently insert and advance the catheter into the tracheostomy tube until resistance is met. Pull the catheter back slightly. *Do not apply suction during insertion.*

11. If secretions are particularly thick/tenacious, instill 3 to 5 ml of sterile normal saline before inserting the catheter.

12. Apply suction as you withdraw the catheter with a gentle rotating motion.

12. Gentle rotation of the catheter reduces mucosal irritation and maximizes secretion removal.

13. While suctioning, observe the patient for
    a. hypoxia (yawning, cyanosis, increased restlessness, shortness of breath)

    a. If hypoxia occurs, administer oxygen as prescribed.

    b. bloody secretions; isoproterenol (Isuprel) or red gelatin may cause secretions to be pink tinged

    b. Bleeding can be indicative of infection or mucosal trauma.

    c. coughing.

    c. Administer oxygen as prescribed and allow patient to rest between passes of the catheter.

14. Limit suctioning to 15 seconds or less.

15. Flush the catheter with normal saline/water.

15. Flushing maintains patency of the suction catheter.

16. Repeat steps 10 to 13 until the airway is clear.

16. Instruct the patient to turn his or her head to the left to suction the left bronchus and to the right to suction the right bronchus.

17. Patients on oxygen therapy should be oxygenated, with three hyperinflations of the resuscitator, between passes of the suctioning catheter.

17. Patients with copious secretions should not be oxygenated with a resuscitator. Use their regular oxygen delivery system, increasing the liter flow just before suctioning.

18. Suction the oropharyngeal/nasopharyngeal areas, if necessary.

18. Remind the patient/family that the nose and mouth are considered "dirty" and should be suctioned after the "clean" tracheostomy.

19. Flush the catheter and connecting tubing thoroughly with normal saline/water.

19. This step reduces the possibility of microorganism transmission.

20. Turn off the suction machine and detach the catheter from the connecting tubing.

20. Cover the end of the connecting tubing with a clean gauze pad, secure the pad with a rubber band and hang the tubing with the tip pointing up.

21. Remove and discard your gloves.

UNIT
3

22. Reassess the patient's lung sounds and respiratory pattern.

23. Offer to perform or assist with oral hygiene.
24. Wash your hands.
25. Thoroughly clean reusable equipment with warm soapy water. Dry and store in an accessible place until its next use.
26. Teach/review with the patient/family
    a. importance of maintaining adequate hydration
    b. importance of environmental humidification

    c. importance of keeping adequate/appropriate supplies on hand
    d. indications for suctioning (restlessness, wheezing, ineffective coughing, cyanosis, decreased level of consciousness)
    e. signs/symptoms of respiratory tract infection (fever, increased amount of secretions, change in color of secretions, foul smelling secretions)
    f. when to notify the nurse/physician
    g. need to change the connecting tubing every day
    h. need to empty the collector cannister once a day

    i. to disinfect reusable equipment (collection cannister, connecting tubings, catheters, basin) at least once a week

    j. need to replace hardened/cracked catheters, tubings or canisters
    k. artificial respiration/CPR.

27. Have the patient demonstrate tracheostomy suctioning without nursing assistance.

22. Notify the physician of
    a. worsening respiratory condition
    b. secretions too thick to suction.

25. Use of a small pipe cleaner–type brush may be necessary.

    a. At least eight 8-oz glasses of fluid daily are recommended.
    b. Tracheobronchial secretions can consolidate in airways without adequate humidification.

    d. The patient should be suctioned as necessary and when tracheostomy care is performed.

    h. The Centers for Disease Control suggests that cannisters don't have to be emptied/changed until full.
    i. Boil reusable equipment that has been thoroughly washed for 15 minutes. Let cool. Dry using clean towels. Store in clean plastic bags, fresh jars or freshly laundered towels.

    k. Certification in basic cardiac life support is recommended for family members.

27. Repeat this step on future visits to assess whether the patient has correctly learned and is compliant with the procedure.

28. Teach the procedure for tracheostomy suctioning to at least one other responsible family member.	28. It is important for another family member to know the procedure in the event the patient is unable to do the suctioning.

DOCUMENTATION

1. The teaching, the procedure, the equipment used, the number of times the patient was suctioned, the quality of the return demonstration and the name and relationship of the person taught, if other than the patient.

2. Assessment of the patient's lung sounds/respiratory pattern before and after the suctioning.

3. The color, consistency, odor and amount of suctioned secretions.

4. The patient's/family's response to the procedure.

5. Date, time and details of consultations with the attending physician.

6. Plans for follow-up.

UNIT
3

Tracheostomy Care Procedure

PURPOSE

- To prevent infection.
- To maintain a patent airway.
- To maintain the integrity of the skin around the tracheostomy stoma.

EQUIPMENT

- suctioning equipment (see Suctioning (Tracheostomy) Procedure)
- 2 clean gloves
- clean basin
- hydrogen peroxide
- normal saline or boiled tap water
- clean 4 × 4 gauze pads
- clean cotton-tipped swabs/applicators
- clean pipe cleaners/small brush
- clean tracheostomy ties (twill/bias tape)
- mirror
- clean washcloth
- clean towel
- clean scissors

Special Note. This procedure uses the principles of medical, rather than surgical, asepsis. The decision to teach this procedure as clean or sterile depends on the nurse's assessment of the patient's needs and the patient's/family's capabilities.

Steps	*Key Points*
1. Explain/review the procedure with the patient/family.	1. Knowing what to expect increases patient compliance and allays patient/family anxiety.
2. Help the patient to a comfortable high Fowler position.	2. Positioning the patient in front of a mirror facilitates his or her understanding of the procedure.
3. Wash your hands and put on gloves.	3. Good handwashing is an essential component of clean technique.
4. Complete tracheostomy suctioning.	4. Refer to Suctioning (Tracheostomy) Procedure.
5. Remove the inner cannula.	5. If the tracheal tube does not have an inner cannula, proceed to step 11.
6. Hold the inner cannula over the basin and pour the hydrogen peroxide over and into it.	6. Clean the inner cannula twice a day.
7. Clean the inner cannula with the pipe cleaner/small brush.	7. This removes adhering crusts/secretions.

8. Thoroughly rinse the inner cannula with normal saline/boiled tap water.

9. Shake excess droplets from the cannula and dry it with a clean gauze pad.

10. Replace the inner cannula and lock it in place.

11. Remove the soiled gauze dressing and assess the stomal area for pressure irritation and signs of stomatitis.

12. Clean the exposed outer cannula and stoma area with cotton-tipped applicators soaked in hydrogen peroxide.

13. Use the washcloth and normal saline/boiled water to remove the hydrogen peroxide and clean the skin.

14. Dry the exposed outer cannula and stoma skin with the clean towel.

15. Change the tracheostomy ties.

    a. measure and cut a piece of bias/twill tape long enough to go twice around the patient's neck
    b. lace the tape through one eyelet, around the back of the patient's neck, through the other eyelet and again around the back of the patient's neck
    c. pull the tape snugly and tie a square knot on one side of the patient's neck
    d. remove the old ties.

16. Apply a fresh gauze dressing under the tracheostomy ties and faceplate.

17. Remove and discard your gloves.

18. Thoroughly clean reusable equipment with warm soapy water. Dry and store in an accessible place until its next use.

---

8. If the patient is on a ventilator, clean and replace the inner cannula as quickly as possible.

12. The exposed outer cannula and stoma area should be cleaned at least once a day and as necessary.

UNIT 3

15. The ties should be changed once a day or when they become loose or wet.
    a. Cut the ends on a diagonal to ease eyelet threading of the tape.

    c. There should be enough space for one finger between the tape and the patient's neck.
    d. Do not cut the old ties until the new ones are in place and securely fastened together.

16. Use a 4×4 gauze pad with tape on the cut edges or fold a 4×4 gauze pad to avoid putting frayed edges near the tracheostomy.

19. Teach/review with the patient/family
    a. to disinfect reusable equipment at least once a week

    a. Boil reusable equipment that has been thoroughly washed for 15 minutes. Let cool. Dry using clean towels. Store in clean plastic bags, fresh jars or freshly laundered towels.

    b. signs/symptoms of stomatitis (hard, red, tender stomal area; foul smelling secretions; change in color of secretions; increased amount of secretions)

    b. An antibacterial solution can be requested from the physician. Ointments are a reservoir for microorganism growth and are not recommended.

    c. importance of keeping the stomal skin clean and dry
    d. importance of environmental humidity

    d. Tracheobronchial secretions can consolidate in airways without adequate humidification.

    e. importance of avoiding bronchopulmonary irritants

    e. Irritants can cause/aggravate respiratory distress.

    f. significance of avoiding water sports and showers
    g. value of wearing an emergency medical identification tag/bracelet
    h. importance of keeping an emergency tracheostomy set and portable suction near the patient

    h. Travel is possible as long as the appropriate equipment is taken along.

    i. when to notify the nurse/physician
    j. artificial respiration/CPR

    j. Certification in basic cardiac life support is recommended for the family members.

    k. signs/symptoms of respiratory distress (tachypnea, restlessness, anxiety, cyanosis, yawning, nasal flaring, retractions, diaphoresis)
    l. need to change the tracheostomy tube if a mucus plug cannot be removed by suctioning
    m. need to loosely cover the tracheostomy with a scarf when going out on a cold day.

    m. Cold atmospheric air can be very irritating to the tracheal mucosa.

20. Have the patient demonstrate the tracheostomy care without nursing assistance.

20. Repeat this step on future visits to assess whether the patient has correctly learned and is compliant with the procedure.

21. Teach the tracheostomy care to at least one other responsible family member.

21. It is important for another family member to know the procedure in the event the patient is unable to do the suctioning.

DOCUMENTATION

1. The teaching, the procedure, the quality of the return demonstration and the name and relationship of the person taught, if other than the patient.
2. Assessment of the stomal area.
3. The color, consistency, odor and amount of secretions.
4. The patient's/family's response to the procedure.
5. Date, time and details of consultation with the attending physician.
6. Plans for follow-up.

PEDIATRIC CONSIDERATIONS

1. Encourage parents to notify the local police department, rescue squad and utility company that there is an infant/child with a tracheostomy in the home.
2. Trachea collars are particularly effective for providing humidification during naps or at night. Scrupulous cleaning/drying is required, however, to prevent skin breakdown.
3. "Fast" mist can be provided by turning on the shower in a bathroom and letting the room fill with steam.
4. Small, thin play objects as well as fuzzy toys, clothing and blankets should be removed from the infant's/child's play areas.
5. Interaction with the infant/child should be as normal as possible. Read stories and show picture books to the infant/child. A bell tied on the infant's/child's ankle can alert the parents to the infant's/child's excitement. An older child can use a note pad, magic erase slate, a horn or a bell. Remember that the infant's/child's "silent cry" can produce extremely high parental anxiety.
6. The need for constant supervision by an adult of an infant/child with a tracheostomy cannot be emphasized enough. Intercom systems may help facilitate supervision of the infant/child if the infant/child wears a bell on his or her ankle.
7. A bib is essential when feeding the infant/child with a tracheostomy.
8. Infants/young children may need to be restrained to prevent pulling at the tracheal tube. Elbow restraints are preferred to wrist restraints. Place a padded cardboard cylinder over the infant's/child's shirt and secure it with ties or tape to prevent it from slipping off. Avoid pressure at the axillae and at the wrists.

UNIT 3

Tracheostomy Tube Changing Procedure

PURPOSE

- To maintain a patent airway.
- To prevent infection.

EQUIPMENT

- sterile/disinfected tracheostomy tube with obturator
- clean tracheostomy ties (bias/twill tape)
- clean 4 × 4 gauze pads
- water-soluble lubricant/vegetable oil/olive oil
- clean scissors
- mirror

Special Note. This procedure should be done at least every other day.

Steps

1. Explain the procedure to the patient/family.
2. Help the patient to a comfortable high Fowler position.

3. Wash your hands.

4. Attach the tracheostomy ties to the tracheostomy tube

   a. measure and cut two lengths of twill/bias tape that are long enough to fold in half and fit around the patient's neck
   b. fold one piece of string in half and bring it up through one hole of the faceplate
   c. bring the loose ends of the tape through the loop created by the folded end
   d. pull the loose ends of the tape to tighten the knot on the faceplate
   e. repeat on the other side of the faceplate.
5. Remove the inner cannula of the disinfected tracheostomy tube and insert the obturator.

Key Points

1. Knowing what to expect increases patient/family compliance.
2. Positioning the patient in front of a mirror facilitates his or her understanding of the procedure.
3. Handwashing is an essential component of clean technique.
4. It is essential that the new equipment is prepared and ready for insertion prior to removing the dirty tube.

6. Lubricate the disinfected outer cannula and obturator tip with the water-soluble substance.
7. Cut the dirty tracheostomy ties.
8. Remove the old tube by pulling it steadily downward and outward.

9. Instruct the patient to take a deep breath as you insert the disinfected tube.

6. Do not use mineral oil, as it may irritate the lungs.

8. Removal may trigger a coughing spasm. Halt the procedure until the coughing stops.
9. If the patient begins to cough, hold the new tube in place until the coughing subsides.

Special Note. If you are unable to insert the new tube, reposition the patient's head and try again. If unsuccessful, try to reinsert the old tube. If unable, insert a suction catheter into the stoma, and cut it off about 6 in above the stoma. *Do not let go of the catheter.* Notify the physician or bring the patient to the emergency room. *Do not leave the patient alone.*

UNIT 3

10. Remove the obturator.
11. Tie the twill/bias tape.

11. Pull the tape snugly and tie a square knot on one side of the patient's neck. There should be enough space for one finger between the tape and the patient's neck.

12. Insert the inner cannula and lock it in place.
13. Apply a fresh gauze dressing under the new tracheostomy ties and faceplate.

13. Use either a 4×4 gauze dressing with tape on the cut edges or fold a 4×4 gauze dressing to avoid pulling frayed edges near the tracheostomy.

14. Teach/review with the patient/family how to clean and disinfect tracheostomy tubes

14. Reinforce with the patient/family the importance of keeping an adequate supply of ready-to-use equipment on hand.

   a. metal tubes—wash with soap, water, pipe cleaners and brush. Remove tarnish with silver polish. Rinse well with running tap water and pipe cleaners. Boil the cleaned tracheostomy tube pieces for 15 min. Drain the water and let the pieces cool. Store in a clean jar with a lid.
   b. plastic tubes—wash with soap, water, pipe cleaners and toothbrush. Rinse well with running tap water. Soak in hydrogen peroxide for 8 hours or overnight. Rinse with rubbing alcohol. Rinse well with boiled tap water. Dry with a clean towel. Store in a clean jar with a lid.

15. Have the patient demonstrate tracheostomy tube changing procedure without nursing assistance.

15. Repeat this step on future visits to assess whether the patient has correctly learned and is compliant with the procedure.

16. Teach the procedure for tracheostomy tube changing to at least one other responsible family member.

16. It is important for another family member to know the procedure in the event the patient is unable to do the suctioning.

DOCUMENTATION

1. The teaching, the procedure, the quality of the return demonstration, the name and relationship of the person taught, if other than the patient.

2. The patient's/family's response to the procedure.

3. Unexpected outcomes and nursing actions.

4. Time and details of consultation with the attending physician and other medical personnel.

5. Plans for follow-up.

PEDIATRIC CONSIDERATIONS

1. Two individuals are necessary when changing the tracheostomy tubes of infants and small children. One person is responsible for holding the old tracheostomy tube in place after its ties are cut, removing the tube and securing the new ties. The other person is responsible for cutting the old ties, inserting the new tube and holding the new tube in place until its ties are secured.

2. Infants and small children must be restrained during a change of tracheostomy tubes.

3. A rolled towel under the infant's/child's shoulders will extend the infant's/child's neck and facilitate insertion.

4. Most pediatric tracheostomy tubes do not have inner cannulas.

Resources

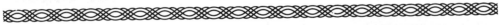

Croup Assessment/ Intervention

Differentiation of Croup Symptoms*

	Acute Tracheobronchitis	Spasmodic Croup	Acute Epiglottitis
Age	<3 years	1 to 4 years	>3 years
History	Gradual onset; preceded by upper respiratory infection	Child awakens during the night with symptoms	Sudden onset; symptoms worsen over a few hours
Symptoms	Fever (<40°C); mild to severe respiratory distress at night	Afebrile; mild to moderate respiratory distress	Child's chin may be thrust forward; drooling, difficulty swallowing; epiglottis cherry red; febrile (>40°C)
Comments	Most common	Sometimes relieved by vomiting; asymptomatic during the day; symptoms recur during night	No attempt should be made to visualize child's epiglottis; child should be kept calm; emergency tracheotomy may be needed; high morbidity

*The progression of symptoms should be reported immediately to the physician.

ASSESSMENT OF RESPIRATORY DISTRESS

The following scoring system provides a method of determining the severity of respiratory distress without the need for arterial blood gas values.

	0	1	2
Inspiratory breath sounds	Normal	Harsh with rhonchi	Delayed
Stridor	None	Inspiratory	Inspiratory and expiratory
Cough	None	Hoarse cry	Bark
Retractions and flaring	None	Flaring and suprasternal retractions	As under 1, plus subcostal and intercostal retractions
Cyanosis	None	In air	In 40% O_2

Score	Nursing Interventions
<4	1. Provide warm mist. 2. Instruct parents to stay with child. 3. Notify physician.
4 to 6	1, 2, 3 as above. 4. Coordinate transportation to physician's office or hospital.
≥7	1, 2, 3 as above. 4. Arrange for ambulance transportation to hospital. 5. Initiate respiratory resuscitation (if necessary).

Suction Catheter Sizes

Suction Catheter Sizes

Age	Size (French)*
Infant	5–8
Child	8–10
Adult	12–18

*Use a size that is half the diameter of the tube/naris to be suctioned.

Suction Vacuum Settings

Suction Vacuum Settings

Age	Setting (mm Hg)
Infant	3–5
Child	5–10
Adult	7–15

Vital Signs: Normal Pediatric Values

Vital Signs: Normal Pediatric Values

Age	Temperature (°C)	Pulse	Respirations	Blood Pressure (mm Hg)
Birth–6 months	36.5–37.0 (rectal)	110–140	30–50	60/40
6–12 months	37.6 (rectal)	105–115	25–35	90/60
1–6 years	37.6 (rectal)	90–110	20–30	100/65
6–12 years	37 (oral)	80–95	15–25	105/68
12–16 years	37 (oral)	75–85	15–20	115/70

Water Requirements for Children

Water Requirements for Children

Age	Average Body Weight (kg)	Total Water in 24 Hours (ml)	Water/Kg Body Weight in 24 Hours (ml)
3 days	3.0	250–300	80–100
10 days	3.2	400–500	125–150
3 months	5.4	750–850	140–160
6 months	7.3	950–1100	130–155
9 months	8.6	1100–1250	125–145
1 year	9.5	1150–1300	120–135
2 years	11.8	1350–1500	115–125
4 years	16.2	1600–1800	100–110
6 years	20.0	1800–2000	90–100
10 years	28.7	2000–2500	70–85
14 years	45.0	2200–2700	50–60
18 years	54.0	2200–2700	40–50

UNIT 3

Bibliography

Abman, S. et al. Experience with Home Oxygen in the Management of Infants with Bronchopulmonary Dysplasia. Clinical Pediatrics, 23(9): 1984, pp. 471–476.

Ahman, E. Home Care for the High Risk Infant. Rockville, Maryland: Aspen Systems, 1986.

Berkemeyer, S. and Hutchins, K. Home Apnea Monitoring. Pediatric Nursing, 12(4): 1986, pp. 259–304.

Carroll, P. Home Care for the Ventilator Patient: A Checklist You Can Use. Nursing, 17(10): 1987, pp. 82–83.

Chu, M. Continuing Care of a Total Laryngectomy Patient. Home Healthcare Nurse, 3(4): 1985, pp. 37–39.

Crow, S. Tips for Successful Respiratory Suctioning. RN, April 1986, pp. 31–33.

Czarniecki, L. Caring for a Young Child With a Tracheostomy. Caring, 4(5):, 1985, pp. 30–32.

Davido, J. Pulmonary Rehabilitation. Nursing Clinics of North America, 16(2): 1981, pp. 275–283.

Feinberg, E. Family Stress in Pediatric Home Care. Caring, May 1985, pp. 38–41.

Feinstein, D. What to Teach the Patient Who's Had a Total Laryngectomy. RN, 50(4): 1987, pp. 53–57.

Fischer, A. Long-term Management of the Ventilator Patient in the Home. Cleveland Clinic Quarterly, 52(3):1985, pp. 303–306.

Fox, J. Chronic Respiratory Patient: A New Challenge for Home Health Nursing. Home Healthcare Nurse, 3(2): 1985, pp. 13–16.

Frace, R. Home Ventilation: An Alternative to Institutionalization. Focus on Critical Care, 13(6): 1986, pp. 28–34.

Hazinski, M. Pediatric Home Tracheostomy Care: A Parent's Guide. Pediatric Nursing, 12(1): 1986, pp. 41–48, 69.

Hughes, C. et al. Caring for Ventilator Dependent Patients. Caring, January 1985, pp. 41–46.

Jackson, D. Nursing Care Plan: Home Care Management of Children with B.P.D. Pediatric Nursing, 12(5): 1985, pp. 342–348.

Kennelly, C. Tracheostomy Care: Parents as Learners. MCN, 12(4): 1987, pp. 264–267.

McCarthy, M. A Home Discharge Program for Ventilator-Assisted Children. Pediatric Nursing, 12(5): 1986, pp. 331–335, 380.

McDonald, G. A Home Care Program for Patients with Chronic Lung Disease. Nursing Clinics of North America, 16(2): 1981, pp. 259–274.

Sexton, D. Chronic Obstructive Pulmonary Disease: Care of the Child and Adult. St. Louis, The C. V. Mosby Co., 1981.

Sjoberg, E. Nursing Diagnoses and the COPD Patient. American Journal of Nursing, 83(2): 1983, pp. 245–248.

Votava, K. et al. Home Care of the Patient Dependent on Mechanical Ventilation. Home Healthcare Nurse, 3(2): 1985, pp. 18–25.

White, K. and Perez, P. Your Ventilator Patient Can Go Home Again. Nursing 86, pp. 54–56.

Mental Health Alterations

Care Plans
- Alcohol Abuse Care Plan
- Bereavement Care Plan
- Depression Care Plan
- Schizophrenia Care Plan
- Sudden Infant Death Syndrome (SIDS) Care Plan
- Spiritual Distress Care Plan

Procedures
- Domestic Violence Assessment/Intervention Procedure

Resources
- Mental Health Assessment/Intervention Guide
- Mental Illness Warning Signs
- Suicidal Patient: Indications for Requesting Hospitalization

Care Plans

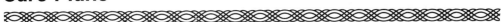

Alcohol Abuse Care Plan

CROSS REFERENCES

Constipation Care Plan
Generic Cardiac Care Plan
Hepatic Cirrhosis Care Plan

Domestic Violence Assessment/Intervention
  Procedure

Home Safety Procedure

Gum Disease Warning Signs
Mental Health Assessment/Intervention Guide

**UNIT
4**

NURSING DIAGNOSES

1. Self-care deficit (feeding, hygiene, grooming, toileting) related to
   a. disordered thought patterns
   b. neuromuscular impairment
   c. preoccupation with alcohol
   d. other.
2. Alteration in oral mucous membrane related to
   a. vitamin deficiencies
   b. dehydration
   c. inadequate oral hygiene
   d. malnutrition
   e. other.
3. Alteration in nutrition (less than body requirements) related to
   a. poor eating habits
   b. gastrointestinal malabsorption
   3. anorexia
   4. other.
4. Potential or actual fluid volume deficit related to
   a. hyperventilation
   b. diarrhea
   c. vomiting
   d. diuresis
   e. other.
5. Alteration in fluid volume (excess) related to compromised regulatory mechanism.
6. Alteration in bowel elimination (diarrhea) related to irritation/malabsorption of bowel.
7. Alteration in bowel elimination (constipation) related to
   a. less than adequate dietary intake and bulk
   b. less than adequate physical activity
   c. neuromuscular impairment
   d. personal habits
   e. dehydration
   f. other.

8. Sleep pattern disturbance related to
    a. anxiety/depression
    b. altered levels of brain biochemicals
    c. other.
9. Potential for injury related to
    a. increased susceptibility to infection
    b. increased susceptibility to uncontrolled bleeding
    c. peripheral neuropathy
    d. alcoholic stupor
    e. weakness/reduced sensation of lower extremities
    f. other.
10. Alteration in health maintenance related to lack of ability to make deliberate and thoughtful judgments.
11. Social isolation related to
    a. embarrassment/shame
    b. unaccepted social behavior
    c. stigma associated with alcoholism
    d. other.
12. Potential for violence (self-directed or at others) related to
    a. misinterpretation of other's behaviors/intentions
    b. misperception of environment
    c. severe anxiety/panic state
    d. inability to tolerate personal feelings
    e. other.
13. Ineffective family coping (compromised/disabling) related to
    a. ambivalent family relationships
    b. exhausted supportive capacity among family members
    c. financial stress
    d. other.
14. Knowledge deficit (alcoholism; physical, legal, social, financial effects; treatment; concept of enabling; nutritional maintenance; community resources; personal hygiene techniques; methods of infection control; signs/symptoms of infection) related to
    a. cognitive limitation
    b. lack of readiness to learn
    c. denial
    d. other.

PROCESS INDICATORS

1. The patient's physical health is maintained.
Indicators
    a. no signs/symptoms of infection
    b. no signs/symptoms of dehydration
    c. no signs/symptoms of anemia
    d. no signs/symptoms of cardiomyopathy
    e. weight gain/stabilization
    f. bowel/bladder patterns are regular and continent
    g. patient's personal hygiene is adequate
    h. patient/family validate a balanced rest/nutrition/exercise program for the patient

i. family verbalization of a method for preventing the patient from driving/having access to car keys when he or she is drinking
j. patient does not engage in self-destructive behaviors
k. patient/family recall how alcohol interacts with the patient's medications
2. The patient's/family's psychosocial integrity is maintained.

Indicators

a. patient/family identifies the relationship between their social, financial, legal and physical problems and the patient's alcohol abuse
b. patient/family expresses feelings in an outwardly appropriate manner
c. familial feedback reflects that members are emotionally supportive of each other
d. familial feedback reflects accurate knowledge about alcoholism, its process and available treatments
e. familial feedback demonstrates an accurate understanding of enabling behaviors
f. familial feedback indicates that members have relinquished their feelings of self-blame
g. familial feedback shows that members are not trying to control the patient's drinking behaviors
h. patient/family maintains satisfactory levels of social/community/occupational inter-actions
i. patient/family participates in self-help groups.

NURSING INTERVENTIONS

1. Assess the patient.
   a. frequency/pattern, amount and duration of alcohol use
   b. frequency/pattern, amount and duration of other substance use
   c. cardiovascular status
   d. pulmonary status
   e. signs/symptoms of pancreatitis (severe constant upper abdominal pain, tenderness radiating to the back)
   f. signs/symptoms of liver damage/disease (hepatomegaly, protruding abdomen, systemic jaundice, peripheral edema)
   g. signs/symptoms of esophagitis/gastritis
   h. signs/symptoms of gastrointestinal bleeding
   i. signs/symptoms of dehydration or fluid retention
   j. signs/symptoms of peripheral neuropathy (loss of sensation, unsteady gait, impaired balance)
   k. signs/symptoms of anemia (pallor, weakness, fatigue, headache, tinnitus, palpitations, vertigo)
   l. signs/symptoms of urinary tract infection (fever, pain, cloudy urine, foul odor)
   m. nutritional status/appetite
   n. bowel/bladder elimination patterns
   o. level of personal and oral hygiene
   p. injuries suggestive of alcoholic stupor (cigarette burns on chest and between index and middle fingers, contusions and bruises, wounds at various stages of healing)
   q. psychological status (anger, hostility, denial, depression, feelings of failure)
   r. pattern of contact/interaction with nuclear/extended family and significant others
   s. social, financial, occupational, legal, personal consequences of alcohol use
   t. readiness/motivation to learn

     u. cognitive ability

     v. topics of conversation (i.e., to what extent does the patient talk about alcohol-related topics).

2. Assess
    a. how the family members are coping with the alcohol abuse
    b. each family member's degree of social isolation
    c. each family member's degree of denial
    d. what problems (personal, social, occupational, legal, financial) the family attributes to living with an alcoholic
    e. interactions among family members
    f. patient's/family's financial status
    g. environmental factors/situations that facilitate the patient's alcohol abuse
    h. patient's/family's understanding of alcoholism
    i. family's understanding of enabling behaviors
    j. each family member's perception/description of the patient's pattern/history of alcohol use.

3. Teach the patient about
    a. personal hygiene techniques
    b. importance of engaging in physical activities
    c. importance of maintaining an adequate daily fluid intake (at least 3000 ml per day, if not contraindicated) using juices, Gatorade, water and bouillon
    d. techniques to promote sleep
    e. importance of balancing rest, nutrition and exercise
    f. the signs/symptoms of constipation.

4. Teach the patient/family about
    a. alcoholism as a disease
    b. physical consequences of alcohol abuse
    c. relationship between social, financial, occupational, personal, legal problems and alcohol abuse
    d. necessity of abstinence for recovery
    e. sobriety being a choice only the patient can make
    f. treatability of alcoholism
    g. available treatment programs
    h. drug and alcohol interactions
    i. importance of avoiding products containing alcohol (cough syrups, after-shave lotion, mouthwash, astringents)
    j. signs/symptoms of infection
    k. methods to promote bowel regularity/avoid constipation
    l. stress management techniques
    m. importance of setting short-term, realistic goals.

5. Provide instruction to the family about
    a. therapeutic communication techniques (do not be drawn into arguments with the patient; do not talk about feelings/treatments when the patient is intoxicated; do not moralize or chastize the patient; avoid ideological/theoretical discussions with the patient regarding the alcohol use; focus on concrete and current issues)
    b. how to refocus the patient when he or she begins to ruminate
    c. importance of consistently providing positive feedback for the patient's successes
    d. importance of making commitments to the patient that only can be met realistically
    e. enabling behaviors (any behavior that covers up/hides the patient's alcohol use and its consequences)
    f. making the home environment safe

g. recognizing signs of impending assault or violent behavior

h. importance of keeping emergency numbers (crisis intervention unit, police, rescue squad, nurse, physician) next to the telephone or in an easily accessible place.

6. Monitor
    a. fluid and electrolyte balance
    b. liver enzyme results
    c. serum magnesium levels
    d. serum calcium levels
    e. serum glucose levels
    f. serum iron levels
    g. platelet counts
    h. white blood cell counts.

7. Refer to and coordinate interventions with
    a. social worker
    b. physical therapist
    c. occupational therapist
    d. vocational rehabilitation counselor
    e. dentist
    f. psychiatric liaison nurse
    g. dietician and coordinate the patient's/family's utilization of the dietician's teaching to promote/maintain the patient's nutritional status.

8. Refer the patient/family (provide telephone numbers, locations and meeting times; do not make contact for the patient/family) to
    a. Alcoholics Anonymous
    b. Alanon
    c. Alateen
    d. treatment programs/centers
    e. counselling services
    f. National Council on Alcoholism.

9. Create situations that encourage the patient/family to express their thoughts and feelings.

10. Provide opportunities that facilitate the patient's/family's independent action/decision-making.

11. Request/obtain orders for medications, blood levels, hospitalization and so forth, as necessary, from the attending physician.

12. Provide progress notes and a discharge summary to the attending physician.

THERAPEUTIC ACHIEVEMENT

- The patient and/or family identifies and talks about the problem with alcohol.
- The family unit is maintained.

RELATED PATIENT INSTRUCTIONS

Antibiotic Medications

Anticonvulsant Medications

Comfort Measures for Dehydration

Diuretic Medications

Guidelines for Describing Seizure Activity

Healthy Heart

Heart Medications

Infection Control for the Home

Making the Home Environment Safe

Management of Seizure Activity

Medication Compliance

Reality Orientation

Seizure Precautions

Skin Care

When to Call for Help

UNIT 4

Bereavement Care Plan

CROSS REFERENCES

Alcohol Abuse Care Plan
Depression Care Plan
Spiritual Distress Care Plan

Telephone Contact with Patient/Family
  Procedure

Suicidal Patient: Indications for Requesting
  Hospitalization
Mental Health Assessment/Intervention Guide

NURSING DIAGNOSES

1. Grieving related to
  a. anticipated/actual loss of significant other/object
  b. anticipated/actual body system alteration
  c. other.
2. Complicated grieving related to
  a. prolonged/stressful anticipatory loss
  b. lack of adequate support systems
  c. unfinished business with the deceased
  d. overidentification with the deceased
  e. multiple losses
  f. secondary gains from grieving
  g. concurrent life crises
  h. other.
3. Disturbance in self-esteem related to
  a. loss of role as caregiver/spouse/parent
  b. threat of change in daily routine
  c. other.
4. Fear related to
  a. increased financial/legal responsibilities
  b. increased decision-making responsibilities
  c. lack of support system
  d. perceived lack of control
  e. other.
5. Self-care deficit (feeding, hygiene, grooming) related to
  a. depression
  b. anxiety
  c. fatigue
  d. other.
6. Sleep pattern disturbance related to
  a. depression
  b. anxiety
  c. life-style disruption
  d. other.
7. Social isolation related to
  a. loss of a significant other/object
  b. depression

c. anxiety

d. loss of usual means of transportation

e. other.

8. Alteration in nutrition (more/less than body requirements) related to

a. emotional stress

b. social isolation

c. anxiety

d. depression

e. loneliness

f. guilt

g. other.

9. Alteration in family process related to

a. anticipatory grief

b. exhausted interdependent supportive capacity

c. family disorganization/role changes

d. guilt

e. anxiety

f. hostility

g. ambivalence

h. economic crisis

i. difficulty in expressing/listening to thoughts/feelings of grief

j. other.

PROCESS INDICATORS

1. The survivor accepts the reality of the death.

Indicators

a. survivor's verbalizations about the personal meaning of the patient's death

b. survivor's constructive progression through the stages of grieving (denial, anger, bargaining, realization of the loss, acceptance, reintegration)

c. survivor's verbalization of acceptance of the loss.

2. The survivor adjusts to an environment in which the deceased is missing.

Indicators

a. survivor's participation in decision-making for the future

b. survivor's initiation of social contacts and interactions

c. progression through the use of linking objects (possessions of the deceased that the survivor needs to always know whereabouts of or will experience severe anxiety), transitional objects (similar to linking objects but without the invested emotional attachment) and keepsakes (possessions of the deceased that are kept as a reminder but that are not essential for the survivor's emotional equilibrium).

3. The survivor physically recuperates from the stress of loss and grieving.

Indicators

a. maintenance of an adequate balance of nutrition, hydration, elimination, rest and exercise

b. maintenance of personal hygiene and grooming at the same or higher level demonstrated prior to the loss

c. lessening/elimination of physical exhaustion, sleep disturbances, restlessness, agitation, digestive alterations and anorexia.

4. The survivor copes with legal and financial obligations.

UNIT
4

Indicators
   a. fulfillment of occupational responsibilities
   b. formulation of a realistic budget
   c. coordination of financial/legal agencies (Social Security, attorneys, probate, deceased's employer, insurance company)
   d. survivor validation (verbally or nonverbally) that the anxiety associated with legal/financial activities and decision-making is controlled.

NURSING INTERVENTIONS

1. Assess
   a. each survivor's stage of grieving
   b. each survivor's behavioral and physical responses to the loss
   c. nature of the loss to each survivor
   d. each survivor's previous pattern of coping with loss
   e. reaction of significant others to each survivor's response to loss
   f. each survivor's psychological status (guilt, anger, depression, loneliness, suicidal ideation, conversational themes, thought context)
   g. degree of each survivor's participation in/accomplishment of the activities of life
   h. extent and quality of each survivor's support system
   i. each survivor's degree of preparation for the loss (e.g., sudden death versus terminal illness)
   j. which survivors desire bereavement intervention
   k. each survivor's risk for complicated grieving (poor relationship with the deceased, social isolation/poor social network, history of multiple losses, history of maladaptive coping strategies, concurrent life crises, traumatic death experience)
   l. family unit's risk for complicated grieving (children/adolescents in immediate family, handicapped/sick/elderly family members, loss of financial provision, feared/actual loss of home, family/marital discord, communication difficulties, inflexible family function).
2. Provide instruction to the survivors about
   a. problem-solving skills
   b. normal process of grieving
   c. signs of complicated grieving (hallucinations, delusions, social withdrawal, prolonged denial, regression, excessive guilt, excessive idealization of deceased, prolonged anxiety, prolonged depression, delayed grief reaction)
   d. stress management/relaxation techniques.
3. Create situations that encourage the survivors to express (verbally and nonverbally) their thoughts and feelings.
4. Coordinate referrals to bereavement groups, social service personnel, pastoral care advisors and other appropriate community agencies.
5. Consult with the attending physician about a referral for psychiatric therapy, if complicated grieving is problematic.
6. Support
   a. realistic goal setting for the future
   b. contact with attorneys, insurance companies, financial institutions, deceased's employer, as needed
   c. reminiscing
   d. expression of angry/ambivalent feelings about the deceased

    e. strengths of each survivor
    f. survivor's cultural, religious and social customs of grieving.
7. Discourage
    a. use of medications as a primary method of coping with grief
    b. use of hospitalization or nonstop activity as a means of coping with grief
    c. immediate decisions regarding assets (home, stocks, bonds).

THERAPEUTIC ACHIEVEMENT

- The survivor emotionally withdraws from the deceased so that his or her emotional energies are free for investment in present and future activities.

UNIT 4

Depression Care Plan

CROSS REFERENCES

Alcohol Abuse Care Plan

Spiritual Distress Care Plan

Telephone Contact with Patient/Family
Procedure

Mental Health Assessment/Intervention Guide

Suicidal Patient: Indications for Requesting
Hospitalization

NURSING DIAGNOSES

1. Sleep pattern disturbance related to
   a. guilt/worry
   b. wish to escape
   c. medication
   d. other.
2. Self-care deficit (feeding, bathing/hygiene, dressing/grooming, toileting) related to
   a. psychological immobility
   b. feelings of worthlessness
   c. other.
3. Alteration in nutrition (less/more than body requirements) related to
   a. agitation
   b. feelings of worthlessness
   c. psychological immobility
   d. medication side effect
   e. other.
4. Potential for injury related to
   a. feelings of worthlessness/guilt
   b. medications
   c. suicidal ideation
   d. psychological immobility
   e. inability to protect self/remove self from danger
   f. other.
5. Alteration in bowel elimination (constipation/diarrhea) related to
   a. medication
   b. inadequate fluid intake
   c. other.
6. Ineffective individual coping related to
   a. situational crisis of physical illness/disability
   b. psychological immobility
   c. poor nutritional status
   d. inadequate support system
   e. disordered thoughts
   f. other.
7. Noncompliance related to
   a. impaired insight
   b. negative expectations of self/future

    c. lack of environmental controls

    d. other.

8. Impaired physical mobility related to psychological withdrawal.

9. Impaired home maintenance management related to

    a. psychological immobility

    b. inadequate finances

    c. lack of support system

    d. other.

10. Potential for self-directed violence related to

    a. anger/hostility

    b. panic state

    c. delusions

    d. toxic reaction to medication

    e. suicidal ideation

    f. other.

11. Social isolation related to

    a. fear of intensity of feelings

    b. poor personal hygiene

    c. feelings of worthlessness

    d. wish to escape

    e. other.

12. Alteration in thought processes related to

    a. pathophysiological change

    b. substance abuse

    c. psychological conflict

    d. medication

    e. perceived/actual loss

    f. traumatic life event

    g. other.

13. Knowledge deficit (medications, reality orientation techniques, limit setting, safety, recognizing suicidal risk/environmental hazards) related to

    a. cognitive/perceptual impairment

    b. unfamiliarity with information resources

    c. lack of/inadequate recall

    d. other.

UNIT 4

PROCESS INDICATORS

1. The patient's physical health is maintained.

Indicators

    a. personal hygiene is adequate

    b. weight is stabilized

    c. bowel elimination pattern is regular

    d. patient/family validates a balance among the patient's rest, exercise and nutrition

    e. no engagement in self-destructive behaviors

    f. patient/family recalls the purpose, side-effects, precautions and administration of prescribed medications.

2. The patient's psychosocial integrity is supported.

Indicators

    a. verbalizes positive statements about self and future

    b. expresses satisfaction with his or her life experiences

    c. expresses anger/hostility in an outwardly appropriate manner
    d. maintains a satisfactory level of social/community/occupational interaction
    e. spontaneously shares his or her thoughts and feelings
    f. patient/family participation in self-help groups/mental health counselling
    g. patient/family feedback reflects an accurate understanding of the relationship between situational crises and depressive symptomatology.

NURSING INTERVENTIONS

1. Assess the patient
   a. life-threatening/self-destructive behaviors and suicidal ideation
   b. suicidal risk
   c. level of personal hygiene/grooming
   d. pattern of bowel elimination
   e. patterns of food/fluid intake
   f. recent weight changes
   g. patterns of rest and activity
   h. presence/degree of regressive behaviors
   i. psychomotor activity level
   j. pattern of medication use
   k. presence/degree of medication side effects
   l. signs/symptoms of ensuing physical disorders
   m. extent of withdrawal from family, friends, activities of life
   n. sensorium/orientation to time, place, person, event.
2. Assess
   a. interactions between patient and family members
   b. environmental factors/situations that facilitate patient's self-destructive behaviors
   c. patient's/family's understanding of depression
   d. availability/reliability of support systems.
3. Provide information to the patient/family about
   a. importance of long-term therapy
   b. relationship between situational crisis and depressive symptomatology
   c. importance of early recognition of depressive symptomatology (minimizes the severity and duration of an acute episode)
   d. symptoms of depression (apathy, feelings of worthlessness/hopelessness, change in sleep/eating habits/patterns, avoidance of simple problems, reductions in activity or ceaseless activity, irritability, recurrent thoughts of/focus on suicide/death, tearfulness, sex drive disturbances, weight loss/gain)
   e. stress management/relaxation techniques
   f. methods to induce/promote sleep (decrease environmental stimuli, do not sleep for long hours during the day, limit caffeine intake)
   g. personal hygiene/grooming
   h. the importance of adhering to medication administration schedules
   i. medications (purpose, side effects, administration)
   j. need to avoid tyramine or dopa-containing foods (bananas, avocados, cheese, wine, yeast, beer, yogurt, pickled herring) when the patient is receiving monoamine oxidase inhibitors
   k. how to record intake and output
   l. methods to promote bowel regularity/avoid constipation

m. setting graded, realistic goals
n. importance of socialization for the patient
o. value of exercise/physical activity.
4. Teach the family
a. reality orientation techniques
b. importance of providing a safe environment for the patient
c. how to modify environmental factors that facilitate successful self-destructive behaviors
d. importance of spending time with the patient
e. how to set realistic limits on the patient's behavior
f. how to avoid arguments/moral judgments regarding what the patient should/should not do
g. how to refocus the patient when he or she begins ruminating
h. how to use firm guidance when the patient hesitates to do things for himself or herself
i. psychodynamics and prognosis of depression
j. importance of consistently providing positive feedback for the patient's successes
k. how to role play/rehearse activities of life situations with the patient to give him or her practice with self-assertive behavior, decision-making and independence.
5. Request/obtain orders, as necessary, for medication, blood levels, hospitalization and so forth from the attending physician.
6. Refer to and coordinate interventions with
a. social worker
b. occupational therapist
c. physical therapist
d. mental health counsellor/psychiatric liaison nurse
e. dietician.
7. Provide opportunities that facilitate the patient's independent action and/or decision-making.
8. Create situations that encourage the patient/family to express their thoughts and feelings.
9. Provide progress reports and a discharge summary to the attending physician.

**UNIT
4**

THERAPEUTIC ACHIEVEMENT

- The patient participates appropriately, constructively and meaningfully in the activities of life.

RELATED PATIENT INSTRUCTIONS

A Daily Food Guide—Four Basic Food Groups
Medication Compliance
When to Call for Help

Schizophrenia Care Plan

CROSS REFERENCES

Alcohol Abuse Care Plan

Constipation Care Plan

Domestic Violence Assessment/Intervention Procedure

Telephone Contact with Patient/Family Procedure

Medication Compliance/Management Guidelines

Mental Health Assessment/Intervention Guide

NURSING DIAGNOSES

1. Alteration in health maintenance related to
   a. inability/difficulty initiating purposeful activity
   b. retarded/hyperactive psychomotor activity
   c. disordered thought processes
   d. other.
2. Alteration in bowel elimination (constipation) related to
   a. inadequate dietary intake
   b. medications
   c. other.
3. Alteration in nutrition (less than body requirements) related to
   a. retarded/hyperactive psychomotor activity
   b. suspiciousness
   c. reliance on a junk food diet
   d. medications
   e. other.
4. Alteration in nutrition (more than body requirements) related to retarded/hyperactive psychomotor activity.
5. Sleep pattern disturbance related to
   a. medications
   b. psychomotor agitation/retardation
   c. misperception/misinterpretation of environment
   d. hallucinations/delusions
   e. other.
6. Self-care deficit (feeding, bathing, hygiene, dressing, grooming, toileting) related to
   a. disordered thought processes
   b. misinterpretation/misperception of environment
   c. other.
7. Impaired home maintenance management related to
   a. insufficient finances
   b. disordered thought processes
   c. unfamiliarity with neighborhood resources
   d. inadequate or lack of support systems
   e. other.
8. Noncompliance in medication regimen related to
   a. suspiciousness
   b. limited insight about disease process
   c. unpleasant side effects
   d. other.

9. Social isolation related to unusual/unacceptable social behavior.
10. Potential for violence (self-directed/directed at others) related to
    a. severe anxiety/panic state
    b. toxic reaction to medication
    c. misperception/misinterpretation of environment or other's behaviors or intentions
    d. inadequate/inappropriate response to patient's threatening behaviors
    e. other.
11. Knowledge deficit (schizophrenia, medications, community resources, safety hazards, personal hygiene, therapeutic communication) related to
    a. sociocultural differences
    b. information misinterpretation
    c. cognitive limitation/impairment
    d. lack of motivation for learning
    e. unfamiliarity with information resources
    f. other.
12. Ineffective family coping related to
    a. patient's unpredictable behavior
    b. chaotic household
    c. financial stress
    d. ambivalent family relationships
    e. familial fear of the patient
    f. other.

UNIT 4

PROCESS INDICATORS

1. The patient's physical health is maintained.
Indicators
    a. bowel/bladder patterns are regular and continent
    b. personal hygiene is adequate
    c. patient/family validates a balance in regard to the patient's rest, exercise and nutrition
    d. home environment is rearranged to eliminate known safety hazards
    e. patient/family validates that the patient is not using illicit drugs/alcohol
    f. patient/family validates adherence to the prescribed medical regimen
    g. patient/family recalls purpose, side effects and precautions for prescribed medications.
2. The patient participates in the activities of life to the extent of his or her capabilities.
Indicators
    a. patient completes simple tasks with no or a minimum of guidance/supervision
    b. patient is oriented to time, place, person, and event
    c. patient identifies tasks at which he or she is successful
    d. family identifies parameters indicating the patient's need for increased guidance/supervision/assistance.
3. The patient's psychosocial health is maintained.
Indicators
    a. demonstrates control over his or her emotional behavior
    b. initiates interactions with others
    c. tolerates physical closeness to others for sustained periods of time
    d. expresses his or her feelings in a socially acceptable manner
    e. states a plan for coping with hallucinations

     f. communicates effectively/appropriately with others

     g. attends/participates in group/individual mental health counselling sessions

     h. maintains his or her occupational responsibilities

     i. appropriately uses community resources.

4. The family's psychosocial equilibrium is maintained.

Indicators

     a. recalls appropriate response to the patient's disturbing behaviors

     b. feedback reflects that members are emotionally supportive of each other

     c. feedback reflects accurate knowledge about schizophrenia

     d. identifies the signs/symptoms of schizophrenic decompensation

     e. appropriately uses community resources

     f. each member's involvement in self-help groups/professional counselling.

NURSING INTERVENTIONS

1. Assess the patient for
   a. nutritional/fluid intake status/habits
   b. bowel/bladder elimination pattern
   c. presence of side effects from prescribed medications
   d. symptoms of ensuing physical disorders
   e. current/potential level of adaptive functioning
   f. psychological status (anger, depression, anxiety)
   g. response to physical touch
   h. sensorium/orientation to time, place, person and event
   i. cognitive/intellectual abilities
   j. physical ability for self-care activities
   k. ability to control behavioral symptoms
   l. what meaning the patient attaches to his or her behavior
   m. extent of socialization/social isolation
   n. motivation/readiness to learn
   o. presence/degree of alcohol/illicit drug use.

2. Assess the patient for signs/symptoms of schizophrenic deterioration
   a. overextension (feeling overwhelmed, increasing anxiety/irritability, poor concentration ability, pressured speech, altered sleep patterns)
   b. restricted consciousness (apathy, withdrawal, decreased energy/activity, regression, flat/blunted affect, disheveled appearance, helplessness/extreme dependency)
   c. psychotic disorganization (loss of identity, magical thinking, looseness of associations, depersonalization, cryptic language, impulsive/uninhibited behavior)
   d. delusions/hallucinations.

3. Assess
   a. availability/reliability of support systems
   b. environmental hazards to patient/others
   c. interactions among the patient and family members
   d. factors in the home environment that might impede the patient's participation in activities of life/daily care
   e. family's understanding of schizophrenia
   f. what meaning the patient/family attaches to schizophrenia
   g. patient's age in relation to the primary care giver's age (the older the primary care giver, the greater the negative impact on the primary care giver's perception of his or her quality of life with the schizophrenic)
   h. each family member for signs of psychological/physical stress.

4. Differentiate between the symptoms related to physical deterioration and the behavioral symptoms related to schizophrenia.
5. Provide instruction to the patient/family/home health aide about
   a. psychopathology and symptomatology of schizophrenia
   b. how to structure and organize the patient's day-to-day activities
   c. making the home environment safe
   d. stress management/relaxation techniques
   e. importance of balancing rest, exercise and nutrition
   f. personal hygiene/grooming techniques
   g. medications (purpose, side effects, precautions, administration, interactions)
   h. signs/symptoms of constipation
   i. personal hygiene/grooming techniques.
6. Provide instruction to the family/home health aide about
   a. importance of supervision that is vigilant but does not suffocate the patient's self-care
   b. reality orientation techniques
   c. recognizing signs of impending assault/violent behavior (sarcasm, obscenities, threats, references to previous violent behavior, angry face, clenched fist, pacing, rigid posture, impaired sense of orientation, inappropriate response to environmental stimuli)
   d. importance of explaining change in routine to the patient
   e. recognizing the signs/symptoms of schizophrenic decompensation
   f. importance of not making demands the patient can't meet
   g. differentiating between demanding a response from the patient and consistently trying to help the patient formulate a response or drawing the patient into a response
   h. setting limits on the patient's behavior
   i. need to make only promises/commitments to the patient that can be met realistically
   j. value of their physical presence when the patient is frightened
   k. therapeutic communication techniques (speak in simple declarative statements; when necessary, repeat using same words or other more simple words; do not argue with patient; do not give support to misperceptions/delusions; avoid ideological/theoretical discussions with the patient; avoid use of long sentences; focus on concrete and current issues)
   l. importance of keeping emergency numbers next to the telephone (crisis intervention unit, rescue squad, police, physician, nurse).
7. Refer to and coordinate interventions with
   a. social worker
   b. occupational therapist
   c. vocational counsellor/rehabilitation service
   d. dietician
   e. mental health clinic/therapist
   f. crisis intervention service
   g. recreational/social activities (church, service clubs, senior citizen groups)
   h. shelter for the homeless
   i. food stamp services
   j. respite volunteer
   k. medication clinic
   l. self-help groups
   m. Alcoholic/Narcotics Anonymous.

UNIT 4

8. Monitor the patient's compliance with the prescribed medical regimen.
9. Assist the patient/family to organize daily patterns of living.
10. Provide opportunities that facilitate the patient's independent action and/or decision-making.
11. Create opportunities that encourage family members to express
    a. their fears and concerns
    b. their uncertainty about the future.
12. Provide progress reports and a discharge summary to the primary physician.

THERAPEUTIC ACHIEVEMENT

- The patient accomplishes self-care activities independently or with limited assistance or guidance.
- The family adapts to the life style changes induced as a result of living with a schizophrenic.
- The family unit is preserved.

RELATED PATIENT INSTRUCTIONS

A Daily Food Guide—Four Basic Food Groups
Medication Compliance
Reality Orientation
When to Call for Help

Sudden Infant Death Syndrome (SIDS) Care Plan

CROSS REFERENCES

Bereavement Care Plan
Depression Care Plan
Spiritual Distress Care Plan

Mental Health Assessment/Intervention Guide

UNIT
4

NURSING DIAGNOSIS

1. Anxiety/fear related to the belief that SIDS is a contagious/inherited disorder.
2. Potential/actual alteration in parenting related to
   a. desire for immediate replacement of the deceased child
   b. interruption in bonding process
   c. lack of support between and from significant others
   d. excessive protectiveness toward any surviving siblings
   e. other.
3. Sleep pattern disturbance related to
   a. guilt
   b. depression
   c. fear/anxiety
   d. other.
4. Knowledge deficit (pathophysiology of SIDS, purpose of autopsy, grief reactions, community resources) related to
   a. information misinterpretation
   b. unfamiliarity with information resources
   c. lack of readiness to learn
   d. cognitive limitation
   e. other.
5. Alteration in family process related to
   a. guilt
   b. anxiety
   c. hostility
   d. family disorganization
   e. exhausted interdependent supportive capacity
   f. difficulty in expressing and/or listening to thoughts/feelings of grief
   g. other.
6. Ineffective family coping (compromised/disabled) related to
   a. highly ambivalent family relationships
   b. inadequate/incorrect understanding about SIDS
   c. rumors/implied accusations of others
   d. other.

PROCESS INDICATORS

1. The family's biopsychosocial integrity is maintained.
Indicators
   a. family exhibits a reduction in anxiety-/guilt-induced thoughts, feelings and behaviors

b. each family member spontaneously shares his or her thoughts/feelings about the infant's death
c. familial feedback reflects that members are emotionally supportive of each other
d. familial feedback reflects accurate knowledge about SIDS
e. each family member's involvement with self-help groups/professional counselling
f. family members identify no sleep pattern disturbance or a return to their previous sleep patterns
g. family maintains its social/occupational responsibilities
h. parents verbalize their recognition that subsequent offspring are not substitutes for the deceased infant
i. parental feedback reflects an accurate understanding of the surviving sibling's age-appropriate reactions to the infant's death
j. parental feedback reflects an accurate understanding about the need for and purpose of autopsy.

NURSING INTERVENTIONS

1. Assess
   a. what each family member has been told about the infant's death
   b. what each family member thinks happened
   c. how each family member is responding to the death (father may have changed by increasing his working hours; mother may still be able to feel the infant and may ache to hold the infant in her arms; sibling reactions are dependent upon their stages of development)
   d. adequacy/appropriateness of the family's coping mechanisms
   e. presence/degree of guilt felt by each family member
   f. verbal/nonverbal interactions among family members
   g. changes in the family's daily pattern of living
   h. each family member's ability/inability to complete/participate in activities of daily life
   i. family's capacity to learn.
2. Provide instruction to the family about
   a. SIDS (it is not contagious/hereditary; the infant's death could not have been foreseen/prevented; the infant did not suffer)
   b. purpose/necessity of autopsy (to make a definitive identification of SIDS to rule out any other underlying disorder/pathology)
   c. being alert to behavioral changes/physical complaints by surviving siblings
   d. possible misinterpretation of the infant's death by surviving siblings
   e. importance of mental health support for surviving siblings/parents and particularly the person who found the deceased infant
   f. normal grief reactions
   g. value of maintaining/encouraging open discussion/communication about the infant's death.
3. Arrange a discussion about the autopsy results for the parents with the physician, pathologist, or medical examiner.
4. Refer to/coordinate interventions with
   a. social worker
   b. pastoral care worker
   c. mental health counsellor.
5. Refer to the local chapter of the National Foundation of Sudden Infant Death.

6. Create situations that encourage the survivors to express their thoughts and feelings.
7. Create situations that encourage the parents to express their thoughts and feelings about subsequent pregnancies.
8. Coordinate, with the parents and attending physician, a plan for notification of the nurse regarding subsequent pregnancies to facilitate counselling the SIDS-at risk follow-up in the prenatal period.
9. Consult with the attending physician about a referral for psychiatric therapy, if grieving is complicated/problematic.
10. Send progress notes and a discharge summary to the attending physician.

THERAPEUTIC ACHIEVEMENT

- The family adapts to the death of the patient.
- The family unit is preserved.

Spiritual Distress Care Plan

CROSS REFERENCES

Telephone Contact with Patient/Family
Procedure

Mental Health Assessment/Intervention Guide
Suicidal Patient: Indications for Requesting
Hospitalization

NURSING DIAGNOSES

1. Spiritual distress related to
   a. challenged belief/value system
   b. stressors associated with everyday life
   c. ambivalent feelings about death
   d. lost belief in diety/religion
   e. moral ethical implications of treatment
   f. intense suffering/pain
   g. inability to engage in usual religious activities
   h. fear of imposing on others with requests for spiritual comfort
   i. embarrassment about religious beliefs/activities
   j. other.

PROCESS INDICATORS

1. The patient demonstrates an absence/reduction of stress-related thoughts/feelings/behaviors.

Indicators
   a. undisturbed sleep
   b. no somatic complaints
   c. demonstration of positive self-esteem
   d. maintenance of an optimistic/happy attitude
   e. initiates interpersonal communication/relationships.
2. The patient demonstrates contentment with his or her personal interpretation of the meaning of life.

Indicators
   a. verbalization of enjoyment of the activities of everyday life
   b. verbalization that he or she accepts his or her past
   c. expression of a sense of achievement in regard to his or her personal goals
   d. development of a constructive philosophy about the meaning of suffering
   e. formulation of realistic hopes/dreams.
3. The patient sustains integration of his or her religious impulse into his or her life experience.

Indicators
   a. participation in usual religious activities
   b. requesting/seeking spiritual guidance
   c. expressing confidence in and adherence to his or her medical regimen.

NURSING INTERVENTIONS

1. Assess
   a. how the patient's religious beliefs affect his or her needs for love, belonging, dependence, purpose and achievement
   b. patient's physical/sensory strengths/deficits (pertains to enjoyment of sacred music, prayers, readings and ceremonies)
   c. aspects of care/treatment that may be contrary to the patient's spiritual beliefs
   d. whether or not the patient regards religion as a supportive resource.
2. Teach the patient to recognize his or her idiosyncratic signs of spiritual distress.
3. Create opportunities that facilitate
   a. patient expression about spiritual issues
   b. patient and family interactions about spiritual issues
   c. patient interaction with others who have similar religious beliefs/affiliations.
4. Initiate and maintain contact with the patient's spiritual advisor as necessary and appropriate.
5. Coordinate the patient, family, spiritual advisor, attending physician and others (e.g., dietician) in order to integrate any spiritual restrictions into the medical regimen.

UNIT 4

THERAPEUTIC ACHIEVEMENT

- The patient affirms life in a relationship with God, self, community and environment that nurtures and celebrates wholeness.

Procedures

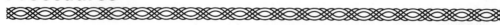

Domestic Violence
Assessment/Intervention
Procedure

PURPOSE

- To meet the biopsychosocial needs of the patient who is a victim of domestic violence.
- To help ensure the safety of the patient and others in the home who are vulnerable.

EQUIPMENT

- None

Special Note. The nurse is strongly encouraged to become familiar with relevant state legislation.

Steps

1. Assess the patient's status
   a. malnourishment/wasting of sub-cutaneous tissue
   b. significant weight loss
   c. dehydration
   d. frequent urinary tract infections
   e. frequent occurrences of fecal impaction
   f. poor oral/personal hygiene
   g. untreated old injuries
   h. multiple injuries (bruises, bites, abrasions, lacerations, burns) in various stages of healing

   i. spotty alopecia
   j. fractures

   k. whiplash-type injury
   l. restraint marks on wrists and/or ankles.
2. Assess the condition and type of the patient's clothing and bed linen and its suitability for existing weather conditions.

Key Points

1 a, b, c, d, e, f, g. These are suggestive of neglect.

h. Common sites of injury in domestic violence are head, face, chest, breasts, abdomen and genitalia.
i. This results from hair pulling.
j. Fractures are especially suspect in nonambulatory patients.
k. This results from severe shaking.

3. Assess the patient's psychosocial status
   a. depression
   b. previous suicidal gestures/attempts
   c. passivity/dependence
   d. infantile behavior
   e. extreme withdrawal or aggression
   f. wariness of contact with others
   g. expression of ambivalent feelings about family.
4. Assess the patient's care givers
   a. ill prepared to provide care to the patient
   b. unrealistic expectations of the patient
   c. increased physical workload
   d. unrelieved responsibility for the patient
   e. resentment toward the patient
   f. financial stress
   g. drug or alcohol abuse/dependency
   h. frustration
   i. low self-esteem
   j. ineffective communication skills
   k. sleeplessness
   l. marital difficulties
   m. intrafamily conflict
   n. lack of external support systems
   o. social isolation.
5. Suspect domestic violence when
   a. patient claims to be physically abused
   b. extent/type of biopsychosocial finding is inconsistent with explanation patient/family gives
   c. patient/family is hesitant/embarrassed/evasive about circumstances leading to/surrounding the biopsychosocial finding
   d. conflicting histories about the biopsychosocial findings are given
   e. patient has a history of frequent emergency room visits
   f. patient has a history of being accident prone
   g. patient/family has a history of domestic violence
   h. family member does not allow private intervention with the patient.

3. The behavior of a patient who is the victim of domestic violence reflects how the patient is coping with a home that is unsafe and unpredictable.

4. Perpetrators of domestic violence are most often family members and close friends or neighbors.

UNIT 4

6. Ask the patient if he or she is being hit, beaten or hurt.

6. The patient is likely to deny domestic violence, if the alleged abuser is present, if privacy is not afforded or if confidentiality is not assured.

Special Note. Most victims of domestic violence respond honestly to a straightforward non-judgmental approach and gentle persistent open-ended questioning. If the patient steadfastly denies being a victim of domestic violence do not pressure him or her to accept help, as forced intervention may put the patient in greater danger. Inform the patient that help is available if needed in the future and give the patient written material about resources. This situation does not, however, relieve the nurse's state-legislated responsibility of mandatory reporting to the appropriate agencies.

7. Assess the present degree of danger to the patient/others who are vulnerable in the home
   a. report of a weapon in the home
   b. report of past use of the weapon or a life-threatening attack
   c. patient statement of fear for his or her life
   d. threats to the patient's life by the alleged abuser
   e. alleged abuser's aggressive behavior toward others.
8. Notify the attending physician of the biopsychosocial findings and, if necessary, coordinate with the physician the patient's transfer/admission to the hospital.
9. Confer and coordinate interventions (including state-legislated mandatory reporting of suspected/actual abuse) with a social worker.

10. Notify the police per agency policy.

7. The possibility of future harm from domestic violence should not be overlooked/minimized.

9. Resources available to victims of domestic violence may include shelters, specialized counselling, legal aid/advocacy and a 24-hour telephone hotline.

DOCUMENTATION

1. Date and time of home visit.
2. Name and relationship of any person with the patient.
3. Biopsychosocial findings of the assessment (be as detailed as possible regarding site, pattern and description; body maps can be useful; avoid subjective interpretation of the data).
4. Discrepancies, inconsistencies or conflicts in the biopsychosocial findings and histories/explanations given by patient/family/caregiver.
5. Statements the patient makes about being a victim of domestic violence (preface statement with "patient states" or "patient alleges"; confine statement to who did what to

the patient and how it was done; do not include circumstances that led up to the domestic violence).

6. Statements the patient makes about weapons/objects used to cause any injuries (preface statements with "patient states" or "patient alleges").

7. If the patient denies being a victim of abuse (but the explanation regarding biopsychosocial findings is inappropriate) include an assessment remark that the findings/injuries are suggestive of battering/abuse/neglect. Do not make a definitive statement that battering, neglect or abuse has occurred.

8. Date, time and content of consultation with the attending physician.

9. Date, time and content of consultation with the social worker.

10. Dates and times of fulfillment of state-legislated notification of protective agencies (include names and titles of persons spoken to).

11. Resource information/materials given to the patient.

12. Date and time of police notification (if applicable).

UNIT 4

Resources

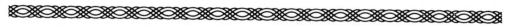

Mental Health Assessment/
Intervention Guide

Has the patient's behavior changed?
↓
YES
↓
Is the behavior change a result of a physiological alteration?

YES ←   → NO

Consult/collaborate with the attending physician regarding further treatment.

Is the patient a danger to himself or herself or others?
↓
NO
↓
Is the patient in need of further treatment?

YES ←

1. Obtain an order for hospitalization from the attending physician.

2. Notify the rescue squad/police department regarding transportation of the patient from home to hospital.

YES   NO
↓

Consult/collaborate with the attending physician regarding
  1. voluntary admission
  2. medication adjustment
  3. referral to therapist clinic/self-help group.

Mental Illness Warning
Signs

1. Marked personality change over time.
2. Confused thinking; strange or grandiose ideas.
3. Prolonged severe depression, apathy, or extreme highs and lows.
4. Excessive anxieties, fears, or suspiciousness; blaming others.
5. Withdrawal from society, friendlessness; abnormal self-centeredness.
6. Denial of obvious problems; strong resistance to help.
7. Thinking or talking about suicide.
8. Numerous, unexplained physical ailments; marked changes in sleeping or eating patterns.

9. Anger or hostility out of proportion to the situation.

10. Delusions, hallucinations, hearing of voices.

11. Abuse of alcohol or drugs.

12. Growing inability to cope with problems and daily activities such as school, job or personal needs.

Suicidal Patient: Indications for Requesting Hospitalization

1. The patient refuses to comply with the plan of treatment.
2. The patient is unable to control his or her self-destructive impulses.
3. The patient refuses to answer questions about his or her self-destructive intentions.
4. The patient lives alone or in a chaotic environment.
5. The patient falls into a high-risk category
   a. previous suicidal attempt
   b. family history of suicide
   c. social isolation/loneliness
   d. recent loss of a significant other
   e. history of impulsive behavior
   f. alcoholism/drug abuse
   g. expression of desire for death
   h. older, single male
   i. severe insomnia
   j. command hallucinations
   k. family in turmoil.

UNIT 4

Bibliography

Baier, M. Case Management with the Chronically Mentally Ill. Journal of Psychosocial Nursing and Mental Health Services, 25(6):1987, pp. 17–20.

Blumenthal, J. and McKee, D. (ed.). Applications in Behavioral Medicine and Health Psychology: A Clinician's Source Book. Sarasota, Florida: Professional Resource Exchange, Inc., 1987.

Borders, C. Alcoholism Rx: How You Can Help. Outpatient Detoxification. Patient Care, 21(1):1987, pp. 85–87.

Borders, C. Identifying and Motivating the Alcoholic. Patient Care, 20(20):1986, pp. 59–61.

Brunger, J. The Young Chronic Client in Mental Health Today. Nursing Clinics of North America, 21(3):1986, pp. 451–460.

Byrne, M. Sr. A Zest for Life. Journal of Gerontological Nursing 11(4):1985, pp. 30–33.

Crosby, R. Community Care of the Chronically Mentally Ill. Journal of Psychosocial Nursing, 25(1):1987, pp. 33–37.

Crovella, A. When Your Patient's an Alcoholic. RN, 47:February 1984, pp. 50–51.

Davidzar, R. and McBride A. Teaching the Client with Schizophrenia about Medication. Patient Education and Counselling, 7:1985, pp. 137–145.

Davis, L. and Brody, E. Rape and Older Women: A Guide to Prevention and Protection. Rockville, Maryland: National Institute of Mental Health, DHEW Pub. No. ADM. 1979.

D'Epiro, P. When Sudden Infant Death Strikes. Patient Care, 18(5):March 15, 1984, pp. 18–20, 22–25, 29, 32, 35, 40–41.

Eells, M. Interventions with Alcoholics and Their Families. Nursing Clinics of North America, 21(3):1986, pp. 493–504.

Field, K. Alcoholism: Helping the Patient Off the Not-So-Merry-Go-Round. Nursing, 14(8):1984, pp. 79–80.

Field, W. Physical Causes of Depression. Journal of Psychosocial Nursing and Mental Health Services 23(10):1985, pp. 7–11.

Fisk, N. Alcoholism: Ineffective Family Coping. American Journal of Nursing, 86(5):1986, pp. 586–587.

Greany, G. Is She a Battered Woman. American Journal of Nursing, 86(6):1984, pp. 725–727.

Grimm, P. Psychotropic Medications: Nursing Implications. Nursing Clinics of North America, 21(3):1986, pp. 397–412.

Harris, P. E. Psychiatric Assessment in the Home: Applications in Home Care. Quality Review Bulletin, 13(4):1987, pp. 131–134.

Hirst, S. and Miller, J. The Abused Elderly. Journal of Psychosocial Nursing, 24(10):1986, pp. 28–34.

Janosik, E. and Davies, J. Psychiatric Mental Health Nursing. Boston: Jones and Bartlett Publishers, Inc., 1986.

Kane, C. The Outpatient Comes Home: The Family's Response to Deinstitutionalization. Journal of Psychosocial Nursing and Mental Health Services, 22(11):1984, pp. 19–25.

Leatherland, J. Do You Know Child Abuse When You See It? RN, 49:1986 , pp. 28–30.

Leonardelli, C. The Process of Developing a Quantifiable Evaluation of Daily Living Skills in Psychiatry. Occupational Therapy in Mental Health, 6(4):1986, pp. 17–26.

Loweree, F., et al. Admitting an Intoxicated Patient. American Journal of Nursing, 84(5):1984, pp. 616–618.

Manderino, M. and Bzdek, V. Mobilizing Depressed Clients. Journal of Psychosocial Nursing, 24(5):1986, pp. 23–28.

Maurer, F. Acute Depression: Treatment and Strategies for this Affective Disorder. Nursing Clinics of North America, 21(3):September 1986, pp. 413–427.

McCandless-Gumcher, L., et al. Use of Symptoms by Schizophrenics to Monitor and Regulate Their Illness. Hospital and Community Psychiatry, 37(9):1986, pp. 929–933.

McCormick, M. Checking Patients for Alcoholism. RN, 47:February 1984, pp. 52–53.

McFarland, G. and Wasli, E. Nursing Diagnoses and Process in Psychiatric Mental Health Nursing. Philadelphia: J. B. Lippincott Co., 1986.

Merker, M. Psychiatric Emergency Evaluation. Nursing Clinics of North America, 21(3):September 1986, pp. 387–396.

Morrison, E., et al. NSGAE: Nursing Adaptation Evaluation. Journal of Psychosocial Nursing and Mental Health Services, 23(8):1985, pp. 10–13.

Norris, J., et al. Mental Health-Psychiatric Nursing. New York: John Wiley & Sons, 1987.

Pfeffer, C. The Suicidal Child. New York: The Guilford Press, 1986.

Roberts, A. (ed.). Battered Women and Their Families. New York: Springer Publishing Company, 1984.

Schultz, J. and Dark, S. Manual of Psychiatric Nursing Care Plans. Boston: Little, Brown and Company, 1986.

Seymour, R., and Dawson, N. The Schizophrenic at Home. Journal of Psychosocial Nursing and Mental Health Services, 26(1):1986, pp. 28–30.

Stark, E., et al. Wife Abuse in the Medical Setting. Rockville, Maryland: National Clearinghouse on Domestic Violence. Monograph Series, No. 7, April 1987.

Steinmetz, S. and Straus, M. Violence in the Family. New York: Harper & Row Publishers, Inc., 1974.

5

Cerebral-Sensory Alterations

**UNIT
5**

Care Plans

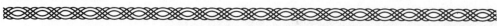

Alzheimer's (Chronic Brain Syndrome) Care Plan

CROSS REFERENCES

Bereavement Care Plan
Bladder Incontinence Care Plan
Depression Care Plan
Generic Cardiac Care Plan
Spiritual Distress Care Plan

Domestic Violence Assessment/Intervention Procedure

Home Health Aide Supervision Procedure
Home Safety Procedure

Gum Disease Warning Signs
Medication Compliance Management Guidelines
Mental Health Assessment/Intervention Guide

NURSING DIAGNOSES

1. Alteration in thought processes related to
   a. memory impairment
   b. cognitive deterioration
   c. sensory overload
   d. lack of environmental consistency
   e. severe/panic level of anxiety
   f. other.
2. Self-care deficit (feeding, hygiene, grooming, toileting) related to
   a. cognitive deterioration
   b. memory loss/impairment
   c. impaired motor coordination
   d. shortened attention span
   e. other.
3. Potential for injury related to
   a. impaired motor coordination
   b. environmental hazards
   c. lack of awareness of safety hazards
   d. wandering
   e. lack of adequate supervision
   f. other.
4. Alteration in family process related to the progressive biopsychosocial deterioration of the patient.
5. Potential for violence related to
   a. panic state
   b. paradoxical reaction to medication
   c. disorientation/confusion
   d. perceptual impairment
   e. cognitive deterioration

    f. frustration

    g. perceived threat to self

    h. other.

6. Alteration in nutrition (less than body requirements) related to

    a. increased caloric needs/hyperactivity

    b. memory impairment/forgetfulness

    c. refusal to eat

    d. denture/dental/oral problem

    e. other.

7. Alteration in bowel/bladder elimination (incontinence) related to

    a. sensorimotor impairment

    b. cognitive deficit

    c. other.

8. Social isolation related to

    a. diminished sense of self-worth

    b. alterations in mental status

    c. deterioration of physical hygiene

    d. unacceptable social behavior

    e. other.

9. Impaired verbal communication related to

    a. cerebral impairment

    b. expressive/receptive aphasia

    c. lack of stimuli

    d. other.

10. Anxiety related to

    a. memory loss

    b. inability to fulfill social/occupational obligations

    c. actual/perceived change in interaction patterns

    d. other.

**UNIT
5**

PROCESS INDICATORS

1. The patient is protected from injury.

Indicators

    a. rearrangement of the home environment to eliminate known safety hazards

    b. an emergency medical identification tag or bracelet is worn

    c. family verbalization of a method for preventing the patient from driving/having access to the car keys.

2. The patient's physical health is maintained.

Indicators

    a. patient's fluid intake is at least 1200 ml per day

    b. patient's personal hygiene is adequate

    c. patient's skin is intact

    d. patient does not experience weight loss/malnutrition

    e. patient's bowel/bladder patterns are regular and continent

    f. family recognizes the signs of physical alterations (cardiovascular, respiratory, urinary tract, dental)

    g. patient/family validates a balance among the patient's rest, exercise and nutrition.

3. The patient participates in the activities of life to the extent of his or her capabilities.
Indicators
  a. patient's disorientation does not increase during the evening
  b. patient completes simple tasks with a minimum of guidance/supervision
  c. patient is oriented to time, place, person and event
  d. patient can identify tasks at which he or she is successful
  e. family can identify parameters indicating the patient's need for increased supervision/guidance/assistance.
4. The patient's psychological health is supported.
Indicators
  a. patient demonstrates control over his or her emotional behavior given the limitations of neurological deterioration
  b. patient expresses satisfaction with life experiences
  c. patient exhibits a reduction of anxiety-induced thoughts, feelings and behaviors
  d. patient spontaneously shares thoughts and feelings about his or her condition, changing lifestyle, losses and so forth
  e. patient participates in an Alzheimer's disease support group.
5. The family's psychosocial equilibrium is maintained.
Indicators
  a. familial feedback reflects that members are emotionally supportive of each other
  b. familial feedback reflects accurate knowledge about Alzheimer's disease, particularly regarding etiology and clinical process
  c. family acclimates to the patient's progressive deterioration
  d. familial feedback indicates acceptance of the possibility/actuality of institutionalization for the patient
  e. each member is involved in a self-help group or in professional counselling
  f. family appropriately utilizes community supports, i.e., respite volunteers.

NURSING INTERVENTIONS

1. Assess
  a. patient's cognitive/intellectual abilities
  b. patient's sensorium/orientation to time, place, person and event (use a mental status questionnaire)
  c. patient's psychological status (anger, depression, anxiety)
  d. interactions among the patient and family members
  e. quality of the patient's communication efforts
  f. extent of the patient's socialization/social isolation
  g. patient's nutritional/fluid intake status/habits
  h. for symptoms of ensuing physical disorders (particularly dehydration, cardiovascular alterations, respiratory alterations)
  i. home environment for factors that might interfere with the patient's ability to participate in activities of life/daily care
  j. family's understanding of Alzheimer's disease
  k. what meaning the patient/family attaches to Alzheimer's disease
  l. each family member for signs of psychological/physical stress
  m. drug interactions specific to the patient's prescribed medications.
2. Differentiate between the symptoms of the disease and the patient's normal behavior.

3. Provide instruction to the patient during the early stages of deterioration and to the family/home health aide about
   a. importance of the patient's wearing a medical emergency tag or bracelet
   b. clinical progression of Alzheimer's disease
   c. importance of supervision that is vigilant but does not suffocate the patient's self-care
   d. reality orientation techniques
   e. recognizing signs of impending assault/violent behavior
   f. simple behavior modification techniques, i.e., positive reinforcement, ignoring undesirable behavior and so forth
   g. monitoring/controlling sensory input to prevent overload and deprivation
   h. verbal/nonverbal therapeutic communication techniques
   i. importance of balancing rest/exercise/nutrition
   j. patient's progressive inability to generalize from one activity to another
   k. breaking tasks down to simple steps
   l. need to allow the patient sufficient time to complete/participate in activities
   m. sunset effect (the patient's confusion increases with the onset of evening)
   n. medications (purposes/side effects/precautions/administration/interactions)
   o. setting a regular schedule for activities of life/daily care
   p. signs of impending physical disorders (particularly cardiovascular, respiratory, urinary tract, dental)
   q. reorganizing the home so that materials for daily care are available and accessible
   r. making the home environment safe
   s. memory aids (clocks, calendars, photographs)
   t. interventions for sleeplessness (warm baths, soft music, warm milk, small amount of wine)
   u. importance of keeping the patient from situations that may be too complex for him or her to cope with
   v. stress management/relaxation techniques
   w. recognizing abrupt changes in the patient's mental status.
4. Create opportunities that encourage the family members to express
   a. their uncertainty about the future
   b. their fears and concerns
   c. their grief
   d. their feelings about actual/potential institutionalization.
5. Coordinate, with the family, neighbors and police, a plan of action for when the patient wanders away from home.
6. Refer to the dietician and coordinate the family's utilization of the dietician's teaching to promote/maintain the patient's nutritional status.
7. Coordinate the family's use of respite volunteers.
8. Coordinate, with the family, occupational therapist and physical therapist, a schedule of activities (dancing, music, art therapy, creative writing, singing, exercising) to promote socialization.
9. Refer the patient/family to
   a. adult day care programs
   b. individual/group therapy
   c. Meals-on-Wheels
   d. Title III nutrition sites
   e. Alzheimer's Disease and Related Disorders Association.
10. Refer to the dentist, as necessary.

UNIT 5

11. Provide opportunities that facilitate the patient's independent action/decision-making.
12. Provide progress reports and a discharge summary to the primary physician.

THERAPEUTIC ACHIEVEMENT

- The patient experiences a deceleration of the degenerative symptomatology.
- The patient's self-esteem and sense of identity are maintained.
- The family unit is preserved.

RELATED PATIENT INSTRUCTIONS

A Daily Food Guide–Four Basic Food Groups
Bladder Retraining
Comfort Measures for Dehydration
Healthy Heart
Infection Control for the Home
Making the Home Environment Safe

Medication Compliance
Range of Motion Exercises
Reality Orientation
Skin Care
When to Call for Help

Cerebral Palsy Care Plan

CROSS REFERENCES

Bladder Incontinence Care Plan
Decubitus Care Plan
Seizure Disorder Care Plan

Assistive Devices Procedure

Home Safety Procedure
Range of Motion Exercises Procedure
Seizure Precaution/Management Procedure

Medication Compliance Management Guidelines

NURSING DIAGNOSES

1. Familial fear/anxiety related to
   a. perceived powerlessness
   b. responsibility of managing the patient at home
   c. threat of hospitalization
   d. other.
2. Patient fear/anxiety related to
   a. loss of control
   b. communication deficits
   c. visual deficits
   d. hearing deficits
   e. dependence on others for care
   f. fear of falling
   g. other.
3. Alteration in nutrition (less than body requirements) related to
   a. dysphagia
   b. athetosis
   c. weakness/fatigue
   d. impaired parent-infant interactions
   e. vomiting
   f. other.
4. Ineffective breathing pattern related to
   a. weakness/fatigue
   b. anxiety
   c. dysphagia
   d. seizures
   e. other.
5. Self-care deficit (feeding, bathing/hygiene, dressing/grooming, toileting) related to
   a. fatigue/weakness
   b. impaired motor control
   c. mental retardation
   d. other.
6. Impaired skin integrity (irritation, breakdown) related to
   a. immobility
   b. brace/splint irritation
   c. other.

7. Potential for injury (falls, infections) related to
   a. impaired skin integrity
   b. impaired motor control/ambulation
   c. seizures
   d. other.
8. Impaired physical mobility related to
   a. spasticity
   b. athetosis
   c. weakness/fatigue
   d. seizures
   e. dependence on others for care
   f. contractures
   g. other.
9. Disturbance in self-concept (body image, self-esteem, sexual identity, role performance, personal identity) related to
   a. loss of body control
   b. dependence on others for care
   c. athetosis
   d. spasticity
   e. drooling
   f. impaired communication abilities
   g. strabismus
   h. other.
10. Potential/actual alteration in parenting related to
    a. lack of support between/from significant others
    b. unmet social needs of parents
    c. no previous model/experience of patient-child interactions
    d. resentment over forced reallocation of family resources/priorities
    e. financial stress
    f. unrealistic expectations of self (parenting figure)/patient/patient's siblings/partner/
       others
    g. limited cognitive ability
    h. dysfunctional grieving
    i. excessive/long-term demands in care of patient.
11. Alteration in bowel/bladder elimination (incontinence) related to poor muscle control.
12. Ineffective individual coping related to
    a. dependence on others for care
    b. multiple/long-term life style adjustments
    c. failure to achieve normal growth
    d. other.
13. Alteration in thought process related to mental retardation.
14. Knowledge deficit (pathophysiology and clinical course of cerebral palsy, therapeutic
    and rehabilitation regimen, diet plan, medications, activity plan, assistive devices, signs
    and symptoms to report, seizure care, normal growth and development) related to
    a. misinterpretation of information
    b. cognitive limitations
    c. lack of readiness to learn
    d. patient's request for no information
    e. other.
15. Alteration in family process related to
    a. situational crisis of a chronically ill family member
    b. disruption of usual pattern of family life

   c. diminished parental focus on healthy siblings
   d. other.
16. Familial grieving related to loss of their perfect/healthy child ideal.
17. Social isolation related to
   a. lack of qualified babysitters
   b. parental anxiety about leaving the patient
   c. patient anxiety about disability
   d. other.
18. Impaired home maintenance management related to
   a. lack of support (family/community/financial)
   b. ineffective individual coping
   c. ineffective family coping
   d. other.
19. Noncompliance with therapeutic regimen related to
   a. knowledge deficit
   b. lack of support (family/community/financial)
   c. difficulty integrating into life style
   d. other.

PROCESS INDICATORS

UNIT
5

1. The patient/family verbalizes an understanding of cerebral palsy and the therapeutic regimen.
Indicators
   a. describe cerebral palsy disease process, therapeutic regimen, rehabilitation plan and strategies to promote independence and to prevent complications
   b. provide a diet plan that promotes adequate nutrition, caloric intake and optimal independence in feeding and compensates for dysphagia
   c. describe action, dose, administration schedule and side effects of medications
   d. verbalize a plan for the patient to receive follow-up care
   e. describe an activity plan that provides for motor development, planned rest and diversional activities that are appropriate for growth and development
   f. demonstrate appropriate safety precautions/modifications in the home
   g. identify community resources
   h. identify signs and symptoms to report.
2. The patient's biopsychosocial integrity is maintained.
Indicators
   a. adequate intake of food/fluid
   b. optimal level of independence is achieved/maintained
   c. health maintenance needs are met (dental care, immunizations, safety)
   d. patient is stimulated/exposed to experiences that foster optimal growth and development
   e. positive/nurturing patient/family relationships (attachment, interaction) are observed
   f. skin integrity is maintained
   g. adequate mobility occurs
   h. seizures are controlled
   i. patient participates in remediation as appropriate for visual needs (corrective glasses), hearing needs, speech/language needs
   j. bowel/bladder control is achieved/maintained
   k. absence of contractures

    l. verbalizes feelings about adapting to cerebral palsy

    m. expresses satisfaction with sexual relationship, if appropriate.

3. The family's psychosocial integrity is maintained.

Indicators

    a. family demonstrates reorganization of roles to adjust to the patient's regimen

    b. family expresses a feeling that the patient's care/needs are manageable.

NURSING INTERVENTIONS

1. Assess the patient for
   a. speech/language/communication abilities/limitations
   b. visual impairments (evidenced through squinting, failure to follow moving object, bringing objects close to the face)
   c. hearing deficits
   d. level of activity/functioning
   e. difficulty in feeding, sucking, swallowing
   f. age-appropriate body weight
   g. presence of listlessness/irritability/weakness
   h. age-appropriate stage of growth and development
   i. motor involvement/type/severity
      - spastic (hypertonicity, persistent infantile reflexes, abnormal postures, unrhythmic/jerking gait or scissoring)
      - athetoxic/dyskinesia (involuntary, uncontrollable, uncoordinated movements exacerbated by emotional stress)
      - ataxia (disturbed balance and gait, nystagmus).
   j. presence of seizures
   k. mental/cognitive limitations (ability to understand disease/treatment, presence of retardation)
   l. bowel and bladder functioning/control
   m. use of assistive devices/mobility aids.
2. Assess the family's
   a. understanding of the disease process and therapeutic regimen
   b. ability to be supportive and to participate in the rehabilitation program
   c. coping with changes
   d. daily pattern of living and changes in the daily pattern
   e. interactional patterns (patient and parents)
   f. verbal/nonverbal interactions with the patient and each other
   g. capacity to learn.
3. Instruct the patient/family/home health aide about the cerebral palsy disease process and the therapeutic/rehabilitation regimen.
   a. correct use of assistive devices/mobility aids for activities of daily living
   b. patterns of growth and development
   c. presence of athetosis or spasticity may not indicate lack of intellectual capacity
   d. seizure management, if appropriate
   e. signs and symptoms to report
      - restlessness/agitation (may indicate infection)
      - appearance of seizures and/or increase in number or severity of seizures.
   f. importance of maintaining the patient's long-term health care plan including immunization schedule and routine dental care

g. maintaining skin integrity through position changes, massage, pressure relief devices and keeping skin clean using warm water (avoid cold or hot water, which increase spasms)
h. bowel/bladder training, if needed
i. breathing exercises, as needed.

4. Instruct the patient/family/home health aide about the medication plan including
    a. name, action, dosage, administration schedule and side effects of prescribed medications
    b. taking medications with foods (apple sauce, mashed potatoes) if permitted
    c. medication dosages increase as the child grows.

5. Instruct the patient/family/home health aide about an activity plan that includes the prescribed exercise/rehabilitation plan.
    a. maximizes the patient's functional abilities
    b. minimizes complications/contractures as the patient grows
    c. incorporates physical therapy into diversional/play activities to the extent possible
    d. incorporates consultation with the physical and occupational therapists, as needed
    e. allows return demonstration for
        • proper body alignment for holding/positioning
        • use of assistive devices and/or mobility aids (splints/casts/braces)
        • age-appropriate infant/child stimulation
    f. includes planned periods of rest particularly before meals and bedtime
    g. plans for frequent change of position for infants.

6. Instruct the patient/family/home health aide about a dietary plan that includes
    a. basic food groups for promotion of general nutrition and adequate caloric intake
        • allows foods that the patient prefers
        • contains foods with the proper consistency in terms of ability to remain on the eating utensil (i.e., mashed potatoes) as well as the patient's ability to swallow
        • permits finger foods for increasing independence in eating
    b. a calm environment at mealtime
        • plan for rest periods before and after
        • minimize sensory stimulation/distractions
    c. position/support for the child to promote optimal independence in eating/feeding
    d. assistive devices/utensils to encourage independent eating
    e. compensate for messy eating
        • in certain situations, it may be necessary to feed the child alone
        • protect the child with a large towel or waterproof bib
        • use newspapers around the feeding chair
    f. cutting food into small pieces
    g. when feeding the patient
        • allow adequate time (a warming tray can be used)
        • prevent hyperactive gag reflex in infants (feed slowly)
        • facilitate swallowing (place food on the back of the tongue)
        • avoid doing so if the child is fatigued
    h. consultation with the dietician, as needed
    i. consultation with the speech therapist for dysphagia assistance, if needed
    j. consultation with the occupational therapist for assistive devices for feeding.

7. Instruct the patient/family/home health aide about a plan to promote patient safety.
    a. protection against falls
        • keep bed in the low position
        • use padded side rails, helmet and other precautions if the patient experiences seizures

UNIT 5

- keep frequently used items within easy reach
- use prescribed braces/supports/shoes/mobility aids
- encourage uncluttered well-lit hallways/rooms and removal of hazards that may cause the patient to trip
- allow adequate time for ambulation/activity; avoid rushing the patient
- use of handrails/safety rails, seat belts

b. guidance in the selection of safe toys.

8. Encourage the patient/family to verbalize their feelings about the diagnoses and the adjustments that are required.
9. Encourage the patient/family to focus on the patient's strengths as a strategy to overcome limitations.
10. Assist the patient/family to establish realistic/achievable short-term and long-term goals.
11. Discuss parenting strategies and the appropriate use of discipline.
12. Assist the parents to cope with a child who is newly diagnosed and to be aware of the potential of grief response.
13. Identify community resources that can facilitate the patient's/family's adjustment to cerebral palsy.
    a. local branch or national office of Cerebral Palsy Association
    b. prevocational and vocational programs
    c. local infant stimulation program or school programs
    d. day care, particularly for periodic respite
    e. state office of handicapped children
    f. counselling/psychological therapy/self-help support groups for patient, parents and siblings
    g. financial counselling services.
14. Coordinate additional members of the health care team, such as the social worker, occupational therapist, physical therapist, speech therapist and registered dietician.
15. Provide progress reports and a discharge summary to the primary physician.

THERAPEUTIC ACHIEVEMENT

- The patient/family adapts to the life style changes induced as a result of cerebral palsy.
- The patient achieves/maintains optimal functional abilities.

RELATED PATIENT INSTRUCTIONS

Anticonvulsant Medications	Oral Suctioning
Bathing the Person in a Chair	Pediatric Diet
Guidelines for Describing Seizure Activity	Range of Motion Exercises
Making the Home Environment Safe	Seizure Precautions
Management of Seizure Activity	Skin Care

Cerebrovascular Accident (CVA) Care Plan

CROSS REFERENCES

Bladder Incontinence Care Plan
Constipation Care Plan
Depression Care Plan
Generic Cardiac Care Plan

Assistive Devices Procedure
Bladder Retraining Procedure
Decubitus Care Procedure
Fecal Disimpaction Procedure
Home Safety Procedure
Range of Motion Exercises Procedure

NURSING DIAGNOSES

1. Ineffective breathing patterns related to
   a. fear/anxiety
   b. impaired chest expansion (decreased mobility and weakened muscles of respiration)
   c. incorrect body positioning and alignment
   d. other.
2. Impaired verbal communication (expressive/receptive aphasia, dysarthria) related to
   a. cerebral ischemia
   b. loss of motor function of muscles of speech articulation
   c. altered thought processes (confusion, decreased attention span)
   d. withdrawal/psychologic impairment
   e. other.
3. Impaired physical mobility related to
   a. weakness/fatigue/unsteadiness
   b. impaired motor-sensory function
   c. fear of injury
   d. visual disturbances
   e. spatial-perceptual alterations
   f. lack of mobility aid (no cane or wheelchair)
   g. lack of motivation/desire or presence of depression
   h. other.
4. Impaired skin integrity (breakdown, irritation, injury) related to
   a. prolonged pressure on tissues due to immobility
   b. neglect of the affected side
   c. frequent contact with irritants (urinary/fecal incontinence)
   d. increased fragility of skin (edema, malnutrition, anticoagulant therapy)
   e. sensory impairment
   f. other.
5. Potential for injury (sensory-perceptual, visual, tactile, proprioceptive and kinesthetic impairments) related to
   a. dizziness/syncope
   b. seizures
   c. visual, spatial-perceptual impairments

UNIT
5

    d. spasticity/flaccidity of extremities (subluxation of shoulder)
    e. altered thought processes (disorientation/confusion, decreased attention span)
    f. impaired swallowing/gag reflexes (aspiration)
    g. immobility (skin breakdown, stasis pneumonia)
    h. gastrointestinal distress (stress ulcer, medication irritation)
    i. weakness of eyelid leading to corneal irritation/abrasion
    j. impaired ambulation (falls)
    k. decreased sensation in affected extremities (burns, abrasions)
    l. environmental hazards/lack of adequate support
    m. other.

6. Alterations in bowel elimination (constipation, incontinence) related to
    a. immobility/decreased activity levels
    b. decreased awareness of and ability to either respond to or control urge to defecate
    c. impaired ability to communicate need to defecate (dependence on others for care)
    d. inadequate dietary intake (due to dysphagia, anorexia, difficulty feeding self)
    e. noncompliance
    f. interactions/side effects of prescribed medications (laxatives, stool softeners) regimen
    g. other.

7. Alteration in comfort related to
    a. stress/anxiety
    b. immobility
    c. uncontrolled pain
    d. skin breakdown
    e. diaphoresis
    f. restlessness
    g. other.

8. Disturbance in self-concept (body image, self-esteem, role performance) related to
    a. change in body image/appearance (hemiplegia, facial droop, ptosis)
    b. feelings of rejection by significant others
    c. dependence on others for care
    d. impaired communication abilities
    e. impaired self-control (automatic speech/emotional lability)
    f. urinary/bowel incontinence
    g. role/life style changes
    h. other.

9. Sexual dysfunction related to
    a. paralysis/hemiplegia
    b. anger
    c. sensory-perceptual alterations
    d. disturbance in self-concept and a fear of rejection
    e. fear of incontinence
    f. inability to express desires or needs
    g. impotence
    h. other.

10. Anxiety related to
    a. lack of understanding of CVA and fear of its recurrence
    b. loss of control, role change and dependence on others for previously independent activities
    c. impaired mobility/fear of falling
    d. financial insecurity/cost of medical care

   e. uncertain prognosis, disease process and rehabilitation end result
   f. alterations in thought processes/inability to communicate thoughts clearly and easily
   g. hospitalization
   h. other.
11. Sleep pattern disturbance related to
   a. paralysis/immobility
   b. incontinence
   c. restlessness
   d. discomfort/inability to change positions without assistance
   e. medication side effects
   f. others.
12. Knowledge deficit (feeding techniques/assistive devices, enteral/parenteral feeding methods, plan for decreasing risk factors for recurrence of CVA, prevention of CVA complications, health care and medical plan for CVA rehabilitation, signs and symptoms to report to the nurse/physician, dysphagia assistance and communication devices) related to
   a. cognitive limitations
   b. alteration in thought processes/misinterpretation of information
   c. lack of readiness to learn
   d. other.
13. Alterations in patterns of urinary elimination (incontinence) related to
   a. intake of high fluid volume/caffeine (diuretic effect)
   b. decreased awareness of and ability to respond to/control urge to void
   c. impaired ability to communicate need to void
   d. dependence on others for assistance
   e. other.
14. Self-care deficit (feeding, bathing/hygiene, toileting, dressing) related to
   a. loss/impaired motor coordination
   b. loss of bladder/bowel control
   c. dependence on others for care
   d. alteration in thought process
   e. visual impairment
   f. apraxia
   g. aphasia
   h. neglect of the affected side
   i. emotional lability
   j. other.
15. Ineffective family coping patterns related to
   a. family disorganization and undefined future role/life style changes
   b. prolonged disability that exhausts supportive capacity of significant others
   c. inadequate financial resources
   d. impaired parenting
   e. hospitalization
   f. impaired verbal communication
   g. social isolation (patient's emotional lability/depression, feeding/toileting problems, impaired communication)
   h. impaired mobility
   i. dysfunctional grieving
   j. alterations in patient's thought process
   k. inability to predict end result of rehabilitative efforts
   l. other.

UNIT 5

16. Noncompliance with therapeutic regimen related to
    a. feelings of worthlessness/depression
    b. impaired mobility
    c. dependence on others for care
    d. cost of care
    e. alteration in thought processes (inability to understand concept of time, decreased attention span)
    f. knowledge deficit
    g. difficulty integrating treatment regimen into life style
    h. inadequate support (family/community/professional)
    i. other.
17. Impaired home maintenance management related to
    a. ineffective individual coping
    b. ineffective family coping/support
    c. motor-sensory losses
    d. demands of rehabilitation plan, dependence of patient stresses family resources (financial, emotional, physical)
    e. changes in family's roles
    f. fatigue/weakness
    g. physical layout/barriers in the home environment
    h. other.

PROCESS INDICATORS

1. The patient/family incorporates the CVA rehabilitation plan into their pattern of daily living.
Indicators
    a. describes a cardiovascular risk factor/life style modification plan that counteracts or reduces atherosclerosis and the risk of recurrent CVA
    b. maintains a satisfactory progressive reintroduction to social/community interactions
    c. adheres to a diet plan that controls dietary fat, calories, stimulants, alcohol and sodium, and accommodates the patient's ability to swallow
    d. maintains an activity plan that promotes the patient's performance of activities of daily living, transfer techniques and ambulation
    e. describes the importance of and a plan for receiving follow-up care
    f. identifies signs and symptoms of exacerbation/complications to report to the physician
    g. describes an appropriate emergency action plan
    h. identifies medications, dosages, administration schedule, side effects, drug interactions and indications for use
    i. identifies community resources that can support adaptation to biopsychosocial/sensory-motor losses
    j. maintains a safe home environment or rearranges the home environment to promote self-care while eliminating known safety hazards.
2. The patient/family demonstrates effective coping patterns.
Indicators
    a. verbalizes acknowledgement that CVA recovery requires long-term adherence to the planned rehabilitation regimen
    b. reorganizes roles and activities to incorporate elements of medication, diet, activity and health care plan compliance

c. expresses satisfactory level of sexual functioning
d. demonstrates satisfactory parenting skills
e. recognizes and uses support systems/resources to assist with adaptation to the CVA
f. communicates thoughts and feelings and effective stress management strategies
g. verbalizes decreased anxiety/fear/depression
h. provides for visual/sensory/psychomotor/cognitive impairments including use of equipment/devices.

3. The patient establishes/maintains a satisfactory level of comfort.

Indicators

a. achieves undisturbed sleep
b. describes satisfactory activity levels with the ability to perform self-care activities
c. expresses satisfaction with the quality of life
d. attains/maintains bladder and bowel control
e. attains/maintains optimal body weight
f. achieves satisfactory defecation pattern
g. expresses absence of uncontrolled pain/discomfort
h. verbalizes/demonstrates that symptoms (dizziness, visual disturbances, motor weakness, irritability and paresthesia) are decreasing in number and/or intensity
i. oriented to time/place/person/events
j. exhibits pulse and blood pressure levels within the patient's normal range.

4. The patient/family demonstrates effective two-way communication.

Indicators

a. correct responses by patient to direct questions
b. communication of abstract thoughts and dialogue
c. successful use of communication devices
d. describes the cause of aphasia or participates in an aphasia rehabilitation plan.

UNIT 5

NURSING INTERVENTIONS

1. Assess, monitor and record the baseline values and subsequent progress of the patient's
   a. motor-sensory alterations performing a complete systems review to include
      - expressive and receptive communication abilities (speech center in the brain is located on the opposite side of the patient's dominant hand; a right-handed person with right hemiplegia may have aphasia since the speech center is on his or her left side)
      - perception of pain, touch, temperature, sensation and posture
      - visual attention to affected side
      - alterations in thought processes/mental acuity/orientation
      - gross and fine motor movements
      - blood pressure levels in both arms supine, sitting and, if possible, standing
      - apical and peripheral pulses
      - lung sounds and respiratory effort.
   b. bladder and bowel control
   c. comfort level and sense of self-esteem
   d. patterns of sleep.
2. Instruct the patient/family/home health aide about a dietary plan that
   a. complies with the prescribed dietary parameters including foods that are
      - compatible with the patient's ability to chew and swallow and promote self-feeding (typically, mechanically soft foods)

- low in sugar, cholesterol, saturated fat and sodium
- low in caffeine and have diuretic effects to promote urinary control and enhanced sleep patterns
- high in fiber, bulk and potassium
- nonirritating to the gastrointestinal tract
- within the patient's cultural/religious/personal preferences.

b. includes a 3-day diet recall completed by the patient/family for calorie count if the patient's nutritional status declines, as defined by percentage weight loss (intake and output recording may also be necessary)

c. includes consultations with the physician and/or dietician, as needed, for inadequate nutritional intake and with the speech therapist for impaired swallowing (dysphagia evaluation)

d. includes the rationale, method and actual administration of enteral or parenteral nutrition, feeding tubes and pumps, as necessary

e. promotes adequate time for meals with rest periods before and after

f. provides written instructions to reinforce verbal instructions and manual demonstrations

g. incorporates strategies to help the patient relearn to swallow, such as
- testing of swallowing with nectar or firm gelatin, then with soft foods
- using a popsicle to promote sucking ability
- avoiding stringy meats, unboned fish and semi-cooked eggs
- giving of foods or fluids on the unaffected side with the patient sitting up; avoiding fluids while solid food is in the patient's mouth; beginning with soft foods
- having the patient flex his or her neck and stroke his or her throat to stimulate swallowing
- giving good oral care after meals (check mouth/gums for trapped food)
- administering medications in liquid form or finely crushed form.

3. Instruct the patient/family/home health aide about
a. cerebrovascular disease, preventing complications, and preventing recurrences
b. cardiovascular risk factor reduction
- maintaining optimal body weight
- maintaining a diet low in cholesterol and saturated fats
- establishing a regular pattern of exercise
- stopping smoking
- controlling blood pressure
- following medical treatment for underlying diseases (diabetes, hypertension).
c. medication regimen
- names, actions, dosages, administration schedule, side and adverse effects and drug interactions
- need to discuss the introduction of any new medications with the physician prior to initiation
- strategies to assist the patient who has an impaired concept of time with adhering to administration schedules.
d. signs and symptoms to report to the physician
- increased weakness or loss of sensation of extremities
- increase in or development of visual disturbances
- greater lethargy, irritability, confusion, emotional lability, vertigo
- increased difficulty in speaking or understanding communications
- more difficulty in swallowing
- suspected or actual seizures.
e. an emergency action plan and obtaining emergency medical identification.

4. Instruct the patient/family/home health aide about promoting a satisfactory defecation pattern.
   a. review signs of constipation
   b. establishing a defecation routine based on the patient's previous elimination patterns and present physical/functional abilities
   c. establishing a signal for the aphasic patient to communicate the need to defecate
   d. maintaining adequate fluid and dietary fiber intake
   e. proper use of mobility aids, such as a walker, bed side commode and toilet handrails.
5. Instruct the patient/family/home health aide about maintaining the skin's integrity.
   a. skin care procedures for urinary/fecal incontinence
   b. turning and positioning schedule as well as proper body alignment for immobilized patients
   c. elevating dependent edematous extremities
   d. utilizing pressure minimizing equipment
   e. maintaining a proper diet
   f. increasing active and/or passive exercise as tolerated.
6. Instruct the patient/family/home health aide about home safety.
   a. completing a home safety assessment with attention to safety/"grab" rails in the bathroom
   b. scheduling a home evaluation with the physical therapist/occupational therapist, as needed
   c. keeping walkways and room well lit and uncluttered
   d. using ambulation aids as needed (walker, cane, wheelchair, eye patch for diplopia)
   e. keeping certain items (telephone, bedpan/commode, personal needs) within reach
   f. planning for supervision and reorientation of the confused patient
   g. teaching thermal injury protection
      • supervision for patient while he or she is smoking, if permitted
      • using a thermometer to check bath water temperature
      • allowing hot foods to cool slightly before eating.
   h. providing safe transfer and ambulation techniques
      • using a transfer safety belt
      • advising the patient to wear shoes with low heels and nonskid soles
      • stabilizing an affected arm with a sling to increase balance when ambulating.
7. Instruct the patient/family/home health aide about a rehabilitation program that
   a. promotes independence in self-care
      • teaching to perform activities of daily living with one hand or with assistive devices
      • consulting with the physical therapist and occupational therapist about utilization of splints, overbed trapeze, 3- or 4-prong cane, wheelchair, ramps, grab rails, raised toilet seat, rocker knife, lipped plate
      • using clothes with Velcro or front fasteners
      • dressing and performing some hygiene tasks while seated
      • allowing for adequate rest periods.
   b. prevents deformities and physical deterioration
      • teaching exercises for gross and fine muscle strengthening/coordination and joint mobility
      • teaching quadriceps setting and gluteal exercises to be done at least 5 times per day
      • using active or passive assistive range of motion exercises at least 4 to 5 times each day
      • teaching the patient to use the unaffected side to exercise the affected side as soon as possible

UNIT 5

- graduating the activity plan for the affected side to incorporate motor/sensory-perceptual alterations (gross movement occurs before fine movement, strategies to overcome neglect of affected side)
- positioning in bed or chair properly to prevent contractures, relieve pressure, maintain good body alignment and promote chest expansion (for more effective breathing patterns)
- teaching coughing and deep breathing to immobile patients

c. includes adaptive strategies for sexual activity
  - adjusting to hemiparesis may require the patient to be supine or to lie on the affected side
  - discussing with the patient and partner alternative ways of expressing caring/affection

d. accomodates for impaired verbal communications
  - encouraging the patient to make lists to compensate for impaired memory
  - providing the patient with taped or written instructions
  - using communication aids such as paper and pencil, letter or picture board, "magic" erasable slate or gestures
  - encouraging the family to respond to the patient's emotional outbursts by distracting him or her by clapping hands or asking the patient to hold his or her mouth open, if crying inappropriately
  - consulting with a speech therapist.

8. Promote urinary control in the patient by
   a. exercising perineal muscles by stopping the flow of urine
   b. using disposable pads in underwear
   c. instituting a bladder training program as needed/if able
   d. limiting fluids 1 to 2 hours before bedtime (also enhances sleep patterns).

9. Encourage the patient/family to verbalize fears/anxieties
   a. consult with the social worker as needed
   b. refer to community resources, vocational rehabilitation, counselling services as needed (such as American Heart Association, self-help stroke support groups, adult day care)
   c. advise the patient/family/home health aide to use the term weak or affected not "bad" side.

10. Coordinate additional members of the health care team such as the social worker, physical therapist, speech therapist, occupational therapist, registered dietician and home health care aide.

11. Provide progress reports and a discharge summary to the primary physician.

THERAPEUTIC ACHIEVEMENT

- The patient achieves optimal biopsychosocial/sensory motor rehabilitation within the limits imposed by the CVA.
- The patient/family adapts to the life style changes induced as a result of the CVA.

RELATED PATIENT INSTRUCTIONS

A Daily Food Guide—Four Basic Food Groups	Mouth Care
Bathing the Person in Bed	Range of Motion Exercises
Bathing the Person in a Chair	Seasonings for Sodium Restricted Diets
Healthy Heart	Warning Signs of a Stroke
High Blood Pressure Medication	Ways to Save Your Energy
Making the Home Environment Safe	

Procedures

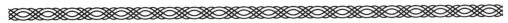

Range of Motion Exercises Procedure

PURPOSE

- To maintain function and/or to improve mobility of a joint.
- To move joints through full range of motion.

IMPORTANT POINTS

1. Types of range of motion exercises
   a. active motion performed independently by the patient
   b. passive motion performed by another person
   c. active assistive motion performed as much as possible by the patient with the help of another person
   d. active, resistive motion performed by the patient working against resistance produced by another person or by mechanical means.
2. Perform exercises in a smooth continuous motion.
3. Avoid pushing the joint past the point of resistance or pain. If the patient complains of pain during an exercise, stop immediately.
4. When muscle spasm is present, move the joint slowly to the point of resistance.
5. If the joint is painful, as in arthritis, supporting the muscular area may be more comfortable for the patient.
6. Contraindications for range of motion exercises include
   a. recent injury/trauma
   b. severe joint inflammation.

<table>
<tr><td>

Steps

1. Verify the physician's order for the type and frequency of the range of motion exercises.
2. Wash hands.
3. Explain the procedure to the patient/family.
4. Position the patient comfortably, providing for privacy as necessary.

</td><td>

Key Points

1. Review the physical therapist's assessment and plan for exercises, if available.

4. Most exercises can be performed with the patient in the supine position. The prone position is necessary for certain joint extension movements. Depending upon the patient's condition, some exercises can be performed with the patient in a sitting position.

</td></tr>
</table>

UNIT
5

Table 5–1
Range of Motion Exercises

Joint	Normal Joint Motion	Part to be Supported/Stabilized	Part to be Moved
NECK	Extension (about 55° from midline)	Head/Chin	Head
	Flexion (about 45° from midline)	Head/Chin	Head
	Lateral flexion (about 30° each way from midline)	Head	Head
	Rotation (about 70° from midline)	Head	Head
SHOULDER	Extension (about 65°)	Shoulder	Arm
	Flexion (about 180°)	Shoulder	Arm
	Abduction (about 180°)	Shoulder	Arm
	Adduction/cross (about 45°)	Shoulder	Arm
	Internal rotation (about 90°)	Shoulder	Arm
	External rotation (about 90°)	Shoulder	Arm
	Hyperextension (about 50°)	Shoulder	Arm
ELBOW	Extension (elbow is straight in normal position)	Upper arm	Forearm
	Flexion (about 160°)	Upper arm	Forearm
WRIST	Pronation (about 90°)	Elbow	Wrist
	Supination (about 90°)	Elbow	Wrist
	Extension (about 70°) from central position	Forearm	Wrist
	Flexion (palmar, about 90°) from central position	Forearm	Wrist
	Ulnar deviation (about 55°) from central position	Forearm	Wrist
	Radial deviation (about 20°)	Forearm	Wrist
FINGERS	Extension (about 12°)	Wrist	Fingers
	Flexion (about 95°)	Wrist	Fingers
	Abduction (about 12°)	Other fingers	One finger
	Adduction (about 12°)	Other fingers	One finger
THUMB	Extension (about 90°)	Fingers	Thumb
	Flexion (about 45°)	Fingers	Thumb
	Opposition (thumb moves toward little finger)	Other fingers	One finger/Thumb
	Abduction (about 90°)	Fingers	Thumb
	Adduction (thumb is straight in neutral position)	Fingers	Thumb
HIP	Extension (about 40°) in prone position	Hip	Leg
	Flexion (about 120°) from straight, extended position	Knee	Leg
	Abduction (about 65°)	Knee	Leg
	Adduction/cross (about 45°)	Leg	Knee
	Internal rotation (about 40°) from straight midline position	Leg	Hip
	External rotation (about 40°) from straight midline position	Leg	Hip
KNEE	Extension (knees straight in neutral position)		
	Flexion (about 130°) from straight extended position	Thigh	Lower leg
ANKLE	Dorsiflexion (about 10° from midline)	Heel	Foot
	Plantar flexion (about 45° from midline)	Heel	Foot
	Eversion (about 20° from midline)	Heel	Foot
	Inversion (about 30° from midline)	Heel	Foot
TOES	Extension (about 90°)	Heel	Toe
	Flexion (about 45°)	Heel	Toes
	Abduction (about 20°)	Other toes	One toe
	Adduction (about 20°)	Other toes	One toe

5. Assist/move each joint through range of motion 3 to 5 times per physician's order.

5. Always consider the normal motion of the joint as well as the bones adjacent to the joint to be moved (Table 5–1). Maintain proper body mechanics as you perform the exercises.

6. Instruct the patient/family to assist with exercises as appropriate.

6. Range of motion exercises typically should be performed at least 2 times per day depending upon the physician's order.

7. Supervise return demonstration by patient/family.

8. Instruct the patient/family concerning safety measures.

8. Safety measures include areas identified in Important Points, as well as patient positioning, body mechanics and indications for calling the nurse/physician.

DOCUMENTATION

1. Type of range of motion exercises and frequency performed at each joint.
2. Patient's tolerance of procedure.
3. Instructions to patient/family.
4. Patient's/family's understanding of/participation in exercises.
5. Consultation with physical therapist, if appropriate.
6. Condition of skin and joints as appropriate.
7. Report to the primary physician.

UNIT
5

Bibliography

Brady, P. Labeling Confusion in the Elderly. Journal of Gerontological Nursing, 13(6): 1987, pp. 29–32.

Bray, G. P. and Clark, G. S. (eds.). A Stroke Family Guide and Resource. Springfield, Illinois: Charles C Thomas, 1984.

Bukowski, L. and Kuhn, M. Interdisciplinary Roles in Stroke Care. Nursing Clinics of North America, 21(2): 1986, pp. 359–374.

Burnside, I. and Moerhrlin, B. Health Care of the Confused Elderly at Home. Nursing Clinics of North America, 15(2): 1980, pp. 389–401.

Campbell, E., et al. After the Fall-Confusion. American Journal of Nursing, 86(2): 1986, pp. 151–154.

Dimental, P. Alterations in Communication. Biopsychosocial Aspects of Aphasia, Dysarthria, and Right Hemisphere Syndromes in the Stroke Patient. Nursing Clinics of North America, June 1986, pp. 321–343.

Dudas, S. Nursing Diagnoses and Interventions for the Rehabilitation of the Stroke Patient. Nursing Clinics of North America, June 1986, pp. 345–357.

Duncan, P. W. and Badke, M. B. Stroke Rehabilitation: The Recovery of Motor Control. Chicago: Year Book Medical Publishers, 1987.

Johnstone, M. Home Care for the Stroke Patient: Living in a Pattern. New York: Churchill Livingstone, 1980.

Kaplan, P. E. and Cerullo, L. J. (eds). Stroke Rehabilitation. Stoneham, Massachusetts: Butterworth, 1986.

Keily, M. Alzheimer's Disease: Making the Most of the Time That's Left. RN, March, 1985, pp. 34–41.

Lubbock, G. (ed.). Stroke Care: An Interdisciplinary Approach. London: Faber & Faber, 1983.

Mace, N. Using Mental Status Tests. Journal of Gerontological Nursing, 13(6): 1987, pp. 33.

Mann, L. Community Support for Families Caring for Members with Alzheimer's Disease. Home Healthcare Nurse, 3(1): 1985, pp. 8–10.

O'Brien, M. T. and Pallett, P. J. Total Care of the Stroke Patient. Boston: Little, Brown, 1978.

Thornton, J., et al. Alzheimer's Disease Syndrome. JPNMHS 24(5): 1986, pp. 16–22.

Endocrine Alterations

Care Plans

Diabetes Mellitus Care Plan

CROSS REFERENCES

Depression Care Plan
Generic Cardiac Care Plan

Blood Glucose Monitoring Procedure

Adult Subcutaneous Injection Sites
Medication Compliance Management Guidelines

NURSING DIAGNOSES

1. Anxiety related to
   a. lack of understanding of diabetes, its treatment and future implications
   b. self-administration of injections
   c. self-blood glucose monitoring (SBGM)
   d. threat to or change in socioeconomic status
   e. sexual functioning, reproductive issues, effect on unborn fetus
   f. dependence on others for care
   g. skin breakdown/poor healing
   h. threat to or change in interactional/social patterns
   i. loss of control
   j. weakness/faintness/unsteadiness
   k. other.
2. Knowledge deficit (nature of diabetes and its treatment, activity/dietary/medication plan, skin/foot care, prevention of hypoglycemia or hyperglycemia) related to
   a. cognitive limitations
   b. denial
   c. patient's request for no information
   d. misinterpretation of information
   e. other.
3. Ineffective patient/family coping patterns related to
   a. grieving
   b. health care beliefs about susceptibility to disease (denial), consequences of disease (indifference), value of treatment (futility) and risks vs. benefits of treatment
   c. substance abuse
   d. feeling overwhelmed because of the extensive information to be learned and the life style modifications to be made
   e. fear or lack of desire to self-administer injections
   f. dependence on others for care
   g. sociocultural implications
   h. cognitive limitations
   i. temporary family disorganization and role changes
   j. exacerbated developmental crisis
   k. other.

UNIT
6

4. Alteration in comfort (burning, numbness, tingling, gastrointestinal fullness/gas pains, fatigue, irritability, weakness, dizziness, blurred vision, nausea/vomiting, infection, polyuria) related to
   a. effects of decreased gastrointestinal mobility
   b. effects of hypoglycemia or hyperglycemia
   c. inadequate adherence to dietary regimen
   d. inadequate adherence to medication regimen
   e. inadequate skin care
   f. lack of follow through to seek medical care
   g. other.
5. Ineffective breathing pattern related to
   a. effects of hypoglycemia or hyperglycemia
   b. effects of gastrointestinal distension
   c. anxiety
   d. weakness/fatigue
   e. other.
6. Impaired verbal communication related to
   a. slurred speech
   b. irritability/emotional lability
   c. drowsiness/confusion/headache
   d. developmental/age-related issues
   e. language barriers
   f. others.
7. Potential fluid volume deficit related to
   a. anorexia
   b. nausea/vomiting
   c. excessive sweating/increased body temperature
   d. polyuria
   e. lack of adequate dietary planning
   f. effects of medication
   g. diarrhea
   h. other.
8. Impaired home maintenance management related to
   a. sociocultural practices/pressures
   b. inadequate support systems and overtaxed family members' responsibilities
   c. lack of knowledge/impaired cognitive ability
   d. dependent on others for care
   e. emotional lability
   f. impaired mobility
   g. fatigue/extreme weakness
   h. substance/drug abuse
   i. lack of necessary equipment, aids, finances
   j. other.
9. Potential for injury related to
   a. denial/refusal to comply with treatment regimen
   b. lack of understanding of treatment regimen
   c. inadequate hygienic techniques/skin care
   d. developmental/age issues
   e. effects of hypoglycemia or hyperglycemia
   f. impaired sense organs (decreased temperature/tactile sensation)
   g. impaired mobility/weakness
   h. other.

10. Impaired physical mobility related to
    a. impaired vision
    b. effects of impaired foot integrity/bulky dressings
    c. lack of understanding or fear about adjusting regimen for activity
    d. effects of muscle cramps
    e. depression/anxiety
    f. effects of orthostatic hypotension
    g. bladder/bowel incontinence
    h. pain/discomfort
    i. effects of neuromuscular impairments
    j. other.
11. Noncompliance with therapeutic regimen related to
    a. fear/lack of desire to self-administer injections
    b. health care beliefs about susceptibility to disease, consequences of disease and risks vs. benefits of treatment
    c. cultural/spiritual beliefs
    d. cognitive limitations/lack of interest in learning
    e. substance abuse
    f. difficulty integrating treatment regimen into life style
    g. insufficient financial resources
    h. dysfunctional grieving
    i. dysfunctional patient-health care provider relationship
    j. lack of individualized health teaching plan
    k. other.
12. Alteration in nutrition (less than body requirements) related to
    a. anorexia
    b. nausea/vomiting
    c. gastric fullness/gas pain
    d. lack of compliance with medical regimen
    e. dietary plan not based upon cultural/personal preferences
    f. need for further adjustment of insulin/oral hypoglycemic agent
    g. insufficient financial resources
    h. substance abuse
    i. growth and development/gestational needs
    j. insufficient support system for shopping and cooking
    k. other.
13. Potential alterations in parenting related to
    a. restriction of spontaneous/strenuous activity
    b. need to plan meals/activities and medications administration daily
    c. lack of family member support
    d. emotional lability
    e. slurred speech
    f. lethargy/weakness
    g. insufficient financial resources
    h. lack of follow through with health care regimen
    i. limited cognitive functioning
    j. sociocultural barriers
    k. other.
14. Self-care deficit (feeding, bathing, dressing, hygiene, toileting, self-administration of medication, blood and urine testing) related to
    a. dependence on others for care
    b. fear/denial/lack of desire

UNIT 6

    c. emotional lability

    d. sensory impairments (visual, psychomotor, cognitive, time/space orientation)

    e. weakness/lethargy

    f. language barrier

    g. cognitive limitations

    h. depression

    i. other.

15. Alterations in sensory perceptual functioning (visual, kinesthetic, tactile) related to
    a. stress/emotional lability/anxiety
    b. altered status of sense organs (temperature, touch, vibration, vision)
    c. pain
    d. effects of hypoglycemia or hyperglycemia
    e. other.

16. Alterations in tissue perfusion (peripheral, gastrointestinal, renal, cardiopulmonary, cerebral) related to
    a. fluid volume deficits
    b. decreased mobility
    c. effects of local allergic reaction to insulin
    d. delayed healing of skin breakdown
    e. other.

17. Potential impairment of skin integrity related to
    a. inadequate injection technique/rotation of sites
    b. altered skin turgor
    c. inadequate foot/skin/mucous membrane hygiene
    d. effects of surgical wound
    e. impaired sense organs (paresthesias)
    f. increased susceptibility to falls/cuts/injury
    g. delayed healing of skin breakdown
    h. impaired bowel/bladder control
    i. effects of local allergic response to insulin injection
    j. decreased mobility
    k. fluid volume deficit
    l. nipple cracking secondary to breast-feeding
    m. other.

18. Sleep pattern disturbance related to
    a. impaired bowel/bladder control
    b. anxiety/restlessness
    c. burning/aching/sensation of cold, pain, especially of lower extremities
    d. nightmares, crying out while asleep, sleepwalking associated with hypoglycemia
    e. effects of tachycardia/palpitations
    f. diaphoresis
    g. nausea/vomiting
    h. polydipsia
    i. other.

19. Alteration in urinary elimination (incontinence) related to
    a. infection
    b. stress
    c. polyuria
    d. dietary intake (caffeine's diuretic effect)
    e. effects of neuropathy/renal dysfunction
    f. other.

20. Alteration in bowel elimination (diarrhea, incontinence, constipation) related to
    a. effects of neuropathy
    b. dietary intake (spicy/gas-producing foods, inadequate bulk)
    c. smoking (stimulates gastrointestinal tract)
    d. fluid intake (inadequate amount)
    e. impaired mobility
    f. effects of medications
    g. other.
21. Potential disturbance in self-concept (body image, self-esteem, role performance, personal identity) related to
    a. embarrassment of incontinence
    b. changes in sexual functioning/infertility
    c. dependence on others to meet self-care needs
    d. changes in life style imposed by diabetes and treatment regimen
    e. stigma/nonacceptance of having a chronic illness
    f. change in social involvement, fear of rejection or adverse reactions by others
    g. substance abuse
    h. other.

PROCESS INDICATORS

1. The patient/family demonstrates core skills to maintain the diabetes regimen.

Indicators
    a. patient/family describes the disease process of diabetes, the treatment regimen and the prevention strategies for common complications
    b. patient/family describes the causes, treatment and prevention of hypoglycemia and hyperglycemia
    c. patient maintains an activity plan which utilizes appropriate caloric expenditures
    d. patient maintains a dietary plan that incorporates the basic food groups, the needs of growth and development, the prescribed caloric parameters, the medication action and activity levels
    e. patient regulates diet and exercise as appropriate to his or her needs
    f. patient/family describes medication action, side effects, administration, interactions with other medications and parameters for adjusting insulin as appropriate
    g. patient/family identifies signs and symptoms to report to the nurse/physician
    h. patient/family correctly demonstrates procedures for blood glucose and/or urine glucose testing
    i. patient monitors blood and/or urine glucose levels as specified
    j. patient demonstrates use of adaptive aids as appropriate.
2. The patient/family demonstrates effective coping patterns.
Indicators
    a. patient/family verbalizes acceptance of diabetes as a chronic disease incorporating religious, cultural, socioeconomic and personal health beliefs
    b. patient/family adapts roles and activities in order to incorporate the diabetic regimen that includes elements of compliance, medication, diet, activity, health care and financial plans
    c. patient/family verbalizes decreased anxiety/depression/fear
    d. patient/family demonstrates satisfactory parenting skills
    e. patient demonstrates adherence to the prescribed medical regimen
    f. patient expresses satisfactory level of sexual functioning

   g. patient does not experience extreme hypoglycemia or hyperglycemia (parameters as defined by physician)
   h. patient/family makes provisions (including equipment/devices) for visual, sensory, psychomotor, cognitive impairments
   i. patient/family utilizes internal/external supports, such as community groups, the American Diabetes Association and the Juvenile Diabetes Association, as appropriate
   j. patient/family identifies that special situations/developmental needs, such as gestational diabetes, pregnancy in diabetes, normal growth and development (type 1 diabetes), surgery, may require adjustment in the regimen by the physician
   k. patient develops a positive relationship with the health care team.
3. The patient establishes/maintains a satisfactory level of comfort.
Indicators
   a. undisturbed sleep
   b. adequate/proper dietary intake
   c. successful coping with stress/anxiety
   d. absence of or controlled pain/burning/numbness
   e. absence of gastrointestinal discomfort (nausea, vomiting, diarrhea, gas pains)
   f. maintenance of blood glucose levels within an acceptable range
   g. maintenance of skin integrity
   h. satisfactory activity levels with the ability to perform self-care activities
   i. expression of satisfaction with quality of life
   j. establishment/maintenance of ideal body weight.
4. The patient/family describes a plan for coping with safety needs.
Indicators
   a. patient carries/wears medical identification at all times
   b. patient carries an acceptable concentrated sugar source at all times
   c. patient adheres to personal hygiene plan including foot/skin care
   d. patient/family expresses understanding of and prevention of potential safety hazards due to paresthesias, delayed wound healing and altered status of sense organs
   e. patient/family describes the causes, treatment and prevention of hypoglycemia or hyperglycemia.

NURSING INTERVENTIONS

1. Assess
   a. patient's/family's understanding of the disease process of diabetes, the treatment regimen and the prevention strategies for common complications including, but not limited to diet, activity and medication compliance
   b. patient's/family's abilities to learn and perform blood glucose monitoring, urine glucose testing and insulin injection, as appropriate, and assessed at the start and at the conclusion of the visit
   c. patient's/family's ability to make adjustments within the diabetic regimen (i.e., balance in diet, medication and exercise)
   d. patient's comfort level and sense of self-esteem
   e. patient's/family's development/awareness of the need for a long-term health care plan and for periodic evaluations to prevent and/or detect complications
   f. patient's/family's plans for safety/injury prevention.

2. Instruct the patient/family/home health aide about an activity program that
   a. utilizes appropriate caloric expenditures
   b. provides for adequate periods of rest
   c. incorporates diet and medication adjustment parameters
   d. begins slowly, is part of a regular exercise program and conditions the cardiovascular system, as appropriate
   e. incorporates use of good supporting shoes, if appropriate.
3. Instruct the patient/family/home health aide about a dietary plan that
   a. meets the prescribed caloric parameters and dietary restrictions
   b. incorporates basic food groups and healthy heart guidelines from the American Heart Association
   c. incorporates sociocultural, religious, economic and personal preferences
   d. avoids foods that irritate gastric mucosa and stimulate the gastrointestinal tract (such as spicy foods, citrus fruits, juices, caffeine-containing items, cabbage, baked beans, carbonated beverages and very hot and very cold foods)
   e. includes a 3-day diet recall completed by the patient/family
   f. for type 1 diabetes, focuses on the type and timing of meals/snacks with insulin injections/peak action and blood glucose testing
   g. for type 2 diabetes, focuses on the nutrient content of foods and weight control in meal planning
   h. includes recording of dietary intake in the patient's log book.
4. Instruct the patient/family/home health aide about glycemic reactions
   a. causes, treatment and prevention of hypoglycemia/hyperglycemia
   b. rebounding (Somogyi effect)
   c. sick day guidelines
   d. exercise and diet implications for hypoglycemia or hyperglycemia
   e. blood glucose and/or urine glucose testing with action steps to prevent or treat hypoglycemia or hyperglycemia.
5. Instruct the patient/family about the medication regimen
   a. type of medication, peak action, adverse reactions
   b. parameters for adjusting the regimen related to blood glucose and/or urine glucose tests
   c. administration procedures including but not limited to injection techniques or an insulin pump
   d. interactions with other medications particularly those that promote hypoglycemia or hyperglycemia.
6. Instruct the patient/family/home health aide about
   a. principles of skin/foot care
   b. prevention of long-term complications and infection
   c. signs and symptoms to report to the physician/nurse including hypoglycemia or hyperglycemia levels outside the parameters established by the physician
   d. supportive equipment/aids/devices to compensate for visual/psychomotor impairments.
7. Assist the patient/family with
   a. safety/injury prevention strategies (particularly thermal/tactile injuries due to impaired sensations)
   b. verbalizing fears and anxieties
   c. strategies to support the patient's adjustment to a chronic illness
   d. use of community resources, educational resources and organizational support (American Diabetes Association)
   e. developing a health care plan for long-term follow-up as well as an emergency action plan.

UNIT 6

8. Assist the patient and family with strategies to promote compliance
   a. establish, with the physician, acceptable parameters for compliance (Requiring total compliance 100% of the time can lead to stress and noncompliance in certain patients.)
   b. assist the patient and family to establish goals.
9. Assist the patient/family to address appropriate life stage/situational needs
   a. growth and developmental needs of a child with type 1 diabetes
   b. diabetics during pregnancy and the implications for the fetus
   c. a diabetic who becomes pregnant
   d. an elderly diabetic with a sensitivity to oral hypoglycemic agents
   e. a diabetic who is experiencing sexual dysfunction.
10. Coordinate additional members of the health care team, such as the social worker, physical therapist, occupational therapist, registered dietician, podiatrist and home health aide.
11. Obtain orders as necessary for medications, laboratory tests, aids/equipment and so forth from the primary physician.
12. Provide progress reports and a discharge summary to the primary physician.

THERAPEUTIC ACHIEVEMENT

- The patient identifies the restoration of a satisfactory quality of life and an adequate level of independence.
- The patient does not demonstrate symptoms of extreme hypoglycemia or hyperglycemia and achieves normal or near normal blood glucose levels.

RELATED PATIENT INSTRUCTIONS

Blood Glucose Monitoring
Calorie Restricted Diets
Foot Care
High Carbohydrate High Fiber Diabetic Diet
How to Take Insulin
Hyperglycemia

Hypoglycemia
Insulin Action
Mixing Insulin
Oral Hypoglycemic Medications
Subcutaneous Injections

Procedures

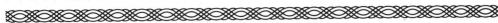

Blood Glucose Monitoring Procedure

PURPOSE

- To optimize control of blood glucose level.
- To monitor changes in blood glucose level.
- To allow the patient/family to make adjustments in the diabetic regimen within prescribed parameters.

EQUIPMENT

- lancet and/or automatic lancet device (optional)
- reagent strips
- cotton (optional for some manufacturers)
- alcohol (considered optional by some authorities)
- reflectance meter (optional)
- watch or clock with second sweep hand
- soap, water and towel

UNIT
6

SPECIAL CONSIDERATIONS

1. Both the visual method and reflectance meter method are included since patients may choose either one or a combination of both methods. For example, some patients may prefer not to take the meter out of the home and may rely on reagent strips for testing during those times when they are away from home.
2. Many diabetic patients could benefit from SBGM. Some diabetics choose to use SBGM to improve their control. Certain categories of diabetic patients are strongly encouraged to use SBGM:
   a. type 1 diabetics, especially those using insulin infusion pumps or those needing multiple insulin injections daily
   b. diabetics who have difficulty with control, particularly those who experience hypoglycemia without warning symptoms
   c. pregnant diabetics, diabetics planning to become pregnant, and gestational diabetics (i.e., pregnant diabetics and implications for the fetus)
   d. diabetics in whom urine testing is neither possible nor reliable.
3. Parameters for adjusting the diabetic's regimen need to be clarified with the primary health care physician or nurse practitioner. SBGM represents only one of the skills needed for self-adjustment of the diabetic's regimen. The patient/family needs to understand the relationship of insulin's peak periods, activity levels and dietary intake to blood glucose levels. Accurate interpretation of blood glucose results and appropriate modifications in the treatment plan require considerable patient/family teaching.

Steps

1. Assess the patient and family for
   a. cognitive ability to understand the procedure, to keep accurate records and to adjust the regimen as appropriate
   b. psychomotor ability to perform the procedure
   c. attitude and motivation for SBGM
   d. any impairments, such as visual acuity, color perception and so forth.
2. Review the package instructions with reagent strips as well as the operating manual of an automated lancet device and/or a reflectance meter.

3. Remove reagent strip from container.
4. Instruct the patient to wash site with warm water and dry thoroughly.

5. Twist off lancet's cap without touching the sterile point. *Option*: If using an automatic device you may desire to wipe the contact site with alcohol prior to inserting the lancet.
6. Wipe the site with alcohol (optional).

7. If using a finger site have the patient lower his or her hand below the level of the heart for about 30 seconds.

Key Points

1. Patient/family ability levels are critical to success with SBGM. Various visual and physical aids are available for patients with impairments. Depending upon the patient's/family's ability levels, the nurse may need to perform/demonstrate the procedure while gradually increasing the patient's/family's level of independence and skill.

2. Reinforce with the patient and family that instructions vary with manufacturers so that reviewing the instructions is an important first step. Instruct the patient/family to check the expiration dates on reagent strips and to discard strips if they are discolored or out of date. Reinforce that reagent strips should be protected from light, moisture and heat.

4. Warm water will increase blood flow to area. Careful drying prevents inaccurate readings due to moisture or sugar from food on the skin. Sites include sides or tips of fingers (not pads) and ear lobes. Toes are not typically preferred sites.
5. Follow the manufacturer's instructions.

6. Follow physician's directions and/or agency's policy concerning alcohol use. This is considered optional by some sources for patient self-testing due to alcohol's drying effect on the skin; repeated use can lead to fissures. If using alcohol, do not puncture the skin until the alcohol dries completely, or the test results may be inaccurate.
7. Efforts are directed to increasing the blood flow.

8. Puncture the skin. *Option*: If using a automated device firmly hold the device against the site and activate.

8. Support the site on or against a firm surface. Use a quick stick and withdraw motion when manually performing the puncture with a lancet. When using an automated device, activate according to manufacturer's instructions.

9. Gently squeeze the site in a downward motion (proximal to distal) to obtain a drop of blood large enough to cover the entire test pad.

9. Allow the blood to accumulate until a large drop hangs from the site. Avoid vigorous "milking," which may cause cell damage and erroneous results.

10. Hold the test strip level and touch the drop of blood to the test pad.

10. Be sure the blood completely covers the pad. Some products do not permit smearing the blood on the pad.

11. Begin timing as soon as the blood is placed on the test pad or as stated in the manufacturer's instructions.

11. Keep the strip level. Timing is critical in obtaining accurate results.

12. Wipe, blot or wash off strip as stated in the manufacturer's instructions.

13. Wait another specified time period.

13. Time period depends upon the manufacturer and method.

Visual Method

14. When timing is complete, match the test pad to the color that most closely matches the color on the scale of the reagent container. The blood glucose level is represented by the number of the matched color.

14. If the test pad color falls between two colors, the blood glucose reading is read as the range between the two numbers; for example, between 80 and 120. Certain brands of test pads can retain color for 4 to 7 days. Patients can be instructed to save test pads in a closed container for review by the nurse/physician. Each strip must be labeled with date and time.

Meter Method

15. When timing is complete, place the test strip in the reflectance meter and follow the manufacturer's instructions to obtain the result.

15. Calibration of the meter may need to be completed prior to starting this procedure. Keeping the unit clean and periodically checking for accuracy are important for valid results.

16. Replace the cap on the lancet and discard. *Option*: If using an automated device remove lancet from the device, replace the cap and discard.

16. Replacing the cap prevents accidental sticks. Do not reuse lancets.

UNIT 6

17. Record the blood glucose result in the patient's log book.

17. Based upon the patient's/family's needs, the log book should include information about the dose of insulin or oral hypoglycemic agent, times for testing blood glucose levels, time of day, dietary intake, including relationship of test to the time of the last meal/activity/exercise, urine glucose tests if performed and symptoms (hypoglycemia or hyperglycemia).

18. Discuss the implications of the blood glucose levels for treatment modification with the patient and family.

18. Notify the primary care physician about results that require adjustments of established parameters.

DOCUMENTATION

1. Patient's/family's skill levels as assessed at the start and at the conclusion of the visit.
   a. careful documentation of the patient's/family's capabilities to perform the procedure and their progress are critical elements for reimbursement
   b. identify achievement of management skills in performing and recording the blood glucose testing results and in understanding the times to perform testing.
2. Type of method used—visual or reflectance meter—as well as the manufacturer of the equipment/strips and any adaptive aids.
3. Results, time and circumstances of the reading. Correlate those areas as applicable from the patient's log book data to demonstrate progress in management of the diabetic.
4. Patient's/family's understanding of the implications of the blood glucose levels in terms of making adjustments in the diabetic regimen within the prescribed parameters.
5. Any adjustments made in the regimen as well as any communications (include dates, times and details of discussions) with the primary physician/members of the health care team.

Resources

Adult Subcutaneous Injection Sites

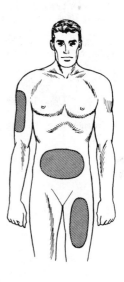

Adult subcutaneous injection sites. (From DuGas, B. Introduction to Patient Care. Philadelphia: W. B. Saunders Co., 1977, p. 463.)

UNIT
6

Bibliography

American Diabetes Association and American Association of Diabetes Educators. Guidelines for Diabetic Care. New York: American Diabetes Association, 1981.

American Diabetes Association. Curriculum for Youth Education. New York: American Diabetes Association, 1981.

American Diabetes Association. The Physician's Guide to Type II Diabetes (NIDDM). New York: American Diabetes Association, 1984.

Bonheim, R. The Second Generation. Diabetes Forecast, March-April 1983, pp. 29–31.

Bovington, M. Neurologic Complications of Diabetes Mellitus. Nursing Clinics of North America, 18(4): 1983, pp 735–747.

Bovington, M., Spies, M. E., Troy, P. Management of the Patient with Diabetes Mellitus During Surgery or Illness. Nursing Clinics of North America, 18(4): 1983, pp. 661–671.

Burns, E. Diabetes Mellitus and Pregnancy. Nursing Clinics of North America, 18(4): 1983, pp. 673–685.

Gavin, James. Diabetes and Exercise. American Journal of Nursing, February 1988, pp. 178–180.

Griffith, HW. Instructions for Patients, 3rd ed. Philadelphia: W. B. Saunders Co., 1982.

Guthrie, D. and Guthrie, R. The Disease Process of Diabetes Mellitus: Definition, Characteristics, Trends, Developments. Nursing Clinics of North America, 18(4): 1985, pp. 617–630.

Heins, J. Dietary Management in Diabetes Mellitus: A Goal-Setting Process. Nursing Clinics of North America, 18(4): 1983, pp. 631–643.

Hoette, S. The Adolescent with Diabetes Mellitus. Nursing Clinics of North America, 18(4): 1983, pp. 763–776.

Hopper, S. Meeting the Needs of the Economically Deprived Diabetic. Nursing Clinics of North America, 18(4): 1983, pp. 813–825.

Jenkins, D. Lente Carbohydrate: A Newer Approach to the Dietary Management of Diabetes. Diabetes Care, 5: 1982, pp. 634.

Jensen, N. and Moore, M. (eds.). Learning to Live Well with Diabetes. Minneapolis: International Diabetes Center, 1987.

Jovanovic, L. Gestational Diabetes. Indianapolis: Boehringer Mannheim Corp., 1986.
Jovanovic, L. Utilizing High Technology to Achieve Optimal Insulin Delivery for Type I Diabetic Patients. Caring, 3:1985, pp. 35–39.
Kilo, C. and Dudley, J. Self Blood Glucose Monitoring. St. Louis: Kilo Diabetes & Vascular Research Foundation, 1984.
Krauser, J. and Madden, P. The Child with Diabetes Mellitus. Nursing Clinics of North America, 18(4): 1983, pp. 749–762.
Marchesseault, L. Diabetes Mellitus with the Elderly. Nursing Clinics of North America, 18(4): 1983, pp. 791–798.
Moorman, M. H. Acute Complications of Hyperglycemia and Hypoglycemia. Nursing Clinics of North America, 18(4): 1983, pp. 707–719.
Popkess-Vawter, S. The Adult Living with Diabetes Mellitus. Nursing Clinics of North America, 18(4): 1983, pp. 777–789.
Price, M. Insulin and Oral Hypoglycemic Agents. Nursing Clinics of North America, 18(4): 1983, pp. 687–706.
Resler, M. Teaching Strategies that Promote Independence. Nursing Clinics of North America, 18(4): 1983, pp. 799–811.
Spies, M. E. Vascular Complications Associated with Diabetes Mellitus. Nursing Clinics of North America, 18(4): 1983, pp. 721–733.
Valenta, C. Urine Testing and Home Blood-Glucose Monitoring. Nursing Clinics of North America, 18(4): 1983, pp. 645–658.
Weinrauch, S. and Tomky, D. Insulin Pump, Update. Diabetes Forecast, May 1986, pp. 35–37.

7

Viral/Communicable Disease Alterations

Care Plans
    Acquired Immune Deficiency Syndrome (AIDS) Care Plan
    Hepatitis Care Plan
    Herpes Simplex (Genital) Care Plan
    Tuberculosis Care Plan
Procedures
    Infection Control Procedure
    Infection Control: AIDS Procedure
    Intradermal Injection Procedure

**UNIT
7**

Care Plans

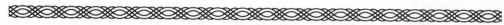

Acquired Immune Deficiency Syndrome (AIDS) Care Plan

CROSS REFERENCES

Bereavement Care Plan
Bladder Incontinence Care Plan
Pain Care Plan
Spiritual Distress Care Plan

Gastric Tube Feeding Procedure
Home Health Aide Supervision Procedure

Home Safety Procedure
Infection Control (AIDS) Procedure
Nasogastric Tube Insertion Procedure
Nasogastric Tube Removal Procedure
Range of Motion Exercises Procedure

Mental Health Assessment/Intervention Guide

NURSING DIAGNOSES

1. Potential/actual impairment of skin integrity related to
   a. inadequate hygiene/skin care
   b. decreased mobility/immobility
   c. emaciation/skeletal prominence
   d. edema (impaired lymphatic flow)
   e. immunological deficit (herpes, Kaposi sarcoma, fungus infection)
   f. diarrhea
   g. bowel/bladder incontinence
   h. other.
2. Alteration in bowel elimination (diarrhea/incontinence) related to
   a. opportunistic bowel infection
   b. intolerance to tube feedings
   c. gastrointestinal malabsorption
   d. neuromuscular impairment
   e. weakness
   f. other.
3. Alteration in nutrition (less than body requirements) related to
   a. anorexia
   b. dysphagia
   c. nausea
   d. diarrhea
   e. gastrointestinal malabsorption
   f. oral/esophageal lesions
   g. depression
   h. other.
4. Potential/actual fluid volume deficit related to
   a. diarrhea
   b. vomiting

    c. anorexia
    d. persistent fever
    e. other.
5. Ineffective airway clearance related to
    a. weakness
    b. tracheobronchial infection
    c. copious/thick sputum production
    d. other.
6. Activity intolerance related to
    a. disease progression
    b. weakness
    c. pulmonary insufficiency
    d. other.
7. Alteration in pattern of urinary elimination (incontinence/retention) related to
    a. neuromuscular impairment
    b. weakness
    c. other.
8. Alteration in thought process related to
    a. neurological impairment
    b. severe/panic level anxiety
    c. belief that contracting AIDS is a punishment
    d. other.
9. Alteration in comfort (pain) related to
    a. neuromuscular impairment
    b. dyspnea
    c. immobility
    d. edema (impaired lymphatic flow)
    e. immunological deficit (herpes, Kaposi sarcoma, fungus infection)
    f. persistent fever
    g. other.
10. Alteration in self-esteem related to
    a. stigma of AIDS
    b. surfacing of internalized homophobia by patient
    c. self-condemnation
    d. other.
11. Anticipatory/actual grieving related to
    a. loss of job/income/insurance coverage/home/career
    b. loss of significant others
    c. chronic fatal illness
    d. other.
12. Social isolation related to
    a. fear of transmitting AIDS
    b. depression
    c. rejection associated with homosexual/illicit drug activities
    d. abandonment by significant others
    e. weakness
    f. other.
13. Anxiety/fear related to
    a. pain
    b. disfigurement
    c. threat of opportunistic infections

UNIT
7

  d. financial stress
  e. knowledge deficit
  f. other.
14. Powerlessness related to chronic fatal illness.
15. Impaired physical mobility related to
  a. neuromuscular impairment
  b. musculoskeletal impairment
  c. weakness
  d. pain
  e. depression
  f. decreased endurance
  g. other.
16. Impaired home maintenance management related to
  a. disease progression
  b. lack of adequate support system
  c. insufficient financial resources
  d. knowledge deficit
  e. cognitive impairment
  f. other.
17. Knowledge deficit (symptoms of infection, prevention of disease transmission, nutritional maintenance, skin care, community resources, mouth care, personal energy conservation methods, medications, etiology of AIDS, pulmonary toileting) related to
  a. cognitive limitation/impairment
  b. misinterpretation of information
  c. lack of motivation for learning
  d. unfamiliarity with information resources
  e. denial
  f. patient's request for no information
  g. other.

PROCESS INDICATORS

1. The patient is protected against opportunistic infection and injury.
Indicators
  a. patient/family recalls the signs/symptoms of infection
  b. patient/family idenitifies the adoption of household precautions/modifications to protect the patient.
2. The patient's biopsychosocial integrity is maintained.
Indicators
  a. no skin irritation/breakdown
  b. intact oral mucosa
  c. weight is maintained
  d. arterial blood gas values are within normal limits
  e. patient is not dehydrated
  f. patient/family recalls purpose, side effects and precautions for prescribed medications
  g. patient/family maintains a satisfactory level of social/community interaction
  h. patient's independent performance of the activities of daily living are realistically commensurate with his or her capabilities

    i. patient participates in mental health counselling/self-help support groups

    j. patient verbalizes incorporation in his or her life of techniques to prevent AIDS transmission.

3. The family's psychosocial equilibrium is maintained.

Indicators

    a. each member's verbalizations of thoughts and feelings about the proximity of AIDS

    b. each member's participation in the patient's care

    c. familial feedback reflects an accurate understanding about the etiology/pathology of AIDS

    d. familial feedback reflects an accurate understanding about modes of contact with the patient that do not transmit AIDS

    e. each member's participation in mental health counselling/self-help support groups.

NURSING INTERVENTIONS

1. Assess the patient.
   a. skin integrity
   b. bowel/bladder elimination pattern
   c. pulmonary status
   d. signs/symptoms of infection
   e. signs/symptoms of dehydration
   f. nutritional status/appetite
   g. patterns of food consumption/fluid intake
   h. level of comfort/discomfort
   i. neurological status
   j. psychological status
   k. readiness/motivation to learn
   l. cognitive ability.

2. Assess
   a. availability/reliability of support systems
   b. environmental hazards to patient/others.

3. Provide instruction to the patient/family/home health aide about
   a. pulmonary toilet (incentive spirometry, humidified air, oxygen therapy, pursed-lip breathing, postural drainage)
   b. skin care
   c. personal hygiene
   d. positioning techniques
   e. active/passive range-of-motion exercises
   f. reality orientation techniques
   g. stress management techniques
   h. importance of engaging in physical activity and building endurance
   i. signs/symptoms of infection (fever, chills, shortness of breath, dry hacking cough, dysuria, inflammation of skin/oral mucosa, diarrhea, deterioration of mental status, purple blotches/bumps on skin, anus and nose and in mouth)
   j. comfort measures (soft/loose fitting clothes/shoes/slippers, sponge baths, soaks with Burow solution, sitz baths, massage/back rubs, frequent linen changes)
   k. techniques to conserve personal energy (pacing activities, sitting instead of standing)
   l. importance of not obtaining patient's temperature rectally

UNIT
7

    m. importance of checking oral/axillary temperature at the same time of day each day

    n. importance of maintaining an adequate daily fluid intake (at least 3000 ml, if not contraindicated, of juices, Gatorade and bouillon)

    o. need to adhere to medication administration schedules

    p. medications (purpose, side effects, administration)

    q. how to care for oral lesions/sores (rinse with saline or a 1:1 saline/hydrogen peroxide mixture at least every 2 hours, use of a topical anesthetic, avoidance of smoking/alcohol, use of soft toothbrush/toothette at least twice a day, avoid extremely hot/cold foods, use of soft foods with low-acid content)

    r. importance of taking daily weights (on the same scale)

    s. techniques of care for edema (elevation of affected extremity/head of bed, wearing of elastic support hose, application of cool moist tea bags for facial edema)

    t. environmental modifications for home safety

    u. techniques to stimulate appetite (eating at the table, serving food at room temperature or chilled, drinking high-calorie, protein supplements served over ice or with flavor added, eating at least a third of the day's total dietary requirements at breakfast, eating frequent small meals/snacks throughout the day)

    v. lesion/decubitus care

    w. use of a condom

    x. the known etiology/pathophysiology of AIDS.

4. Teach the patient/family/home health aide techniques to prevent AIDS transmission.

    a. avoid donating blood/plasma, body organs/parts, sperm

    b. do not share needles/syringes/personal care items

    c. engage only in safe sex (monogamy, masturbation, body rubbing, massage, petting, hugging)

    d. avoid unsafe sex practices (anal/vaginal intercourse with/without a condom, fellatio/orogenital contact, swallowing body secretions/excretions, anonymous sexual contacts, use of small rodents, insertion of foreign objects into rectum, games/practices that cause mouth/genital trauma, wet/French kissing)

    e. do not use recreational drugs

    f. alert health care providers to the presence of AIDS.

5. Teach the patient/family/home health aide precautions for protecting the patient against infections.

    a. well-ventilated rooms

    b. good personal hygiene

    c. choose/prepare foods to minimize bacterial contamination (canned foods, cook all raw fruits/vegetables before eating, peel fruits, cook meat well before eating, use only pasteurized dairy products)

    d. avoid contact with animal/pet excreta

    e. consult with the physician about having a pet

    f. adequate environmental cleaning.

6. Teach the patient/family/home health aide routine precaution techniques.

    a. handwashing

    b. wash dishes/utensils between use; do not share them until washed

    c. launder the patient's clothes/linens separately using household detergent

    d. clean household surfaces/durable medical equipment/reusable items with a 1:10 bleach/water solution

    e. wear a mask if the patient has a productive cough

    f. wear gloves when handling urinal/bedpan

    g. keep clothes/linens soiled by patient in a plastic bag until laundered

    h. double bag soiled dressings/trash and discard with household trash

    i. put needles/syringes/sharp items in puncture-proof container prior to disposal

    j. dispose of contaminated materials/cleaning fluids in toilet

    k. use disposable items whenever practical/feasible.

7. Help the patient/family identify/eliminate foods/habits that exacerbate diarrhea.

8. Request/obtain orders, as necessary, for medications, arterial blood values, nasogastric tube, urinary catheter and so forth from the attending physician.

9. Refer to and coordinate nutrition-based interventions with the dietician.

10. Monitor/adjust, in collaboration with the attending physician and the dietician, the rate and concentration of tube feedings.

11. Coordinate referrals, as necessary, to social worker, physical therapist, occupational therapist, durable medical equipment supplier, spiritual adviser, respite volunteer and legal aid and hospice workers.

12. Refer the patient/family to
    a. AIDS support/self-help groups
    b. United States Public Health Service/local health department
    c. Centers for Disease Control
    d. AIDS hotlines.

13. Provide opportunities that facilitate the patient's independent action/decision-making.

14. Create situations that encourage the patient/family to express their thoughts and feelings.

15. Assess the family/household members
    a. signs/symptoms of infection
    b. signs/symptoms of AIDS, herpes, Kaposi sarcoma
    c. degree of increased/high-risk exposure to AIDS virus.

16. Encourage family/household members at high risk to seek follow-up HTLV-III (human T-cell leukemia virus) testing and, if positive, refer to a support group/counsellor.

17. Refer to/coordinate public health follow-up of the family/household members after the patient's death.

18. Send progress notes and a discharge summary to the attending physician.

UNIT 7

THERAPEUTIC ACHIEVEMENT

- The patient/family adapts to the life style changes induced as a result of AIDS.

RELATED PATIENT INSTRUCTION

AIDS: Precautions for the Home	Making the Home Environment Safe
Bronchopulmonary Health	Measuring Liquid Intake and Output
Care for the Patient Confined to Bed	Nasogastric, Orogastric, Nasointestinal Tube
Comfort Measures for Dehydration	Feedings
Clinical Signs of Imminent Death	Oxygen Therapy
Diuretic Medications	Pain Medications
General Comfort Measures	Reality Orientation
Healthy Heart	Skin Care
Heart Medications	Ways to Save Your Energy
High Calorie High Protein Diet	When to Call for Help

Hepatitis Care Plan

CROSS REFERENCES

Infection Control Procedure

NURSING DIAGNOSES

1. Anxiety/fear related to
   a. potential transmission of disease
   b. unemployment
   c. change in appearance (jaundice)
   d. altered social interactions
   e. other.
2. Knowledge deficit (prevention/causes of hepatitis, program for alcohol/drug rehabilitation, sexual activity guidelines, medication/activity/dietary regimen) related to
   a. cognitive limitations
   b. lack of interest in learning
   c. substance abuse
   d. unfamiliarity with information resources
   e. other.
3. Alteration in nutrition (less than body requirements) related to
   a. anorexia
   b. nausea/illness
   c. abdominal pain/dyspepia
   d. dependence on others for shopping/cooking
   e. other.
4. Activity intolerance related to
   a. fatigue
   b. generalized malaise
   c. nausea/vomiting
   d. abdominal pain
   e. other.
5. Disturbance in self-concept (body image, self-esteem, role performance) related to
   a. change in appearance (jaundice)
   b. change in social involvement
   c. dependence on others for care
   d. unemployment
   e. activity intolerance
   f. therapeutically restricted environment/isolation
   g. sexual activity restrictions
   h. impaired ability to fulfill parent role
   i. other.
6. Impaired skin integrity related to
   a. impaired nutritional state (anorexia)
   b. impaired mobility (bed rest)
   c. altered metabolic state resulting in skin itchiness
   d. increased risk of bleeding
   e. inadequate hygiene/skin care
   f. other.

7. Ineffective individual/family coping related to
    a. isolation
    b. fatigue
    c. irritability/malaise
    d. unemployment
    e. financial demands
    f. dependence on others for care
    g. change in family role and responsibilities
    h. other.
8. Self-care deficit (feeding/bathing/grooming/hygiene/toileting) related to
    a. dependence on others for care
    b. fatigue/activity intolerance
    c. malaise/anorexia
    d. other.
9. Social isolation related to
    a. fear of transmitting hepatitis
    b. depression
    c. rejection associated with homosexual/illicit drug activities
    d. abandonment by significant others
    e. fatigue
    f. other.

PROCESS INDICATORS

1. The patient's biopsychosocial integrity is maintained.
Indicators
    a. no skin irritation or breakdown
    b. patient performs self-care/activities of daily living as appropriate with his or her capability/activity tolerance
    c. adequate personal hygiene
    d. patient/family validates balance among the patient's rest, activity and nutrition
    e. patient/family maintains a satisfactory level of social/community interaction
    f. patient/family utilizes community resources as needed
    g. patient expresses satisfaction with quality of life.
2. The patient/family adapts to the hepatitis regimen for convalescence and for the prevention of disease transmission.
Indicators
    a. patient maintains satisfactory nutritional status, maintains acceptable body weight, eats small frequent meals and takes vitamin supplements as prescribed
    b. patient/family explains the purpose, administration schedule and adverse effects of prescribed medications
    c. patient/family identifies the need to avoid taking any medication, including over-the-counter medications, without physician's prior approval
    d. patient/family identifies signs and symptoms to report to the physician/nurse
    e. patient maintains an activity plan that includes planned rest periods
    f. patient/family follows precautions to prevent transmission of disease.

NURSING INTERVENTIONS

1. Assess the patient
    a. skin integrity, ecchymosis, pruritus and areas of bleeding (including gums)

UNIT
7

      b. nutritional status/appetite (nausea, vomiting, anorexia)
      c. patterns of food consumption/frequency of meals
      d. level of comfort/discomfort (abdominal pain or tenderness, epigastric discomfort)
      e. bowel/bladder patterns and color of stool/urine
      f. current level of activity/tolerance (fatigue)
      g. psychological state (changing mentation, irritability, substance abuse).

2. Assess
      a. availability/reliability of support systems
      b. patient's/family's understanding of causes, treatment and prevention of transmission of hepatitis
      c. public and home sanitation
      d. patient's/family's awareness of community resources (homemakers, unemployment/disability process, drug/alcohol treatment programs as appropriate)
      e. patient's/family's/contact's risks of exposure.

3. Instruct the patient/family/home health aide about an activity plan that includes
      a. gradual increase in activities as ordered
      b. resting before and after activities
      c. restricting activities when fatigued.

4. Instruct the patient/family/home health aide about signs and symptoms to report to nurse/physician.
      a. increasing anorexia
      b. change in mentation (confusion)
      c. vomiting or diarrhea (increasing frequency)
      d. increasing jaundice
      e. skin breakdown and/or increasing skin rash/itching
      f. sudden increase or occurrence of abdominal pain/tenderness
      g. bruises, petechiae, bleeding (gums, skin)
      h. blood in stool, tarry stool
      i. asterixis (metabolic tremors)
      j. increase or occurrence of edema/ascites.

5. Instruct the patient/family/home health aide about skin care/management pruritus.
      a. keep the skin moist and clean
         • use tepid water and baking soda or emollient baths daily
         • avoid soap, particularly alkaline soap
         • apply emollient lotions daily and as needed
         • apply lotions, such as calamine, if ordered.
      b. treat skin breakdown immediately to prevent infection
      c. keep the environment cool
      d. linens should be soft (cotton) and changed when wet
      e. wear loose soft clothing
      f. prevent skin trauma by using an electric razor and a soft-bristled toothbrush
      g. review medications prescribed to decrease skin itching
      h. review strategies to minimize skin scratching
         • plan diversional activities
         • keep nails clean, short/trimmed
         • use knuckles to apply pressure to an itching site
         • give soothing massages
         • avoid heavy top bed linens
         • for patients who scratch in their sleep or for confused patients, encourage them to wear clean white gloves.

6. Discuss strategies with the patient/family/home health aide to promote patient self-esteem and successful patient/family coping.
   a. encourage the patient/family to verbalize feelings/concerns
   b. encourage the patient to perform daily grooming
   c. explain that wearing yellow or green clothing may increase the appearance of the yellow skin tone (red, blue or black clothing may be better)
   d. explain that changes in appearance are usually temporary
   e. assist the family to explore methods to enhance the patient's appearance
   f. assist the patient/family to plan sensory stimulation/diversonal activities/relaxation strategies.
7. Instruct the patient/family/home health aide about the medication regimen (antihistamines, tranquilizers/sedatives, cholestyramine analgesics, antiemetics, antacids).
   a. names of drugs
   b. actions/indications for use
   c. dosages
   d. schedule of administration
   e. possible side effects
   f. adverse effects to report to the physician
   g. avoiding any medications without prior approval of the physician, including over-the-counter medications, such as acetylsalicylic acid (ASA) and birth control pills, and hepatotoxic drugs
   h. including vitamin or mineral supplements as prescribed.
8. Instruct the patient/family/home health aide about a dietary plan that
   a. includes techniques to stimulate appetite
      • eating while sitting up, in a pleasant environment (preferably at the table)
      • giving oral hygiene before and after meals to decrease the unpleasant mouth taste
      • eating small meals 4 to 5 times every day
      • incorporating patient food preferences as permitted
      • eating fresh or canned fruits or juices between meals to minimize the unpleasant mouth taste (hard candy may not be recommended because of its effect of decreasing the appetite).
   b. maintains weekly weight monitoring
   c. incorporates feeding supplements as prescribed
   d. incorporates a balanced diet within prescribed parameters for percentages of protein, carbohydrate and fat.
9. Instruct the patient/family/home health aide about techniques to prevent hepatitis transmission.
   a. avoid donating blood/plasma and sperm
   b. identify contacts at risk who need to seek medical follow-up
   c. do not share needles/syringes/personal care items/cigarettes
   d. engage only in safe sex (condoms, body rubbing, massage, hugging)
   e. avoid unsafe sex practices (wet/French kissing, anal/vaginal intercourse without a condom, orogenital contact, swallowing body secretions/excretions)
   f. do not use recreational drugs.
10. Instruct the patient/family/home health aide about techniques of routine precautions.
   a. handwashing with soap and warm water after toileting and contact with body fluids/excretions
   b. washing dishes/utensils between use; do not share them until washed
   c. launder the patient's clothes/linens separately using household detergent

UNIT 7

   d. clean household surfaces/durable medical equipment/reusable items with a 1:10 bleach/water solution

   e. wear gloves when handling urinal/bedpan/soiled linens

   f. keep clothes/linen soiled by the patient in a plastic bag until laundered

   g. double bag soiled dressings/trash and discard with household trash

   h. dispose of contaminated materials/cleaning fluids in the toilet as appropriate

   i. put needles/syringes/sharp items in puncture-proof container prior to disposal

   j. use disposable items whenever practical/feasible.

11. Instruct the patient/family about

   a. need to eliminate patient alcohol intake until approved by the physician

   b. recording the color of urine/stool if ordered.

12. Follow your agency's policy for notification/follow-up of a reportable disease.

13. Request/obtain orders, as necesary for blood work, medications, vitamin K.

14. Test urine/feces for blood as ordered.

15. Coordinate referrals, as necessary to

   a. social worker

   b. occupational therapist

   c. self-help/community resources

   d. drug/alcohol rehabilitation programs

   e. financial counseling services

   f. dietician.

16. Provide progress reports and a discharge summary to the primary physician.

THERAPEUTIC ACHIEVEMENT

- The patient adheres to convalescence regimen without transmitting the disease.

RELATED PATIENT INSTRUCTIONS

A Daily Food Guide—Four Basic Food Groups	Pain Medications
Bathing the Person in a Chair	Skin Care
Infection Control for the Home	Ways to Save Your Energy

Herpes Simplex (Genital) Care Plan

CROSS REFERENCES

Constipation Care Plan
Depression Care Plan
Pain Care Plan

Bladder Retraining Procedure
Infection Control Procedure

Cancer Warning Signs

NURSING DIAGNOSES

1. Potential/actual activity intolerance related to
   a. weakness/malaise
   b. complicating infection/inflammation
   c. other.
2. Alteration in comfort (pain) related to
   a. herpes lesions
   b. prodromal symptomatology (itching, burning, sacral neuralgia, myalgia)
   c. lymphadenopathy
   d. headaches
   e. dysuria
   f. pharyngitis
   g. febrile episodes
   h. other.
3. Potential/actual impairment of skin integrity related to
   a. prodromal symptomatology
   b. herpes lesions
   c. inadequate skin care/hygiene
   d. other.
4. Alteration in pattern of urinary elimination or retention related to
   a. urethritis
   b. cystitis
   c. other.
5. Powerlessness related to a chronic disease.
6. Anxiety/fear related to
   a. change in health status
   b. threat to self-concept
   c. threat to or change in patterns of sexual/intimate interactions
   d. pain
   e. knowledge deficit
   f. other.
7. Knowledge deficit (pathophysiology of herpes simplex, prevention of disease transmission, medications, community resources, modification of predisposing factors) related to
   a. denial
   b. patient's request for no information

UNIT
7

   c. misinterpretation of information
   d. cognitive limitation/impairment
   e. unfamiliarity with information resources
   f. other.
8. Sexual dysfunction related to the disease process.

PROCESS INDICATORS

1. The patient and sexual partner accept and use techniques to prevent transmission of the herpes simplex virus.
Indicators
   a. feedback reflects an accurate understanding about the mode of transmission
   b. verbalization that techniques to prevent herpes simplex transmission have been incorporated into their lives
   c. recall of how to modify predisposing factors
   d. patient does not exhibit signs/symptoms of complicating infections/inflammations
   e. verbalizations of thoughts and feelings about herpes simplex.

NURSING INTERVENTIONS

1. Assess the patient
   a. skin integrity
   b. signs/symptoms of infection (aseptic meningitis, pelvic cellulitis, yeast vaginitis)
   c. level of comfort/discomfort
   d. previous history/treatment of sexually transmitted disease
   e. patterns of sexual activity
   f. psychological status
   g. readiness/motivation to learn
   h. cognitive ability.
2. Provide instructions to the patient about
   a. lesion care (keep outbreak areas clean and dry)
   b. medications (purposes, side effects, administration, precautions, interactions)
   c. stress management techniques
   d. importance of balancing rest, nutrition and exercise
   e. methods to promote voiding
   f. importance of maintaining an adequate fluid intake
   g. sitz baths/care of equipment
   h. necessity of informing sexual partners/contacts that they need to be examined/treated
   i. need to avoid alcohol during the treatment period (causes genitourinary irritation, interacts with medications).
3. Assist the patient to develop a clear truthful explanation about herpes simplex for presentation to sexual partners/contacts.
4. Identify the patient's sexual partners/contacts from the present to 3 months before the onset of symptoms.
5. Provide instruction to the patient/sexual partner about
   a. pathophysiology of herpes simplex
   b. complications of herpes simplex (mild photophobia, constipation, yeast vaginitis, pelvic inflammatory disease, urethritis, cystitis, dyspareunia)

    c. prevention of disease transmission (avoid oral, genital and anal sexual contact from onset of prodromal symptoms to 10 days after lesions have healed; limit number of sexual partners; wash with soap and water before and immediately after sexual contact; urinate immediately after sexual contact; use a condom)

    d. how to use a condom

    e. high frequency of recurrence

    f. lack of a uniform pattern of recurrence

    g. potential precipitating factors of recurrence (stress, menses, heat, moisture, climate change, pregnancy, oral contraceptive use, illness)

    h. the importance of regular checkups for sexually transmitted disease.

6. Counsel the female patient to

    a. have a routine Papanicolaou (PAP) smear every 6 months to a year (because of increased risk for cervical cancer)

    b. alert her gynecologist/obstetrician about the presence of herpes simplex (because of the transmission of the disease to the neonate during birth).

7. Create opportunities that encourage the patient/family/sexual partner to express their thoughts and feelings.

8. Refer to

    a. American Social Health Association

    b. American Council for Healthful Living

    c. self-help support groups

    d. family counseling

    e. mental health counselling (individual/group).

9. Request/obtain orders from the attending physician for topical anesthetics, antibiotics, acyclovir and cultures as necessary.

10. Send progress notes and a discharge summary to the attending physician.

**UNIT
7**

THERAPEUTIC ACHIEVEMENT

- The patient/family adapts to the life style changes induced as a result of herpes simplex.

RELATED PATIENT INSTRUCTIONS

Antibiotic Medications
Bladder Retraining
Constipation

General Comfort Measures
Infection Control for the Home
Skin Care

Tuberculosis Care Plan

CROSS REFERENCES

Depression Care Plan

Home Health Aide Supervision Procedure

Infection Control Procedure

Telephone Contact with Patient/Family Procedure

Medication Compliance Management Guidelines

NURSING DIAGNOSES

1. Alteration in nutrition (less than body requirements) related to
   a. nausea
   b. anorexia
   c. depression
   d. fatigue
   e. other.
2. Alteration in comfort (pain) related to
   a. inflammatory process
   b. persistent fever
   c. other.
3. Ineffective airway clearance related to
   a. thick/copious secretions
   b. weakness
   c. minimally productive cough
   d. other.
4. Activity intolerance related to
   a. inadequate nutritional status
   b. pulmonary insufficiency
   c. weakness/fatigue
   d. other.
5. Sleep pattern disturbance related to
   a. pain/discomfort
   b. nocturnal diaphoresis
   c. anxiety
   d. other.
6. Noncompliance (medication regimen, public health surveillance) related to
   a. denial
   b. anxiety
   c. patient/family value system
   d. other.
7. Knowledge deficit (tuberculosis, prognosis, disease transmission, infection control methods, importance of compliance, nutritional maintenance, medications) related to
   a. cognitive limitation/impairment
   b. misinterpretation of information
   c. denial
   d. lack of motivation/readiness for learning
   e. other.

8. Anxiety related to
   a. occurrence of hemoptysis
   b. chest pain
   c. knowledge deficit
   d. financial stress
   e. myths about tuberculosis
   f. other.
9. Alteration in self-esteem related to stigma of tuberculosis.
10. Social isolation related to
    a. fear of transmitting tuberculosis
    b. weakness
    c. embarrassment
    d. depression
    e. other.
11. Potential for injury related to peripheral neuropathy.

PROCESS INDICATORS

1. The patient's/family's biopsychosocial integrity is maintained.
Indicators
   a. patient's weight is maintained or there is a gain
   b. balance among rest, nutrition and exercise is validated
   c. vital signs and laboratory values are within normal limits
   d. patient validates (verbally/nonverbally) that pain/discomfort are controlled/minimized
   e. patient demonstrates/verbalizes increased tolerance for exercise/activity
   f. patient/family validates adherence to prescribed medical regimen
   g. patient/family recalls the importance of compliance with follow-up public health surveillance
   h. patient/family recalls the purpose, side effects and precautions associated with prescribed medications
   i. patient/family identifies the adoption of household measures/precautions to prevent disease transmission
   j. patient/family recalls signs/symptoms of respiratory deterioration
   k. patient maintains a satisfactory level of social/community interaction
   l. patient/family utilizes community resources
   m. patient/family verbalize thoughts and feelings about tuberculosis and its associated life style changes.

UNIT 7

NURSING INTERVENTIONS

1. Assess the patient
   a. signs/symptoms of tuberculosis (progressive cough, weight loss, unresolved or poorly resolved respiratory infection, aching chest pain, hemoptysis, persistent fever, anorexia, nocturnal diaphoresis, fatigue)

    b. history (recent or past exposure to tuberculosis; travel to or residence in a country with high incidence of tuberculosis; vaccination with bacille Calmette-Guerín (BCG); substance abuse)

    c. degree of pain/discomfort

    d. pattern of physical activity

    e. pattern of sleep/rest

    f. nutritional status/appetite

    g. cardiorespiratory status

    h. coexisting health problems

    i. current laboratory values and x-ray studies.

2. Assess

    a. what meaning the patient/family assigns to tuberculosis

    b. changes in the patient's/family's routine

    c. availability/reliability of support systems

    d. cognitive abilities of each family member.

3. Provide instruction to the patient/family/home health aide about

    a. pathophysiology and course of tuberculosis

    b. importance of long-term compliance with the prescribed medication regimen

    c. medications (purposes, side effects, administration, precautions)

    d. how to control/minimize medication side effects

    e. importance of not running out of medication

    f. signs of respiratory deterioration

    g. need to balance rest, nutrition and exercise

    h. methods to induce sleep

    i. techniques to stimulate appetite

    j. importance of engaging in physical activity/endurance building

    k. personal energy conservation techniques

    l. time restriction on activities and social interactions

    m. personal hygiene

    n. mode of tuberculosis transmission (droplet)

    o. measures to prevent disease transmission (handwashing, well-ventilated rooms, covering nose and mouth, disposal of tissues)

    p. importance of compliance with follow-up public health surveillance

    q. proper sputum collection procedure.

4. Monitor the patient for side effects of the medications (peripheral neuropathy, liver dysfunction, gastrointestinal disturbance, rash)

5. Monitor the patient, with the physician, for parameters indicating the need for hospitalization (acute illness, high-risk living conditions, noncompliance).

6. Request/obtain orders, as necessary, from the attending physician for sputum cultures, chest x-rays, medications, hospitalization and so forth.

7. Refer to and coordinate nutrition-based interventions with the dietician.

8. Coordinate referrals, as necessary, to the public health department, social worker, physical therapist, American Lung Association.

9. Provide opportunities that facilitate the patient's independent action and/or decision-making.

10. Create situations that encourage the patient/family to express their thoughts and feelings.

11. Assess family/household members/others at high risk (close proximity to patient for long durations in areas with poor ventilation) for signs/symptoms of tuberculosis.

12. Supervise, perform, or refer to the public health department high-risk contacts for follow-ups.
13. Send progress notes and a discharge summary to the attending physician.

THERAPEUTIC ACHIEVEMENT

- The patient/family adapts to the life style changes induced as a result of tuberculosis.

RELATED PATIENT INSTRUCTIONS

A Daily Food Guide—Four Basic Food Groups
Antibiotic Medications
General Comfort Measures

Infection Control for the Home
Medication Compliance
Ways to Save Your Energy

UNIT
7

Procedures

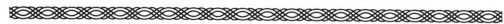

Infection Control
Procedure

PURPOSE

- To decrease the risk of microorganism transmission.

EQUIPMENT

- None

Steps

1. Assess the home environment for factors that facilitate the spread of infection.
   a. poor personal hygiene
   b. infrequent/superficial handwashing
   c. inadequate environmental cleaning
   d. exposure to contaminated household/medical equipment
   e. exposure to individuals with infectious diseases
   f. exposure to stagnant water
   g. exposure to pet excreta.
2. Alert the patient/family/home health aide to the identified factors.
3. Teach the patient/family/home health aide how to correct the situation/prevent the spread of infection (Table 7–1).
4. Teach the patient/family/home health aide about infection control measures necessitated by the patient's disease.
5. Reassess the home environment for correction/implementation of the identified factors/measures during the next visit.

Key Points

1. A methodical assessment is easily achieved when a checklist is used.

3. Be specific when teaching. Useful materials can be obtained from the local health department.

4. Specific measures depend on the patient's medical problems and related nursing diagnoses.

DOCUMENTATION

1. The assessment of the home environment for factors that allow for the spread of infection.

Table 7–1
Infection Control

Factors that Facilitate the Spread of Infection	Precautionary/Corrective Measures
POOR PERSONAL HYGIENE	Regular bathing/hair washing. Daily oral hygiene. Dental care once or twice a year. Weekly trimming finger/toe nails. Wearing clean/laundered clothes. Change soiled clothing as soon as it is noticed.

INFREQUENT HANDWASHING	Wash hands *before*
	    food preparation
	    eating food
	    serving food.
	Wash hands *after*
	    toilet use
	    contact with own/another's body fluids
	    blowing/wiping nose
	    outside activities.

SUPERFICIAL HANDWASHING	Wet hands with plenty of soap and warm water. Work up a lather over hands and wrists. Rub the palm of one hand over back of the other and rub together several times. Repeat for other hand. Interlace fingers of both hands and rub back and forth. Clean under fingernails with a nail brush or an orange stick. Rinse hands thoroughly under warm running water. Dry hands and wrists thoroughly.
INADEQUATE ENVIRONMENTAL CLEANING	Avoid environmental clutter. Thoroughly ventilate with fresh air. Clean kitchen counter with scouring powder. Dust and vacuum weekly. Mop kitchen/bathroom floors weekly and when spills occur. Clean inside of refrigerator weekly with soap and water.
EXPOSURE TO CONTAMINATED HOUSEHOLD/MEDICAL EQUIPMENT	Scrub medical equipment with 70% alcohol solutions or a solution of 1 part bleach to 30 parts water or 1 to 2% iodine solution. Clean soap dishes, denture cups and so forth weekly. Do not use the same sponge to clean the bathroom and kitchen. Do not pour mop water down kitchen sink. Do not clean sponges/rags at kitchen sink. Disinfect mops and sponges weekly by soaking in a 1 part bleach to 9 parts water solution for 5 minutes. Flush body wastes down toilet. Do not clean bedpan, potty seats and so forth in kitchen sink. Do not share towels, washcloths, lingerie/undergarments and toothbrushes.
EXPOSURE TO STAGNANT WATER	Add a teaspoon of bleach to each quart of water used for flower vases to prevent development of microorganisms. Add a teaspoon of vinegar to each quart of water/saline used for respiratory equipment/humidifier/dehumidifier.
EXPOSURE TO PET EXCRETA	Immunosuppressed individuals should not clean bird cages, aquariums, litter boxes and so forth and should avoid areas where dogs are walked. Wear gloves when cleaning bird cages, litter boxes, aquariums and so forth.
EXPOSURE TO PEOPLE WITH INFECTIOUS DISEASES	Avoid crowds. Avoid individuals who have been recently vaccinated. Avoid individuals with bacterial infections, cold sores, shingles, influenza, colds, chicken pox, measles and so forth. Cover mouth with tissue/hand when sneezing/coughing. Do not share food/drink. Do not lick fingers or taste from mixing spoon while cooking.

UNIT 7

2. The identified factors.

3. The teaching done pertinent to correction of the identified factors.

4. The teaching done about infection control measures necessitated by the patient's disease.

5. The patient/family/home health aide's response to the teaching.

6. The reassessment for correction of identified factors and/or implementation of disease-specific infection control measures.

Infection Control: AIDS Procedure

PURPOSE

- To decrease the risk of AIDS transmission.

EQUIPMENT

- nonsterile disposable gloves
- heavy duty latex gloves
- plastic garbage bags
- coverall gown
- disposable mask
- goggles
- household bleach
- soap
- hot water

GENERAL GUIDELINES FOR THE NURSE

1. Wear nonsterile disposable gloves when handling the AIDS patient's blood specimens, body fluids, secretions and excretions, as well as surfaces, materials and objects contaminated with these fluids.

   Special Note. Persons who care for AIDS patients should avoid direct skin contact (particularly if their skin is chapped or broken) with the blood and body fluids of patients with AIDS.

2. Wear gown, mask and goggles when clothing, eyes and face may be exposed to body fluids, blood secretions or excretions of an AIDS patient (e.g., when doing a venipuncture, when cleaning an incontinent patient).

   Special Note. Persons who care for AIDS patients should avoid direct contact of the mucous membranes and clothing with the blood and body fluids of the AIDS patients. (Direct or indirect transmission may otherwise occur.)

3. Double bag soiled disposable equipment, using plastic garbage bags, tie the bags securely and discard with the household trash.

   Special Note. If using a nondisposable gown, keep it in a plastic bag until laundered.

4. Wash your hands thoroughly with soap and hot water after caring for an AIDS patient.

5. If any surface or container becomes visibly contaminated with an AIDS patient's blood, put on heavy duty latex gloves and clean the contaminated area with a 1:10 bleach:water solution.

   Special Note. The AIDS virus is fragile and can be easily destroyed by a mixture of household bleach and water.

UNIT
7

Steps	Key Points
1. Assess the home environment for factors that facilitate the transmission of AIDS (see also Spread of AIDS and Precautionary Measures, which follows).	1. A methodical assessment is easily achieved when a checklist is used.

1. Assess the home environment for factors that facilitate the transmission of AIDS (see also Spread of AIDS and Precautionary Measures, which follows).
   a. poor personal hygiene
   b. infrequent/superficial handwashing
   c. unsafe sexual practices
   d. inadequate environmental cleaning
   e. exposure to contaminated body fluids
   f. exposure to contaminated household/medical equipment.
2. Assess the home environment for factors that place the AIDS patient at greater risk for opportunistic infections (see also Spread of AIDS and Precautionary Measures, which follows).
   a. poor personal hygiene
   b. inadequate environmental cleaning
   c. inappropriate/inadequate food selection/preparation
   d. exposure to individuals with infectious diseases
   e. exposure to pet excreta.
3. Alert the patient/family to the identified factors.
4. Teach the patient/family how to correct the situation/prevent the transmission of AIDS.
5. Teach the patient/family how to decrease the risk of opportunistic infection.
6. Reassess the home environment for correction of the identified factors and implementation of AIDS-specific infection control measures during the next visit.

Key Points

4. Be specific when teaching. Useful materials can be obtained from the local health department.

DOCUMENTATION

1. The assessment of the home environment for factors that facilitate the transmission of AIDS and that place the AIDS patient at greater risk for opportunistic infections.
2. The identified factors.
3. The teaching done pertinent to the correction of the identified factors.
4. The patient's/family's response to the teaching.
5. The precautions used by the nurse during the visit, the patient's/family's response to them and the nurse's subsequent interventions.
6. The reassessment for correction of identified factors and implementation of AIDS-specific infection control measures.

Spread of Aids and Precautionary Measures

Factors that Facilitate the Spread of AIDS/ Increase the Risk of Opportunistic Infection	Precautionary/Corrective Measures
POOR PERSONAL HYGIENE	Regular bathing/hair washing Daily oral hygiene Dental care yearly/twice a year/more often, as needed Weekly trimming finger/toe nails Wearing clean/laundered clothes Changing soiled clothing/linen as soon as it is noticed.
INFREQUENT HANDWASHING	Wash hands *before* food preparation eating food serving food. Wash hands *after* toilet use contact with own/another's body fluids blowing/wiping nose outside activities.
SUPERFICIAL HANDWASHING	Wet hands with plenty of soap and water. Work up a lather over hands and wrists. Rub the palm of one hand over the back of the other and rub together several times. Repeat for other hand. Interlace fingers of both hands and rub back and forth. Clean under fingernails with a nailbrush or an orange stick. Rinse hands thoroughly under warm running water. Dry hands and wrists thoroughly.
UNSAFE SEXUAL PRACTICES	Engage only in safe sex (monogamy, masturbation, body rubbing, massage, petting, hugging). Use a condom when engaging in intercourse. Avoid unsafe sex (anal or vaginal intercourse with/ without a condom, fellatio/orogenital contact, swallowing body secretions/excretions, anonymous sexual contacts, use of small rodents, insertion of foreign objects into rectum, games/practices that cause mouth/genital trauma, wet/French kissing). Avoid use of recreational drugs.
INADEQUATE ENVIRONMENTAL CLEANING	Avoid environmental clutter. Thoroughly ventilate with fresh air. Clean kitchen counter with scouring powder. Dust and vacuum weekly. Mop kitchen/bathroom floors weekly and when spills occur. Clean inside of refrigerator weekly with soap and water. Add a teaspoon of bleach to each quart of water used for flower vases to eliminate growth of microorganisms. Add a teaspoon of vinegar to each quart of water/ saline used for respiratory equipment/humidifier/ dehumidifier.

Table continued on following page

UNIT 7

Spread of Aids and Precautionary Measures Continued

Factors that Facilitate the Spread of AIDS/ Increase the Risk of Opportunistic Infection	Precautionary/Corrective Measures
INAPPROPRIATE/INADEQUATE FOOD SELECTION/ PREPARATION	Use canned foods. Cook all raw fruits and vegetables before eating. Peel fruits. Cook meat well before eating. Use only pasteurized dairy products. Avoid foods that exacerbate diarrhea. Do not share food and drink. Do not lick fingers or taste from mixing spoon while cooking.
EXPOSURE TO CONTAMINATED BODY FLUIDS	Avoid donating blood/plasma, body organs/parts and sperm. Others to wear a mask if the patient has a productive cough. Wear gloves when handling urinal/bedpan. Cover mouth with tissue or hand when sneezing/ coughing.
EXPOSURE TO CONTAMINATED HOUSEHOLD/MEDICAL EQUIPMENT	Scrub medical equipment with a 1:10 bleach:water solution or with a 70% alcohol solution. Clean soap dishes, denture cups and so forth weekly. Do not use the same sponge to clean the bathroom and kitchen. Do not pour mop water down the kitchen sink. Do not clean sponges/rags at the kitchen sink. Disinfect mops and sponges weekly by soaking in a 1:10 bleach:water solution for 5 minutes. Flush body wastes down the toilet. Do not clean bedpan/potty seats in the kitchen sink. Do not share towels, washcloths, lingerie/ undergarments and toothbrushes. Wash dishes/utensils between use and do not share them until washed. Launder the patient's clothes/linens separately using household detergent. Keep clothes/linens soiled by the patient in a plastic bag until laundered. Double bag soiled dressings/trash and discard with household trash. Put needles/syringes/sharp items in puncture-proof container prior to disposal. Flush contaminated cleaning fluids down the toilet. Use disposable items whenever possible/practical.
EXPOSURE TO PEOPLE WITH INFECTIOUS DISEASES	Avoid crowds. Avoid individuals who have recently been vaccinated. Avoid individuals with bacterial infections, cold sores, shingles, influenza, colds, chicken pox, measles and so forth.
EXPOSURE TO PET EXCRETA	Immunosuppressed persons should not clean bird cages, aquariums, litter boxes and so forth and should avoid areas where dogs are walked. Wear gloves when cleaning bird cages, litter boxes, aquariums and so forth.

Intradermal Injection Procedure

PURPOSE

- To conduct tuberculin skin testing.

EQUIPMENT

- tuberculin syringe 3/8- to 5/8-in, 26- or 27-gauge needle
- alcohol swabs
- vial/ampule of skin testing solution

Steps	Key Points
1. Explain the procedure and its purpose to the patient.	1. Knowing what to expect increases patient compliance.
2. Draw up the solution into the syringe.	2. Be sure to check the vial/ampule against the physician's order.
3. Have the patient sit facing you.	
4. Determine the injection site (Fig. 7–1) on the patient's inner forearm by placing one of your hands, palm down, on the patient's wrist and the other hand on the antecubital space of the patient. The area between your hands provides acceptable injection sites.	4. Select a site that has no scars or lesions and is not inflamed or hairy, since these interfere with accurate reading of the skin's reaction.
5. Have the patient flex his or her elbow and rest his or her forearm on a flat surface.	5. This step provides stability of the forearm.
6. Wipe the selected site with an alcohol swab.	
7. Stretch the skin of the selected site.	
8. Hold the syringe between your thumb and index finger with the needle at a 10- to 15-degree angle to the skin. Make sure the bevel is up.	8. The skin testing solution is less likely to be deposited in the tissue below the dermis when the bevel is up.
9. Insert the needle just under the skin's surface.	9. The needle can be seen through the skin.
10. Do not aspirate.	10. The dermis is relatively avascular.
11. Slowly inject the solution.	11. If resistance is felt, the needle is correctly inserted. The needle is probably too deeply inserted if the solution flows in easily.

UNIT 7

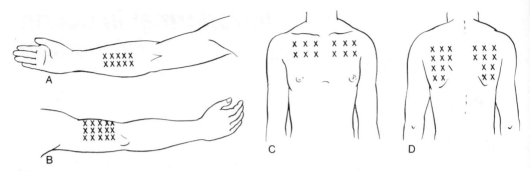

Figure 7–1. Intradermal injection sites. (From K. Sorensen and J. Luckmann, Basic Nursing, 2nd ed. Philadelphia: W. B. Saunders Co., 1986, p. 1080.)

12. During the injection, observe the injection site for balancing and for a wheal that is about 0.5 cm in diameter.
13. Withdraw the needle.
14. Do not massage the site.

15. Draw a circle around the perimeter of the wheal.
16. Instruct the patient
    a. not to wash the circle off
    b. not to cover the site with a bandage
    c. that a positive result does not necessarily mean tuberculosis
    d. that his or her physician may order further tests, e.g., a chest x-ray and sputum cultures, if the result is positive
    e. when you will return to read the skin's reaction.
17. Evaluate the skin's reaction 48 to 72 hours after the injection.
18. Measure any area of induration in millimeters at the largest diameter.
19. Report your findings to the attending physician.

12. If no wheal appears, the solution is probably in the subcutaneous tissue. The test is invalid, and the procedure must be repeated.

14. Massaging the site could distort the reading.

DOCUMENTATION

1. The type and amount of skin testing solution used.
2. The date and time of the injection.
3. The site of the injection.
4. The instructions given to the patient.

5. The patient's response to the procedure/instructions.
6. The scheduled date to evaluate the skin's reaction.
7. The actual date of evaluation and the test results/findings.
8. Notification of the attending physician of the test results/findings.
9. Date, time and method of the physician's notification.

Bibliography

Boland, M. and Klug, R. AIDS: The Implications for Home Care. American Journal of Maternal Child Nursing, 11: Nov.-Dec. 1986, pp. 404–411.

Coleman, D. How to Care for an AIDS Patient. RN, 1986, pp. 16–21.

Coping with AIDS. Rockville, Maryland: National Institute of Mental Health, 1986, DHHS Pub. No. (ADM) 85–1432.

Greenleaf, J. Infectious Waste From Home Care. Health Watch, 2(1): 1985, pp. 32–35.

Gurevich, I. and Tafuro, P. Nursing Measures for the Prevention of Infection in the Compromised Host. Nursing Clinics of North America, 20(1): 1985, pp. 257–260.

Jones I. You Can Drive Back Infection. Nursing, 1985, pp. 50–51.

LaCamera, D., et al. The Acquired Immunodeficiency Syndrome. Nursing Clinics of North America, 20(1): 1985, pp. 241–256.

Lilliard, J., et al. The Acquired Immunodeficiency Syndrome (A.I.D.S.) in Home Care: Maximizing Helpfulness and Minimizing Hysteria. Home Healthcare Nurse, 1984, pp. 11–16.

Owens, D., et al. Sexually Transmitted Diseases. American Association of Occupational Health Nurses Journal, 34(3): 1986, pp. 126–131.

Pfaff, S. and Terry, B. Infection and Control in the Home. Nursing Clinics of North America, 15(4): 1980, pp. 893–908.

End Stage of Life

Care Plans

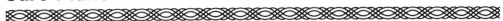

Imminent Death Care Plan

CROSS REFERENCES

Bereavement Care Plan
Bladder Incontinence Care Plan
Constipation Care Plan
Depression Care Plan
Ostomy Care Plan
Pain Care Plan

Spiritual Distress Care Plan
Terminal Illness Care Plan

Decubitus Care Procedure
Fecal Disimpaction Procedure
Post-Mortem Care Procedure
Pronouncement of Death Procedure

NURSING DIAGNOSES

1. Impaired physical mobility related to
   a. decreased strength
   b. pain
   c. neuromuscular/musculoskeletal impairment
   d. perceptual/cognitive impairment
   e. depression
   f. other.
2. Total self-care deficit related to
   a. decreased strength/activity tolerance
   b. pain
   c. neuromuscular/musculoskeletal impairment
   d. depression
   e. comatose/semicomatose state
   f. other.
3. Alteration in oral mucous membranes related to
   a. dehydration
   b. ineffective oral hygiene
   c. mouth breathing
   d. decreased salivation
   e. medications
   f. other.
4. Ineffective airway clearance (death rattle) related to
   a. thick secretions
   b. loss of muscle tone
   c. altered level of consciousness
   d. other.
5. Alteration in bowel/bladder elimination (incontinence) related to
   a. decreased sphincter control
   b. cognitive/perceptual impairment
   c. altered level of consciousness
   d. other.

UNIT 8

6. Alteration in bowel elimination (constipation) related to
   a. loss of muscle tone
   b. low fluid intake
   c. decreased activity
   d. medications
   e. other.
7. Sensory-perceptual alteration (visual, tactile, kinesthetic, gustatory, olfactory) related to
   a. ventilation-perfusion imbalance
   b. social isolation
   c. environmental monotony/complexity
   d. medications
   e. metabolic/neurological impairment
   f. other.
8. Anticipatory grieving of patient/family related to imminent death.
9. Ineffective family coping (compromised) related to
   a. situational crisis of imminent death
   b. inadequate understanding of imminent death
   c. role changes and family disorganization
   d. exhausted supportive capacity
   e. emotional/spiritual conflicts
   f. other.
10. Anxiety/fear of patient/family related to
    a. lack of understanding about clinical process of dying
    b. impending separation from significant other
    c. feeling of powerlessness
    d. other.
11. Knowledge deficit in recognition of imminent death related to
    a. lack of motivation to learn
    b. cognitive limitations
    c. sociocultural differences
    d. low readiness for acceptance of information
    e. other.

PROCESS INDICATORS

1. The patient's biopsychosocial and spiritual comfort will be sustained.
Indicators
   a. moist oral mucous membranes
   b. patient's validation (verbally or nonverbally) that pain/discomfort are controlled/ minimized
   c. elimination/lessening of death rattle
   d. patient's verbalization of thoughts and feelings about the proximity of death
   e. cleanliness of patient/environment.
2. The family will maintain its psychosocial and spiritual equilibrium.
Indicators
   a. each member's verbalization of thoughts and feelings about the proximity of death
   b. each member's participation in the patient's care during and after the period of imminent death
   c. each member's ability to tolerate physical proximity to the patient
   d. familial feedback reflects basic understanding about the clinical process of imminent death.

NURSING INTERVENTIONS

1. Provide instruction to the family/home health aide about
   a. clinical signs of imminent death (twitching, Cheyne-Stokes respirations, death rattle, mottling/cyanosis, cold skin, relaxation of facial muscles, blurred vision, difficulty speaking)
   b. general comfort measures (physical presence, warmth, analgesia, sedation, reality orientation, natural light source/dim lamp, personal hygiene)
   c. comfort measures for hydration (ice chips, cold fruit nectars, bland lip cream, humidifier, frequent oral hygiene, artificial saliva/tears)
   d. comfort measures for impaired mobility (frequent position changes, skin care, bowel/bladder care, positioning in body alignment, passive range of motion)
   e. comfort measures for altered respiration (medication, semi- to high Fowler position, oxygen therapy).
2. Help the family to
   a. reassure the patient through the moment of death (stroke/touch the patient, say goodbye to the patient)
   b. complete the post-mortem care and transfer of the patient
   c. arrange for the return of all medical equipment after death of the patient.
3. Arrange for additional support (home health aide, social worker, clergy, volunteer) as needed.
4. Request, if necessary, a prescription from the physician for atropine 0.4 mg subcutaneously, as needed for death rattle.
5. Provide opportunities that facilitate the patient's independent action/decision making.
6. Create situations that encourage the patient/family to express their thoughts and feelings.
7. Participate in the pronouncement of death according to state regulations.
8. Provide post-mortem care.
9. Initiate bereavement follow-up for the survivors.
10. Alert the physician about the patient's imminent death and provide a discharge summary when the case is closed.

UNIT 8

THERAPEUTIC ACHIEVEMENT

- The family will identify the period of imminent death as a satisfying experience of separation from the patient.

RELATED PATIENT INSTRUCTIONS

Care for the Patient Confined to Bed	Pain Medications
Clinical Signs of Imminent Death	Range of Motion Exercises
Constipation	Skin Care
Comfort Measures for Dehydration	Urinary Catheter Care
Oxygen Therapy	

Terminal Illness Care Plan

CROSS REFERENCES

Bereavement Care Plan
Constipation Care Plan
Imminent Death Care Plan
Pain Care Plan

Domestic Violence Assessment/Intervention
   Procedure
Home Health Aide Supervision Procedure

Home Safety Procedure
Oxygen Therapy Procedure
Range of Motion Exercises Procedure
Telephone Contact with Patient/Family
   Procedure

Medication Compliance Management Guidelines

NURSING DIAGNOSES

1. Alteration in bowel elimination (constipation) related to
   a. loss of muscle tone
   b. low fluid intake
   c. decreased activity
   d. medications
   e. other.
2. Anxiety/fear related to
   a. religious conflicts
   b. isolation/abandonment
   c. the unknown
   d. concern about significant others
   e. pain
   f. other.
3. Alteration in nutrition (less than body requirements) related to
   a. nausea
   b. altered taste sensation
   c. constipation/obstruction
   d. depression/anxiety
   e. anorexia
   f. hypermetabolic demands of disease
   g. other.
4. Grieving related to
   a. loss of self-esteem
   b. loss of functional capacity
   c. anticipated cessation of self
   d. separation from significant others
   e. other.
5. Impaired physical mobility related to
   a. weakness/fatigue
   b. dyspnea
   c. anticipated/actual pain
   d. surgical intervention

    e. anticipation/actual nausea and vomiting

    f. depression

    g. other.

6. Potential/actual impairment of skin integrity related to

    a. inadequate hygiene/skin care

    b. decreased mobility/immobility

    c. cachexia/skeletal prominence

    d. frequent contact with the products of elimination

    e. pruritus

    f. other.

7. Alteration in family process related to

    a. role changes and family disorganization

    b. exhausted supportive capacity

    c. emotional/spiritual conflicts

    d. unpredictable cycle of remission/exacerbation

    e. discrepancy between familial expectations and patient capabilities

    f. familial response to patient's anorexia

    g. other.

8. Alteration in oral mucous membrane related to

    a. inadequate/ineffective oral hygiene

    b. mouth breathing

    c. low fluid intake

    d. medications

    e. oxygen therapy

    f. decreased/lack of salivation

    g. poor fit of dentures

    h. other.

9. Ineffective breathing pattern related to

    a. decreased lung expansion

    b. altered oxygen-carrying capacity of blood

    c. pain

    d. fluid collection in lungs

    e. anxiety

    f. other.

10. Alteration in thought processes related to

    a. touch/tactile deprivation

    b. depression/anxiety

    c. medication

    d. physical exhaustion

    e. other.

11. Potential/actual fluid volume deficit related to

    a. low fluid intake

    b. emesis

    c. diarrhea

    d. medication

    e. hypermetabolic demands of disease

    f. other.

12. Knowledge deficit (skin care, oral hygiene, relaxation/stress management techniques, medications, nutritional maintenance, personal energy conservation methods, comfort

UNIT 8

measures, pulmonary toilet, odor control, bowel/bladder maintenance, pain management, community resources) related to
    a. cognitive limitations
    b. sociocultural differences
    c. low readiness for acceptance of information
    d. misinterpretation of information
    e. denial
    f. other.
13. Potential for injury related to
    a. impaired motor coordination
    b. environmental hazards
    c. lack of awareness of safety hazards
    d. lack of adequate supervision
    e. other.
14. Alteration in comfort (pain) related to
    a. neuromuscular impairment
    b. obstruction
    c. immobility
    d. anxiety/depression
    e. insomnia
    f. other.

PROCESS INDICATORS

1. The patient's biopsychosocial and spiritual discomforts are alleviated.
Indicators
    a. moist oral mucous membranes
    b. bowel/bladder patterns are regular and continent
    c. no skin irritation/breakdown
    d. patient is not dehydrated
    e. patient is alert
    f. patient validates (verbally or nonverbally) that pain/discomfort is minimized/controlled
    g. patient is oriented to time, place, person and event
    h. patient's independent performance of activities of daily living are realistically commensurate with his or her capabilities
    i. patient spontaneously shares thoughts/feelings about his or her condition, changing lifestyle, losses and so forth
    j. patient exhibits a reduction in anxiety-induced thoughts, feelings and behaviors
    k. cleanliness of the patient/environment
    l. patient expresses contentment with his or her personal interpretation of the meaning of life
    m. activity coordinated between the patient's acute care and home care systems.
2. The family's psychosocial and spiritual integrity are supported.
Indicators
    a. each member's participation in the patient's care
    b. each member's verbalization of thoughts and feelings about the patient's final illness
    c. each member's ability to maintain hope within a realistic context.

NURSING INTERVENTIONS

1. Assess the patient
   a. vital signs
   b. skin integrity
   c. bowel/bladder elimination pattern
   d. pulmonary status
   e. signs/symptoms of dehydration
   f. nutritional status/appetite
   g. patterns of food consumption/fluid intake
   h. pattern of sleep/rest/activity
   i. psychological status
   j. level of comfort/discomfort
   k. cognitive ability.
2. Assess
   a. availability/reliability of support systems
   b. interactions between the patient and family members
   c. environmental/safety hazards
   d. each family member's psychological status
   e. each family member for signs of psychological/physical stress
   f. family's understanding of and response to the emotional stages of terminal illness
   g. what meaning the patient/family attaches to the terminal illness
   h. each family member's degree of preparation for the loss
   i. each family member's risk for complicated grieving.
3. Provide instruction to the patient/family/home health aide about
   a. general comfort measures (physical presence, warmth, reality orientation, personal hygiene, back rubs, bland lip cream, humidified air, uncluttered environment, artificial saliva)
   b. skin care
   c. positioning techniques
   d. active/passive range of motion exercises
   e. decubitus care
   f. care for oral ulcerations (rinse with saline or a 1:1 saline/hydrogen peroxide mixture at least every 2 hours, use of a topical anesthetic, avoidance of smoking/alcohol, avoidance of extremely hot/cold foods, use of soft foods with low acid content)
   g. stress management/relaxation techniques
   h. techniques to conserve personal energy
   i. oxygen therapy
   j. medications (purpose, side effects, precautions, administration)
   k. environmental modifications for home safety
   l. importance of supervision that is vigilant but does not suffocate the patient's self-care
   m. interventions for sleeplessness (quiet/darkened environment, warm milk, small amount of wine, warm baths, soft music)
   n. techniques to stimulate appetite (food at room temperature or slightly chilled, use of high-calorie/protein supplements served over ice or with added flavors, eating at least a third of the day's total dietary requirements during breakfast, frequent snacks/small meals throughout the day, socialization during meals)

UNIT 8

    o. clinical progression of terminal illness

    p. odor control techniques (room deodorizer, sprinkle spirits of peppermint/oils of wintergreen on bed linens, regular cleansing of affected area/source of odor, topical application of a multienzyme biocatalytic odor eliminator)

    q. management of pruritus (skin moisturizers, avoidance of perfumed soaps, use of cotton clothes/bed linens, soft/loose fitting clothes/slippers, activities that divert the patient's attention)

    r. bowel/bladder management

    s. pain management techniques (distraction, hypnosis, imagery, therapeutic touch, transcutaneous electrical nerve stimulation (TENS), pharmacological interventions)

    t. the importance of maintaining an adequate daily fluid intake (use of juices, bouillon, water, Gatorade, ice pops and Jello).

4. Refer to the dentist, as necessary.
5. Refer to the dietician and coordinate the patient's/family's utilization of the dietician's teaching to promote/maintain the patient's nutritional status.
6. Coordinate referrals, as necessary, to
    a. social worker
    b. physical therapist
    c. occupational therapist
    d. durable medical equipment suppliers
    e. pharmacists
    f. spiritual advisers
    g. respite volunteers
    h. hospice care workers
    i. self-help support groups
    j. legal aid service
    k. financial counselling service.
7. Provide opportunities that facilitate the patient's independent action/decision making.
8. Create situations that encourage the patient/family to express their thoughts and feelings.
9. Request/obtain orders, as necessary, from the attending physician.
10. Provide progress notes and a discharge summary to the attending physician.

THERAPEUTIC ACHIEVEMENT

- The patient/family demonstrates an adequate ability to cope with the ramifications of catastrophic illness.
- The patient/family verbalizes personal satisfaction with the dying process.
- The patient remains as long as reasonable/feasible in the customary setting of his or her life.

Pediatric Considerations

1. The terminally ill child continues to have developmental needs that must be met.

2. The dying child is often aware of the severity of his or her illness or that his or her illness has a special significance.

3. The child with a life-threatening illness is likely to feel isolated from significant others. Separation anxiety is a critical issue.

Children's Concepts of Death

Age Range	Concepts of Death
Under 2 years	No evidence the child is aware of death.
3–5 years	Perceive death as temporary or as life under different circumstances.
	Intermingle reality and death-related fantasy.
6–10 years	Personification of death as something to be eluded.
	Beginning awareness of the universality of death but do not see death as inevitable.
	Concern about the ceremonial rites for the dead.
11 years to adolescence	Perceive death as a personal and internal phenomenon.
	Understand the permanence of death.
	Understand the universal and inevitable nature of death.
	Interest in the concept of afterlife.

4. The dying child's anxiety can increase to the point of mental and physical exhaustion as his or her perception of death is refined and his or her awareness of future time develops. (Future time has little meaning for children under 7 years old.)

RELATED PATIENT INSTRUCTIONS

Care for the Patient Confined to Bed
Clinical Signs of Imminent Death
Constipation
Comfort Measures for Dehydration
General Comfort Measures
Heparin Lock
Intramuscular Injections

Intravenous Therapy
Oxygen Therapy
Pain Medications
Range of Motion Exercises
Reality Orientation
Skin Care
Ways to Save Your Energy

UNIT 8

Procedures

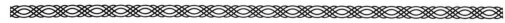

Post-Mortem Care Procedure

PURPOSE

- To prepare the patient for transfer.
- To protect the body prior to final viewing.

EQUIPMENT

- shroud
- gauze rolls
- absorbent pads
- identification tags
- bath equipment

Special Note for Communicable Diseases

1. Obtain/use special post-mortem packs (defined by agency policy).
2. Alert the funeral director/mortician/others who may handle the body of its possible infectiousness.
3. Maintain disease-appropriate precautions while doing post-mortem care.
4. Label the shrouded body "Caution Communicable Disease," specifying the communicable disease present.
5. Secure all patient-contaminated syringes/needles/sharps in a puncture proof container prior to double-bagged disposal.
6. Double-bag all patient-contaminated tubes, drains, dressings and so forth for disposal with the household trash.
7. Bag all patient-contaminated linen and clothing for laundering according to disease-appropriate precautions.

Steps	Key Points
1. Notify the attending physician of the patient's death.	1. During this time, help the family through closure with the patient. Stay physically near, answer their questions, and encourage them to touch or speak to the deceased.
2. Verify the pronouncement of death.	2. Family members who want to participate in post-mortem care should be allowed to do so.
3. Notify the funeral director, religious support person and so forth or delegate this responsibility to the family.	

4. Place the patient in a supine position with the head slightly elevated. Maintain proper body alignment.
5. Place clean dentures in the patient's mouth and close the mouth by applying slight pressure.
6. Close the patient's eyes. Do not use pressure. Apply paper tape or damp cotton balls if needed.
7. Remove all external objects (clothing, tubing, jewelry and so forth).
8. Bathe the patient.
9. Place absorbent pads against the patient's buttocks and any draining wounds.

10. Place one absorbent pad under the patient's chin and secure with gauze. Do not tie tightly.

    10. Avoid creating ridges or marks on the patient's face, neck and hands.

11. Using absorbent pads and gauze, cross and tie ankles.
12. Using absorbent pads and gauze, cross and tie wrists on top of the patient's chest.

    12. Nursing actions should be completed quietly, quickly and with respect. If a family member is assisting, brief explanations about what is being done and reminiscing about the patient are supportive.

13. Attach an identification (ID) tag to the patient's big toe.
14. Place the patient in the shroud.
15. Attach an ID tag to the outside of the shroud.
16. Dispose of used items.
17. Bag and label items that will accompany the patient.
18. Arrange for the return of all medical equipment.
19. Remain with the family until the patient is transferred.

UNIT
8

DOCUMENTATION

1. Circumstances of death event.
2. Time the attending physician was notified of the death.
3. Time that death was pronounced and by whom.
4. Condition of the patient's body.
5. Activities of post-mortem care.
6. Time and destination of the patient transfer.
7. Emotional status of the family.
8. Presence of supportive personnel (clergy).
9. Plans for bereavement contact.

Pronouncement of Death Procedure

PURPOSE

- To make the determination and pronouncement of death.
- To report the patient's death according to state law.

EQUIPMENT

- flashlight
- sphygmomanometer
- stethoscope
- death certificate

Special Considerations. The agency is providing service to the patient. The responsibility for pronouncement has been transferred to the agency by the physician and has been documented by the physician in the chart. The nurse does not suspect or see evidence of foul play at the place of death. Registered nurses may pronounce death by state law in New Jersey and New Hampshire.

Steps	Key Points
1. Go to the patient's place of residence.	

2. Examine the patient and verify
  a. absence of respirations
  b. absence of heartbeat/pulses
  c. absence of blood pressure
  d. fixed, dilated pupils.
	2. If the family is present, explain the procedure. Complete nursing actions quietly, quickly and with respect.

3. If criteria for coroner cases are evident, notify the agency, the attending physician and the coroner.	3. Criteria for coroner cases are state-specific.
4. If the coroner's criteria are not evident, make the pronouncement of death.	
5. Notify the physician of the death.	
6. Notify the funeral director of the death.	
7. Complete the death certificate as specified by state law.	
8. Notify the agency of the death.	

DOCUMENTATION

1. Circumstances of death event.
2. Condition/position of patient's body upon nurse's arrival at place of residence.
3. Date, time and place of death pronouncement.
4. Times the attending physician, funeral director, agency and, if appropriate, coroner were notified.
5. Emotional status of family.

Bibliography

Conrad, N. Spiritual Support for the Dying. Nursing Clinics of North America, 20(2): June 1985, pp. 415–426.

Corr, C. and Corr, D. Pediatric Hospice Care. Pediatrics, 76(5):1985, pp. 774–780.

Gonda, T. and Ruark, J. Dying Dignified: The Health Professional's Guide to Care. Menlo Park, California: Addison-Wesley Publishing Company, 1984.

Green, P. The Pivotal Role of the Nurse in Hospice Care. Ca. A Cancer Journal for Clinicians, 34(4): 1984, pp. 204–205.

Martinson, I. Home Care for the Dying Child: Professional and Family Perspectives. New York: Appleton-Century-Crofts, 1976.

Martocchio, B. Grief and Bereavement: Healing Through Hurt. Nursing Clinics of North America, 20(2):June 1985, pp. 327–341.

Ross-Alaolmolki, K. Supportive Care for Families of Dying Children. Nursing Clinics of North America, 20(2):June 1985, pp. 457–466.

UNIT 8

Impaired Comfort

Care Plans

Pain Care Plan

CROSS REFERENCE

Transcutaneous Electrical Nerve Stimulation
(TENS) Procedure

NURSING DIAGNOSES

1. Alteration in comfort (pain) related to
   a. noxious stimulus
   b. life-threatening stress
   c. psychic conversion
   d. organic trauma
   e. tissue damage
   f. other.
2. Impaired physical mobility related to
   a. anticipation of discomfort
   b. pain
   c. decreased strength/endurance
   d. other.
3. Self-care deficit (feeding, hygiene, grooming, toileting) related to
   a. perceived/actual loss of functional capacity
   b. anticipation of discomfort
   c. decreased strength/endurance
   d. pain
   e. other.
4. Sleep pattern disturbance related to
   a. pain/discomfort
   b. depression
   c. anxiety
   d. other.
5. Knowledge deficit (nutritional maintenance, relaxation/stress management techniques, personal energy conservation methods, medications, pain pathology, comfort measures, personal hygiene) related to
   a. misinterpretation of information
   b. lack of or low readiness to learn
   c. cognitive limitations
   d. sociocultural differences
   e. other.
6. Anxiety/fear related to
   a. dependency
   b. feeling of powerlessness

UNIT 9

    c. belief that the pain is punishment

    d. anticipated suffering

    e. other.

7. Alteration in thought process related to
    a. neurological impairment
    b. severe/panic level anxiety
    c. belief that pain is punishment
    d. pain or reduced pain tolerance
    e. other.

8. Social isolation related to preoccupation with pain.

9. Ineffective individual coping related to
    a. lack of adequate support system
    b. poor nutrition
    c. insufficient financial resources
    d. multiple losses or bereavement overload
    e. unrealistic expectations of self or others
    f. depression
    g. other.

10. Grieving related to
    a. perceived/actual loss of functional capacity
    b. perceived/actual loss of job/income
    c. other.

11. Diversional activity deficit related to
    a. loss of functional ability
    b. lack of environmental stimulation/diversity
    c. other.

12. Spiritual distress related to belief that pain is a punishment.

PROCESS INDICATORS

1. The patient's sensation/perception of pain is modified.

Indicators

    a. utilization of noninvasive techniques of pain control (stress management, relaxation/ autosuggestion, imagery, distraction, hot/cold application, TENS, massage)

    b. identification/reduction/elimination of factors that precipitate his or her pain

    c. verbalization/demonstration of increased tolerance for activity

    d. validation (verbally or nonverbally) that his or her level of comfort is increased

    e. patient/family recalls the purpose, side effects and precautions for prescribed medications/treatments

    f. patient/family demonstrates appropriate use/administration of medications.

2. The patient's biopsychosocial integrity is maintained.

Indicators

    a. realistic identification of his or her physical limitations

    b. demonstration of an adequate/appropriate level of personal hygiene/grooming

    c. bowel/bladder habits are regular and continent

    d. weight loss/malnutrition not experienced

    e. maintenance of his or her social/occupational responsibilities

    f. verbalization of acceptance of/comfort with dependency needs

    g. reduction in anxiety-induced thoughts, feelings and behaviors

    h. demonstration of personal energy conservation techniques

i. the patient/family validates a balance between rest, nutrition and exercise
j. patient/family feedback reflecting an understanding of the pain pathology.

NURSING INTERVENTIONS

1. Assess the patient's pain.
   a. pain behaviors (facial expressions, writhing, splinting, guarding, restlessness)
   b. associated symptoms (weakness, sweating, diarrhea/constipation, nausea, vomiting, tachycardia/bradycardia, increased respiratory rate, pale/ashen face, hypotension, disorientation, shortness of breath, dehydration)
   c. site/location of the pain
   d. timing/frequency/duration of the pain
   e. character/quality of the pain
   f. how/if the pain interferes with safety and performance of activity of daily life
   g. what the pain means to the patient
   h. effects the pain has on the patient
   i. what secondary gains are associated with the pain
   j. behaviors/interventions that relieve the pain
   k. precipitating factors
   l. how the patient talks about the pain.
2. Assess the patient.
   a. activity pattern
   b. sleep pattern
   c. bowel/bladder elimination pattern
   d. level/quality of personal hygiene/grooming
   e. nutritional status/appetite
   f. patterns of food consumption/fluid intake
   g. losses
   h. psychological status
   i. pattern of medication use
   j. side effects associated with the medications
   k. ethnic/cultural factors that influence perception of/reaction to pain.
3. Differentiate among
   a. the pain, depression and functional impairment
   b. the types of pain the patient is experiencing (acute, chronic, progressive).
4. Assess the family.
   a. availability/reliability of support systems
   b. ethnic/cultural factors that influence perception of/reaction to the patient's pain.
5. Teach the patient/family about
   a. medications (purpose, side effects, administration)
   b. comfort measures (loose-fitting/soft clothes, reality orientation, natural light source/dim lamp)
   c. techniques to conserve personal energy
   d. stress management/relaxation techniques
   e. TENS
   f. cutaneous stimulation techniques (back rubs/massages with lotions or menthol creams; hot/cold applications; sponge baths; rhythmic/constant motion of moderate intensity)
   g. importance/value of distraction (television, radio, reading, needlework, music, hobbies, imagery, socialization)

UNIT 9

    h. personal hygiene
    i. positioning techniques
    j. methods to induce sleep
    k. methods to relieve/prevent constipation.

6. Assist the patient/family to develop a schedule of medication administration that satisfies the patient's need for pain management but that creates minimal interference with the patient's alertness and physical strength/safety.
7. Confer and coordinate interventions with
    a. social worker
    b. occupational therapist
    c. physical therapist
    d. pastoral care provider
    e. dietician.
8. Refer the patient/family to
    a. mental health counselor
    b. self-help groups.
9. Provide opportunities that facilitate the patient's independent action/decision-making.
10. Create situations that encourage the patient/family to express their thoughts and feelings about the pain.
11. Request/obtain orders, as necessary, from the primary physician.
12. Send progress notes/discharge summary to the attending physician.

THERAPEUTIC ACHIEVEMENTS

- The patient experiences an alleviation of the pain-related symptomatology.

RELATED PATIENT INSTRUCTIONS

Care for the Patient Confined to Bed	Range of Motion Exercises
General Comfort Measures	Skin Care
Intramuscular Injections	

Procedures

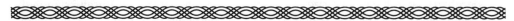

Decubitus Care Procedure

PURPOSE

- To treat open skin areas.
- To promote wound/skin healing.
- To prevent additional skin breakdown.

EQUIPMENT

- solution to clean skin
- skin treatments (protective ointments, prescribed medications or ointments)
- dressings (sterile/clean gauze; transparent, moisture- and vapor-permeable dressing or pouching system)
- adhesive tape
- clean/sterile gloves
- bag for waste

Steps

1. Gather supplies.
2. Wash hands.
3. Explain procedure to patient/family.
4. Position the patient comfortably.

5. If patient has a dressing follow agency policy for its removal.

6. Don clean/sterile gloves.
7. Cleanse the skin with warm water and a nonalkaline, nondrying soap (e.g., Dove, Basis, Purpose, Castile) or skin cleaning solution per physician's order. Clean in a spiral motion from the center out.
8. Pat the skin dry with a cloth or gauze.
9. Clean the decubitus with the solution prescribed by the physician or designated by agency policy. Use a new sterile gauze for each wipe, moving from the center outward.

Key Points

4. Provide for privacy. Expose only the skin area to be treated.
5. A plastic bag must be used for wet dressings. Note the number of saturated dressings.

7. Assess patient's allergies before using any antiseptic. Hydrogen peroxide will loosen dried blood. Gently massage the skin while cleaning.

9. Deep and/or draining wounds may require irrigation.

UNIT
9

10. Assess the condition of the skin and decubitus. Note the wound size (width, length and depth), wound color, skin color (including width of discoloration), drainage color and odor.
11. Pat the decubitus dry with gauze sponges moving from the center outward.
12. Remove gloves and discard in waste bag.
13. Perform prescribed therapy (e.g., wet dressings, medications, ointment and heat).

14. Apply protective ointment to the skin around the decubitus if ordered.
15. Apply the dressing following the physician's and/or agency's policy (e.g., wet dressings, dry sterile, dry unsterile, pouching system or a transparent, moisture- and vapor-permeable dressing).
16. Wash hands.
17. Assist with positioning the patient.

10. The staging method for wound classification provides a useful standardized reference. Each stage has a corresponding treatment goal and a wound-cleansing and wound-dressing set of guidelines.

13. Pressure sore grading provides guidance for successful protocols. (Refer to Pressure Sore Grading Guidelines, which follows.)

Pressure Sore Grading Guidelines

Stage/Skin Appearance

Stage 1
1. Erythema that turns white upon finger pressure.
2. Warmth/tenderness.

Stage 2
1. Distinct break in the skin (excoriation, blistering or slight ulceration; drainage).
2. Skin temperature variable.

Stage 3
1. Broken skin exposing subcutaneous tissue.
2. Infection or cellulitis may be present.

Treatment

1. Lubricating creams.

2. Protective coverings (moisture- and vapor-permeable dressings, hydroactive dressings, vasodilator sprays).
3. Pressure relief devices, massage and turning schedule (appropriate for all stages).

1. Clean the wound prior to treatment.

2. Protective coverings (moisture- and vapor-permeable dressings, hydroactive dressings, vasodilator sprays).

1. Clean the wound prior to treatment, usually with antibacterial agent.
2. Dressings to absorb drainage (granular types, gel-like types).
3. Enzyme medicated ointments.

Stage 4

1. Tissue destruction extends to the level of muscle or bone.
2. Decayed areas may be larger than apparent wound.

1. After medical débridement, clean wound as prescribed.
2. See *Stage 3*.

DOCUMENTATION

1. Wound assessment (pressure sore grading, size, width, length, depth, drainage color, odor and number of saturated dressings).
2. Skin color around the decubitus.
3. Cleansing solution and method.
4. Medications/other prescribed therapies.
5. Type of dressing used.
6. Nursing assessment of wound progress.
7. Patient response.
8. Patient's/family's participation in maintaining turning/positioning schedule, nutrition and skin care.
9. Report to the primary physician.

UNIT
9

Suture/Staple Removal Procedure

PURPOSE

* To remove nonabsorable sutures/staples without subcutaneous contamination or dermal irritation.

EQUIPMENT

* suture removal tray/kit
   antiseptic swab
   forceps
   scissors
* sterile gloves if needed
* dressings
* tape
* bag for waste
* staple remover
* wound closure strips

Steps	**Key Points**
1. Confirm the physician's order as to the date and number of sutures to be removed.	
2. Gather supplies.	
3. Wash hands.	
4. Explain the procedure to the patient.	
5. Position the patient comfortably.	5. Assist the patient to assume a position that allows for the best visualization and stabilization of the sutured area. Props or assistance may be required. A small child or a confused adult may need restraint.
6. Prepare sterile area with necessary supplies.	
7. If a dressing is present, follow agency policy for dressing removal.	7. A plastic bag must be used for wet dressings.
8. Inspect the wound.	8. Assess wound healing/integrity of suture line; absence of signs and symptoms of infection.
9. Don sterile gloves, if needed.	
10. Cleanse the suture area thoroughly with an antiseptic swab. Clean from the suture line outward.	10. Assess patient's allergies before using any antiseptic. Hydrogen peroxide will loosen dried blood at the suture line.

For Intermittent Sutures

11. Place gauze by the suture line.
12. Hold the scissors in the dominant hand and the forceps in the non-dominant hand.
13. Grasp the knot of the suture with forceps and gently pull upward.

14. Cut the short end of the suture as close as possible to the skin (between the knot and the skin surface) (Fig. 9–1).

15. Remove the entire suture with the forceps using a continuous smooth action. Pull the suture by the knot upward. Place the suture on the gauze.
16. Observe for any signs of separation of wound edges before removing all sutures.

17. Repeat steps 14, 15 and 16 until all sutures are removed.
18. Refer to Wound Care.

13. Pull the suture away from the skin enough to allow free movement of the scissors.
14. Never snip both ends of the suture.

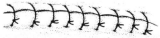

Figure 9–1. Intermittent sutures.

15. Do not pull any part of the suture that is on *top* of the skin's surface, *beneath* the skin's surface (may cause subcutaneous contamination).

16. To better determine the status of questionable wound healing, remove every other suture. Assess if the suture line remains closed before removing all sutures.

For Continuous Sutures

11. Place gauze by the suture line.
12. Hold the scissors in the dominant hand and the forceps in the non-dominant hand.
13. Grasp the knot of the suture with forceps and gently pull upward.
14. Cut the suture at each skin penetration on one side only of the suture line (the side the knot is on should be used) (Fig. 9–2).

15. Grasp the suture with forceps from the opposite side skin opening. Pull the suture out gently.

16. Observe for any signs of separation of wound edges.

17. Refer to Wound Care, which follows.

14. Pull the suture away from the skin enough to allow free movement of the scissors.

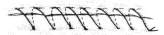

Figure 9–2. Continuous sutures.

15. Avoid subcutaneous contamination. Do not pull any part of the suture that is on *top of* the skin's surface, *beneath* the skin's surface.

16. Assess status of wound healing; wound closure strips may need to be applied.

UNIT 9

For Staple Removal

11. Place a gauze by the suture line.
12. Place the lower tip of the staple remover under the first staple.

13. Hold the hand with the staple remover off the skin surface to prevent contamination and to avoid excessive pressure on the suture line (Fig. 9–3).
14. As soon as both ends of the staple are free from the skin, remove the staple and place on the gauze or in refuse bag.
15. Refer to Wound Care, which follows.

12. Be sure to close the handles completely so that the ends of the staples bend upward and simultaneously exit the insertion sites.

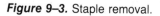

Figure 9–3. Staple removal.

Wound Care

1. Pat the wound site with antiseptic swab.
2. Apply wound closure strips, if needed.
3. Apply a dressing, if needed.
4. Dispose of sutures/staples and other disposable equipment in the refuse bag.
5. Wash hands.
6. Instruct patient/family in proper wound management (dressing change, wound closure strip care, signs and symptoms of infection, when to notify the nurse or doctor).

1. Avoid traumatizing the wound surface.
2. Wound closure strips maintain skin approximation.

DOCUMENTATION

1. Date and time of suture/staple removal.
2. Number of sutures/staples removed, number remaining, if appropriate.
3. Condition of wound and skin prior to and after suture removal.
4. Presence and condition of any drainage devices.
5. Type of dressing and/or wound closure strips, if used.
6. Patient's response and tolerance to procedure.
7. Instructions given to the patient/family regarding wound care.
8. Report to the primary physician procedure performed and any abnormal findings.

Transcutaneous Electrical Nerve Stimulation (TENS) Procedure

PURPOSE

- To relieve the patient's pain.

EQUIPMENT

- TENS stimulator
- batteries/battery pack (per manufacturer's guide)
- electrodes
- conductor gel/pads ⎫
- tape   ⎬ depends on the type of electrode used
- water   ⎭

CONTRAINDICATIONS

- cardiac arrythmia
- myocardia ischemia/infarction
- pacemaker
- pregnancy

Steps

1. Obtain an order for TENS from the attending physician.
2. Explain the procedure and review the equipment with the patient.
3. Select the area for electrode placement.
   a. refer to the manufacturer's guide for suggested sites
   b. directly over the painful area
   c. at trigger points innervated by same spinal cord segment as pain area
   d. along peripheral nerve pathways
   e. at acupuncture/acupressure points.
4. Apply the electrodes.
   a. there must be complete contact between the skin and the electrode
   b. position the electrodes 2 to 18 in apart.

Key Points

2. Knowing what to expect increases patient compliance.
3. Never apply electrodes over the patient's eyes, carotid sinus nerves, pharyngeal/laryngeal muscles, hair, skin prep areas, incisions/sutures, broken skin or irritated skin.

4. Use water or conductive gel/pads as appropriate.

UNIT
9

5. Set the pulse width at midrange and the amplitude at its lowest rate.
6. Have the patient turn on the stimulator and increase the amplitude until stimulation is perceived.
7. Tell the patient to continue increasing the rate until the sensation is slightly uncomfortable; then have him or her reduce the rate to a strong but comfortable level.
8. Ask the patient where the stimulation is felt and what it is he or she feels.

7. The goal is to produce a sensation that is pleasant and that relieves pain. The patient should learn to rely on the feeling rather than on the calibrated rates.
8. If the stimulation is not sensed in the pain area, change the electrode placements and/or increase the pulse widths.

9. Instruct the patient to report any changes in pain characteristics or levels of discomfort.

9. Changes may be indicative of an alteration in the patient's condition, of a potential complication or of another disorder.

10. Teach the patient how to cope with skin irritation.
    a. use hypoallergic tape/Velcro/elastic bandage to secure the electrode
    b. mix cortisone cream with the conductor gel
    c. change brand of gel
    d. clean skin and electrodes (if electrodes are not disposable) frequently with soap and water
    e. reposition electrodes off any irritated areas.
11. Provide instructions to the patient about frequency of use.

11. Frequency of use is individualized and depends upon why the TENS is prescribed.

12. Instruct the patient regarding electrical safety.
13. When no relief is felt by the patient
    a. use another type/brand of stimulator
    b. if using continuous stimulation, try intermittent stimulation or, if using intermittent stimulation, try continuous stimulation
    c. consult with the physical therapist regarding alternative placement of the electrodes
    d. assess for impediments to TENS effectiveness (central nervous system drugs, greater than 20 mg diazepam daily, alcohol abuse, regular use of narcotics).
14. Teach the procedure to at least one other responsible family member.

DOCUMENTATION

1. The teaching, the procedure, the name/relationship of the person taught if other than the patient.
2. The patient's/family's response to the procedure.
3. The patient's behavioral changes secondary to pain relief.
4. The sensations and pain levels during and between TENS treatment.
5. Alternative measures used, if necessary.
6. Brand/type of unit; number, position and type of electrodes; frequency of treatments.
7. The need for continued/reinforced teaching/monitoring until the pain is controlled or the patient is satisfied.

Resources

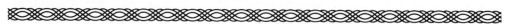

Pain Perception in School-Age Children

Pain Perception in School-Age Children*

5 to 7 years	8 to 12 years
Fears body mutilation	Fears body injury
Cannot localize or describe pain	Can define intensity of pain on scale of 1 to 10; can point to region of pain if pain is not constant.
Pain equated with punishment. Perceives infliction of pain as deliberate and mean.	Understands the reason for pain if it is explained and sees inflicted pain as necessary to improve health.
Not reassured by statements that the pain will be brief.	Understands and is reassured by the time limits of pain.
Determines what is painful and how to react to pain by others' reactions and by the nature of the equipment involved.	Exaggerates every little scratch, tends to brag about his or her hurts and compares them with those of siblings and peers. He or she submerges the fear of pain in bravado or nervous behavior. Fears being treated like a baby or succumbing to tears during pain.
Centers on one object as the source of pain.	Comprehends causes of pain. Pain creates self anger because a child this age dislikes the physical restrictions imposed by pain.

*Tackett, J. M. and Hunsbergher, M. Family-Centered Care of Children and Adolescents. Philadelphia: W. B. Saunders Co., 1978.

Adult Intramuscular Injection Sites

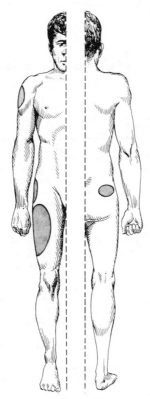

Adult intramuscular injection sites. (From DuGas, B. Introduction to Patient Care. Philadelphia: W. B. Saunders Co., 1977, p. 469.)

Allergies: Telltale Signs

PHYSICAL

- nasal speech
- mouth breathing
- coughing spells followed by wheezing
- repetitive sneezing
- allergic shiners (dark circles under eyes)
- conjunctivitis
- eczema on the edge of the upper eyelid

BEHAVIORAL

- recurrent clearing of throat
- rubbing of eyes and/or nose (allergic salute)
- nocturnal tooth grinding
- listlessness
- weakness
- unnatural fatigue alternating with unpredictable bursts of activity

Itching: Home Remedies

Home Remedies to Relieve the Itch*

Problem	Remedy
BEE/WASP STINGS	Add a little water to meat tenderizer powder and rub into the bite.
JELLYFISH BITES	Urinate on area.
sea anemone stings	Dab mud onto the bite.
	Add a little water to cornstarch and rub into the bite.
POISON IVY	Rub Ban roll-on deodorant onto the rash.
	Wash the rash with brown laundry soap and warm water.
	Apply compresses of Burow's solution.
CHICKENPOX	Spray the lesions with spray starch.
	Strong tea with sugar can be used as a mouthwash or gargle for mouth sores.
	Bathe in a tub of warm water and 4 tablespoons cornstarch.
CHIGGER BITES	Paint each bite with clear nail polish.
	Cover each bite with petroleum jelly.

*Data from McMillan, J. A., Stockman, J. A., and Oski, F. A.: The Whole Pediatrician Catalogue, Vol. 3. Philadelphia: W. B. Saunders Co., 1982, p. 355.

Pediatric Injection Sites

Pediatric Injection Sites. *A*, Vastus lateralis site. The site is located in the midthird of the thigh and is found by dividing the thigh into thirds from the greater trochanter of the femur to just above the knee. The area of insertion within the midthird of the thigh is found midway between imaginary lines midanteriorly and midlaterally. *B*, Deltoid site. The site is located in the lower part of the upper third of the deltoid. The site of insertion is midway between the acromion and the axilla on the lateral surface of the arm. *C*, Ventrogluteal site. The site is located by placing the palm on the greater trochanter, the index finger on the anterior iliac spine (this may be facilitated by flexing of the thigh at the hip); the middle finger is extended along the iliac crest as far as possible, forming a triangle. The injection is given in the center of the triangle or V formed by the hand, with the needle directed slightly upward toward the iliac crest. *D*, Gluteal region. *Injection is given into the gluteus medius.* The site is found by locating the greater trochanter and posterior

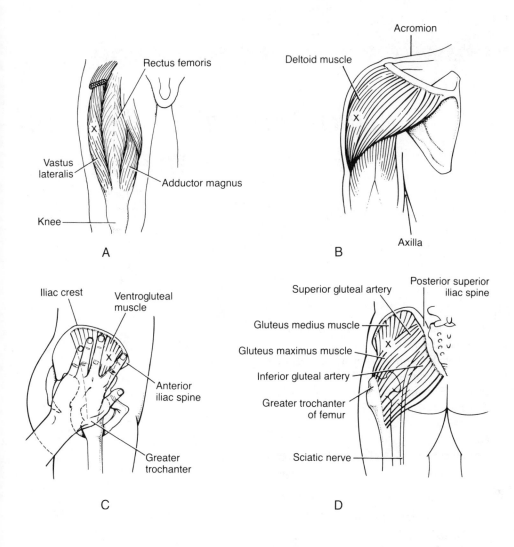

A

B

C

D

iliac spine. Draw an imaginary line between these two points and inject above the line into the gluteus medius. (From Tackett, J. M. and Hunsberger, M. Family-Centered Care of Children and Adolescents. Philadelphia: W. B. Saunders Co., 1978.)

UNIT 9

Bibliography

Baker, C. and Wong, D. Q.U.E.S.T.: A Process of Pain Assessment in Children. Orthopaedic Nursing, 6(1):Jan./Feb. 1987, pp. 11–20.

Barnes, S. Patient/Family Education for the Patient with a Pressure Necrosis. Nursing Clinics of North America, 22(2):June 1987, pp. 463–474.

Byrne, N. and Feld, M. Overcoming the Red Menace: Preventing and Treating Decubitus Ulcers. Nursing 84, 4(14):1984, pp. 55–57.

Fuestel, D. Pressure Sore Prevention. Nursing 82, April 1982, pp. 78–83.

Meinhart, N. and McCaffery, M. Pain: A Nursing Approach to Assessment and Analysis. Norwalk, Connecticut: Appleton-Century-Crofts, 1983.

Meyer, T. TENS: Relieving Pain Through Electricity. Nursing 82, 12(9):1982, pp. 57–59.

Olsson, G. and Parker, G. A Model Approach to Pain Management. Nursing 87, 17(5):1987, pp. 52–57.

Sebern, M. Home-Team Strategies for Treating Pressure Sores. Nursing 87, April 1987, pp. 50–53.

Taylor, A., et al. How Effective is TENS for Acute Pain. American Journal of Nursing, 83(8):1983, pp. 1171–1174.

Neuro-Musculo-Skeletal Alterations

Care Plans

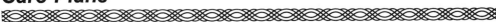

Amyotrophic Lateral Sclerosis Care Plan

CROSS REFERENCES

Bereavement Care Plan
Constipation Care Plan
Decubitus Care Plan
Depression Care Plan
Imminent Death Care Plan
Spiritual Distress Care Plan
Terminal Illness Care Plan
Ventilator Care Plan

Assistive Devices Procedure
Home Safety Procedure
Oxygen Therapy Procedure
Post-Mortem Care Procedure
Pronouncement of Death Procedure
Range of Motion Exercises Procedure
Suctioning (Oronasopharyngeal) Procedure
Suctioning (Tracheostomy) Procedure
Tracheostomy Care Procedure
Tracheostomy Tube Changing Procedure

NURSING DIAGNOSES

1. Anxiety/fear related to
   a. life style changes resulting from progressive nature of disease
   b. fear of death
   c. powerlessness/hopelessness
   d. financial demands of treatment
   e. dependence on others for care
   f. dysphagia
   g. dysarthria
   h. other.
2. Ineffective breathing pattern related to
   a. neuromuscular impairment
   b. decreased energy and fatigue
   c. other.
3. Ineffective airway clearance related to
   a. inadequate cough reflex
   b. dysphagia
   c. ineffective suctioning of tracheostomy
   d. other.
4. Impaired physical mobility related to
   a. neuromuscular impairment (spasticity/atrophy)
   b. depression
   c. anxiety
   d. decreased energy and fatigue
   e. other.
5. Alteration in nutrition (less than body requirements) related to
   a. dysphagia
   b. inadequate support systems (cooking /shopping)
   c. weakness/fatigue
   d. other.

UNIT 10

6. Impaired verbal communication related to
   a. neuromuscular impairment
   b. tracheostomy
   c. other.
7. Ineffective individual coping related to
   a. dependence on others
   b. multiple life changes
   c. dysfunctional grieving
   d. uncontrolled affective outbursts (laughing /crying)
   e. feelings of powerlessness/hopelessness
   f. other.
8. Ineffective family coping related to
   a. progressive/terminal disease process
   b. dysfunctional grieving
   c. family disorganization and role changes
   d. other.
9. Self-care deficit (feeding, bathing /hygiene, dressing /grooming, toileting) related to
   a. progressive muscular spasticity/atrophy
   b. depression
   c. dependence on others for care
   d. immobility
   e. weakness/fatigue
   f. dysphagia
   g. other.
10. Impaired skin integrity related to
    a. immobility
    b. inadequate nutritional intake
    c. inadequate personal hygiene
    d. other.
11. Alteration in bowel elimination (constipation) related to
    a. inadequate fluid /delivery intake
    b. immobility
    c. muscle wasting
    d. other.
12. Social isolation related to
    a. impaired verbal communication
    b. drooling
    c. uncontrolled affective outbursts (laughing /crying)
    d. impaired mobility
    e. other.
13. Potential for injury (falls, infection, aspiration) related to
    a. impaired mobility/muscular control
    b. impaired skin integrity
    c. difficulty chewing /swallowing
    d. other.
14. Impaired home maintenance management related to
    a. loss of control/spasticity
    b. progressive physical decline
    c. lack of support (family/community/financial)
    d. ineffective patient/family coping
    e. other.

15. Patient/family grieving related to progressive/terminal disease process.
16. Disturbance in self-concept (body image, self-esteem, role performance, personal identity) related to
    a. loss of body function/control
    b. change in role/job/life style
    c. dependence on others for care
    d. drooling
    e. uncontrolled affective outbursts (laughing/crying)
    f. other.
17. Sexual dysfunction related to
    a. immobility
    b. weakness/fatigue
    c. other.
18. Knowledge deficit (nature of disease process, treatment regimen, signs/symptoms to report) related to
    a. cognitive limitations
    b. lack of readiness to learn
    c. patient's request for no information
    d. other.
19. Noncompliance with the therapeutic regimen related to
    a. lack of support (family/community/financial)
    b. difficulty integrating regimen into lifestyle
    c. other.

PROCESS INDICATORS

1. The patient/family verbalizes an understanding of amyotrophic lateral sclerosis and the therapeutic regimen.

Indicators

   a. describes amyotrophic lateral sclerosis disease process, therapeutic/palliative regimen and strategies to promote independence and to prevent complications
   b. describes a diet plan that promotes adequate nutrition and caloric intake, optimal independence in feeding and compensates for dysphagia
   c. describes medication's action, dose, administration schedule and side effects
   d. describes an activity plan that maintains range of motion and mobility to the extent possible, avoids overexertion, demonstrates transfer techniques and use of mobility aids and includes diversional activities
   e. demonstrates appropriate safety precautions/modifications in the home
   f. demonstrates proper techniques/procedures for patient treatments (i.e., suctioning, gastrostomy care, tube feedings, tracheostomy care)
   g. verbalizes a plan for the patient to receive follow-up care
   h. identifies appropriate community resources
   i. identifies signs and symptoms to report to the nurse and/or physician.
2. The patient's biopsychosocial integrity is maintained.

Indicators

   a. airway/adequate ventilation is maintained
   b. adequate intake of food/fluid to maintain nutritional status
   c. optimal level of independence is maintained/adjusted as disease progresses
   d. skin integrity is maintained
   e. absence of contractures

UNIT 10

f. satisfactory defecation pattern
g. bladder control is achieved/managed (including use of urinary catheter)
h. absence of evidence of aspiration
i. presence of an effective communication system
j. absence of infection (respiratory, urinary tract, wound/skin breakdown sites)
k. performs self-care/activities of daily living as appropriate with functional ability.
3. The family's psychosocial integrity is maintained.

Indicators

a. family demonstrates reorganization of family roles to adjust to the patient's regimen
b. family expresses an ability to cope with patient's needs
c. family prepares for the end stage of the disease.

NURSING INTERVENTIONS

1. Assess the patient for
   a. degree of muscle weakness/atrophy, spasticity, fasciculations, range of motion and presence of contractures
   b. level of activity/functioning
   c. respiratory rate/pattern /effort /effectiveness
   d. adventitious breath sounds
   e. temperature, pulse, blood pressure readings
   f. speech/communication abilities/limitations
   g. ability to chew and swallow
   h. body weight
   i. presence of/extent of drooling
   j. bowel/bladder functioning /control
   k. use of assistive devices/mobility aids
   l. expressions of fear, anxiety, depression, grief and satisfaction with quality of life
   m. signs of infection (respiratory tract, urinary tract, wound /skin breakdown sites)
   n. affective behavior (outbursts of laughing /crying)
   o. understanding of the disease process.
2. Assess the family's
   a. understanding of the disease process
   b. reorganization of roles/activities
   c. ability to be supportive and to participate in/plan for the patient's care needs
   d. verbal /nonverbal interactions among family members and the patient.
3. Instruct the patient /family/home health aide about the amyotrophic lateral sclerosis disease process and the therapeutic /supportive regimen.
   a. correct use of assistive devices/mobility aids for activities of daily living and hygiene
   b. proper techniques for tube feedings as needed
   c. proper techniques for dressing care as needed
   d. proper techniques for perineal care and maintaining an indwelling urinary catheter system as needed
   e. proper technique for tracheostomy care as needed
   f. strategies to prevent skin breakdown
      • keeping skin clean and dry
      • use of massage
      • use of pressure relief devices
      • repositioning schedule

    g. strategies to promote patient safety
- use of hand rails/safety rails, seat belts
- keeping items within easy reach
- preparation of the patient /family for the need to adapt to the progressive nature of muscle weakness
- use of rubber soled shoes

    h. strategies to prevent and treat constipation

    i. medications including name, dosage, action, administration schedule and side effects of prescribed medications
- medication route may need adjustment based upon the patient's ability to swallow
- review proper procedure for medication administration through a tube, as appropriate.

4. Instruct the patient /family/home health aide about signs and symptoms to report.
    a. respiratory infection
    b. urinary tract infection
    c. difficulty breathing /signs of respiratory failure
    d. skin breakdown/irritation (including sites such as tracheostomy and gastrostomy)
    e. feeding tube difficulties (questionable placement /tube falls out)
    f. tracheostomy tube falls out.

5. Instruct the patient /family/home health aide about strategies to maintain airway/ ventilation.
    a. performance of oral suctioning to remove the copious oral secretions to minimize choking
    b. use of oxygen as prescribed
    c. care of tracheostomy and techniques of tracheostomy suctioning as appropriate
    d. use of pulmonary equipment, such as incentive spirometry, as needed
    e. avoiding irritants, such as smoke/perfume, which can stimulate coughing
    f. strategies to prevent respiratory infections
- abdominal breathing exercises to minimize the effects of respiratory decompensation
- postural drainage to loosen and raise secretions
- avoiding crowds during flu season and avoiding anyone with a cold

    g. care of the patient when using a ventilator as needed
    h. advising the patient /family to notify the fire and electric companies that life-sustaining equipment is in the home
    i. use of a battery backup for equipment such as a suction pump or a ventilator
    j. consult with the respiratory therapist as needed.

6. Instruct the patient /family/home health aide about a dietary plan that complies with prescribed parameters.
    a. basic food groups for promotion of general nutrition and adequate caloric intake
    b. proper positioning, such as the high Fowler position, with the neck slightly flexed (chin pointed toward chest) for eating and drinking
    c. use of a neck brace, soft cervical collar or small pillows to support head while eating as per physician prescription
    d. ways to minimize aspiration
- instruct the patient to concentrate on eating and to avoid laughing and talking while eating
- eat soft foods that tend to hold together such as soft-boiled eggs, casseroles, stews
- cut food into small pieces
- minimize/avoid drinking fluid with solid food in the mouth

UNIT
10

    e. keep oral suction available for immediate use

    f. schedule small frequent meals to avoid fatigue and to enhance nutritional intake

    g. limit mucus-producing foods (such as milk)

    h. offer very warm or very cold foods/drinks (stimulate swallowing)

    i. consult with the dietician and/or physician for use of liquid supplements and/or alternate feeding methods to maintain nutrition (tube feedings/hyperalimentation) as needed

    j. maintain adequate hydration to avoid thick tenacious secretions

    k. use of assistive devices/utensils to encourage independence in eating/feeding

    i. include foods with high fiber

    m. consult with the speech therapist for techniques/exercises to minimize dysphagia.

7. Instruct the patient/family/home health aide about an activity plan that attempts to maintain function and mobility.

    a. maximizes the patient's functional abilities

    b. includes range of motion exercises to prevent contractures

    c. incorporates diversional strategies

    d. plans activities (such as swimming or stationary bicycling) to strengthen uninvolved muscles

    e. includes return demonstration for
  - proper positioning using pillows to support limbs and to prevent contractures as a result of head drooping
  - use of assistive devices and/or mobility aids to help with activities of daily living, to employ energy saving techniques and to provide for safety (includes use of electric toothbrush, raised toilet seat, Velcro closures)
  - use of equipment (hospital bed, mechanical lift)
  - proper transfer techniques

    f. includes repositioning at least every 1 to 2 hours for immobile patients

    g. incorporates consultation with the physical therapist and/or occupational therapist as needed

    h. includes planned periods of rest and avoiding fatigue.

8. Instruct the patient/family/home health aide about communication strategies.

    a. keep communication devices within easy reach

    b. consult with a speech therapist as early as possible

    c. patients with impaired speech may need further assistance
  - voice amplification (microphone, telephone voice piece)
  - electrolarynx

    d. patients without speech may benefit from
  - hand signals
  - communication board
  - eye movement as a communication system
  - computer assisted communication where messages can be typed on the screen using a control switch attached to any functional muscle (e.g., in the eyebrow area)
  - voice synthesizers can be used in conjunction with computers.

9. Promote the patient's/family's coping abilities.

    a. encourage the patient/family to express feelings (frustrations, helplessness, hopelessness)

    b. encourage the patient/family to focus on the patient's strengths as a strategy to overcome limitations

    c. reinforce that the patient remains alert and intelligent despite physical limitations/inability to respond

    d. identify that affective outbursts may be involuntary and unrelated to the patient's mood

    e. include the patient in decision making/planning

    f. encourage the patient to make choices concerning activities that will be performed independently and those in which assistance will be accepted

    g. assist with grooming and hair care to enhance the patient's self-esteem

    h. identify sources for diversional activities (talking library, tapes, radio, automatic page tuner, television)

    i. assist the patient/family in setting appropriate goals that are attainable and adjustable

    j. assist the patient/family in making a weekly checklist (including frequency) for managing care activities

    k. encourage the patient and sexual partner to discuss ways of expressing affection

    l. assist the patient/family with the grieving process

    m. assist the patient/family with plans for long-term care, hospice care and living will.

10. Identify community resources that can facilitate the patient's/family's adjustment to amyotrophic lateral sclerosis.

    a. local branch or national office of the Amyotrophic Lateral Sclerosis Association

    b. counselling, psychological therapy and self-help support groups

    c. financial counselling services.

11. Coordinate additional members of the health care team such as the occupational therapist, physical therapist, speech therapist, social worker, registered dietician and respiratory therapist.

12. Provide progress reports and a discharge summary to the primary physician.

THERAPEUTIC ACHIEVEMENT

- The patient/family adapt to the life style changes induced as a result of amyotrophic lateral sclerosis.
- The patient maintains optimal functional abilities appropriate to the disease stage.

RELATED PATIENT INSTRUCTIONS

A Daily Food Guide—Four Basic Food Groups
Care for the Patient Confined to Bed
Comfort Measures for Dehydration
Constipation
General Comfort Measures
Making the Home Environment Safe
Nasogastric, Orogastric, Nasointestinal Tube
  Feedings

Oral Suctioning
Ostomy Tube Feedings (Adult)
Range of Motion Exercises
Skin Care
Tracheostomy Care
Tube Feeding—Special Conditions
Ventilator Care
Ways to Save Your Energy

UNIT
10

Arthritis (Rheumatoid) Care Plan

CROSS REFERENCES

Constipation Care Plan
Decubitus Care Plan
Depression Care Plan
Joint (Hip/Knee) Replacement Care Plan
Pain Care Plan

Assistive Devices Procedure
Home Safety Procedure

Range of Motion Exercises Procedure
Transcutaneous Electrical Nerve
 Stimulation (TENS) Procedure
Crutch Walking

Medication Compliance Management Guidelines
Vital Signs: Normal Pediatric Values

NURSING DIAGNOSES

1. Alteration in comfort (joint inflammation/pain/stiffness, muscle spasms) related to
   a. chronic progressive nature of disease
   b. inadequate daily exercise
   c. other.
2. Impaired physical mobility related to
   a. fatigue
   b. joint inflammation
   c. joint pain/stiffness
   d. joint deformity/subluxation
   e. muscle atrophy
   f. prescribed activity restrictions
   g. other.
3. Anxiety related to the chronic progressive nature of disease.
4. Ineffective individual/family coping related to chronic progressive disabling nature of disease.
5. Disturbance in self-concept (body image, self-esteem, role performance, personal identity) related to
   a. joint deformity
   b. dependence on others for care
   c. progressive disability
   d. other.
6. Sleep pattern disturbance related to
   a. joint pain/stiffness
   b. muscle spasms
   c. other.
7. Self-care deficit (feeding, bathing/hygiene, dressing/grooming, toileting, ambulating) related to
   a. fatigue
   b. joint deformity/subluxation
   c. joint pain/stiffness
   d. muscle spasms
   e. other.

8. Knowledge deficit (disease process, treatment regimen of diet/activity/medications, strategies to prevent complications, signs and symptoms to report) related to
   a. misinterpretation of information
   b. cognitive limitation
   c. lack of readiness to learn
   d. patient's request for no information
   e. other.
9. Noncompliance with treatment regimen related to
   a. chronic progressive nature of disease
   b. no known disease cure but with highly advertised/available unproven remedies (quackery)
   c. other.
10. Impaired home maintenance management related to
    a. fatigue
    b. dependence on others for care
    c. chronic progressive nature of disease
    d. joint pain/stiffness
    e. joint deformity/subluxation
    f. other.
11. Potential impairment of skin integrity related to thinning of the skin.
12. Alteration in bowel elimination (constipation) related to
    a. impaired mobility
    b. inadequate dietary intake
    c. other.
13. Alteration in nutrition (less than body requirements) related to
    a. anorexia
    b. temporomandibular joint pain/stiffness
    c. lack of support systems (cooking/shopping)
    d. other.
14. Sexual dysfunction related to
    a. body image disturbance
    b. depression
    c. pain
    d. deformity
    e. fatigue
    f. other.

UNIT 10

PROCESS INDICATORS

1. The patient/family verbalizes an understanding of rheumatoid arthritis and the therapeutic regimen.
Indicators
   a. describes the rheumatoid arthritis disease process, therapeutic regimen and strategies to prevent complications
   b. describes an activity/exercise plan that maintains joint function and promotes mobility
   c. describes a diet plan that includes basic food groups, promotes achievement/ maintenance of optimal weight and promotes bowel elimination
   d. identifies signs and symptoms to report to the nurse and/or physician
   e. verbalizes a plan for receiving follow-up care

   f. identifies appropriate community resources
   g. demonstrates proper use of assistive devices/mobility aids.
2. The patient's biopsychosocial integrity is maintained.
Indicators
   a. exhibits minimal joint deformity
   b. maintains proper positioning during all activities
   c. demonstrates optimal joint function
   d. does not exhibit fever
   e. verbalizes decrease in/relief of fatigue
   f. verbalizes/demonstrates optimal ability to be mobile and engage in self-care activities
   g. achieves/maintains optimal weight
   h. maintains a satisfactory defecation pattern
   i. expresses satisfaction with sexual relationships, as appropriate
   j. patient /family verbalizes feelings about adapting to arthritis.
3. The patient establishes/maintains satisfactory level of comfort.
Indicators
   a. verbalizes/exhibits an absence of uncontrolled pain/discomfort/stiffness
   b. verbalizes/exhibits successful coping with anxiety
   c. expresses satisfaction with the quality of life
   d. reports undisturbed sleep.

NURSING INTERVENTIONS

1. Assess the patient for
   a. current ability to perform activities of daily living
   b. joint size, shape, color, and symmetry noting
      • joints involved
      • joint mobility, function, range
      • joint swelling, redness, warmth, tenderness, irregularity, subluxation
   c. description of pain (quality, severity, location at onset, duration, exacerbating and alleviating factors)
   d. description of location of stiffness (localized or generalized), time (morning, night, all day) and duration of stiffness, exacerbating and alleviating factors of stiffness
   e. presence of fatigue, weakness, fever, malaise
   f. skin integrity/presence of taut shiny skin over joints
   g. presence of adjacent muscle atrophy/flexion contractures involving the joint
   h. level of muscle strength/function/spasm
   i. quality of peripheral pulses
   j. presence of subcutaneous nodules over bony prominences (particularly the elbows)
   k. medication side effect (e.g., bleeding, cushingoid features)
   l. current sleep pattern
   m. use of unproven remedies
   n. current body weight and history of weight loss
   o. level of satisfaction with quality of life (assess relationship between potential depression and complaints of fatigue/unhappiness)
   p. level of satisfaction with sexual relationship, as appropriate
   q. pattern of bowel elimination.
2. Assess the patient's/family's understanding of
   a. the disease process and treatment regimen

     b. correct use of assistive devices/mobility aids

     c. signs and symptoms to report.

3. Monitor and record

     a. vital signs

     b. joint status

     c. progression of the disease to the point of involvement of connective tissue in the heart, lungs, eyes, nervous system, blood vessels and muscles

     d. body weight

     e. amount of weakness.

4. Instruct the patient/family/home health aide about rheumatoid arthritis and the therapeutic regimen.

     a. rheumatoid arthritis disease process and the benefits of control despite lack of cure

     b. maintaining comfort through

- proper positioning
- exercising
- use of analgesics 30 to 45 minutes before exercise, if prescribed
- use of massage around joints; never massage acutely inflamed joints
- use of relaxation techniques
- use of transcutaneous electrical nerve stimulation (TENS), if prescribed
- use of bed cradle/footboard to keep bed linens off feet
- use of a firm mattress, bedboard (3/4-in plywood can be used) or pressure relieving devices
- encouraging the patient to allow time to adjust to splints and proper body positioning
- avoiding pain precipitating factors such as emotional stress, dampness, temperature extremes

     c. promoting undisturbed sleep by

- taking a warm 20-minute shower/bath immediately before bedtime
- performing gentle range of motion exercises (after shower/bath) to relieve pain and stiffness
- sleeping in proper position
- using an electric blanket (set on low temperature)
- avoiding stimulating foods (caffeine) and activities before bedtime
- using relaxation techniques
- taking prescribed medications (analgesics, anti-inflammatory agents, sleeping medications) as appropriate

     d. strategies to promote home safety

- allow adequate time for activities
- encourage maintenance of uncluttered well-lit hallways/rooms; eliminate throw rugs and slippery floors
- use of hand rails in showers or tub

     e. strategies to prevent skin breakdown

- avoiding trauma to fragile thin skin
- massage areas around the joints and at contact points for splints/braces
- inspect skin daily, especially at splint/brace contact points

     f. preparing for treatment protocols and/or surgery as defined by the physician (synovectomy, arthroplasty, arthrodesis, joint replacement)

     g. signs and symptoms to report

- decreasing range of motion/function in joints
- skin breakdown

- falls
- unusual/excessive bleeding
- medication side effects

h. achieving/maintaining optimal body weight to minimize stress on the joints
i. maintaining a nutritional diet with
- basic food groups
- adequate fluid intake
- adequate fiber/roughage to promote satisfactory bowel elimination
j. plans to receive long-term follow-up care.

5. Instruct the patient/family/home health aide about an activity plan that
a. maximizes the patient's functional abilities
b. reinforces exercise goals of maintaining joint function, strengthening muscles supporting joints, improving circulation and promoting endurance
c. includes exercise to be performed daily (if inflammation is controlled) in a smooth slow manner, in short frequent sessions
d. reinforces proper body mechanics for lifting, reaching, standing, sitting, lying, transferring, ambulating
- flexing and extending knees several times before standing up after sitting for awhile
- using high firm chairs with armrests
- active positioning and exercising to prevent or possibly correct mild deformities
- use of sandbags, footboards, trochanter rolls to maintain alignment
- when lying in bed use only a small pillow or towel under the head, lie flat on the back with affected joints in position of extension, use a small pillow under the ankles to straighten the knees and use a small pillow/towel under the elbows/wrists for extension (arms with palms up)
e. allows for systemic and total body rest to help control symptoms of rheumatoid arthritis
- increase usual sleep duration by at least 1 hour
- schedule *at least* two, 30-minute uninterrupted rest periods during the day
- encourage the patient to lie prone at least twice per day for at least 15 to 30 minutes
f. allows for articular (joint) rest through use of splints to help prevent deformity and increase function
- splint should not be worn 24 hours per day
- splint should be removed several times to check skin for redness, swelling, and soreness, and to perform range of motion exercises
- patient should contact the nurse/occupational therapist if the splint causes discomfort or does not fit properly
- resting splints are worn at night but can be worn during the day if the part is red, swollen, warm or tender
- working splints are worn when active but can be worn at night when inactive if prescribed
- molded plastic splints should be washed in warm soapy water; avoid hot places and hot water
g. provides strategies for joint protection to reduce stress
- maintaining good posture and body mechanics
- avoiding positions of deformity
- avoiding sitting or standing for long periods of time (a shower chair can be used for 20-minute showers)
- maintaining a balance between work and rest

- stopping activities before tiring and in response to pain; avoiding overdoing on "good days"
- using large joints and strongest muscles to perform tasks

h. includes energy saving techniques
- plan tasks so frequent rest breaks can be taken
- work at an even pace; alternate light and heavy tasks
- avoid extra trips, arrange activities/materials for ready availability

i. includes range of motion exercises to be performed at least 1 to 2 times a day
- moist heat 15 to 20 minutes before exercising helps movement
- move the part as far as it will go
- if supporting a limb, support the muscle area around the joint, not the joint itself
- exercise within the prescribed parameters may decrease the pain/stiffness

j. includes isometric and strengthening exercises
- minimal joint movement is involved if performed properly
- remind the patient to hold the contraction and count to 10 out loud (to avoid Valsalva maneuver)

k. reinforces proper use of assistive devices
- proper fit is essential; devices may need alteration as the disease progresses
- devices compensating for impaired hand grip also protect the joint from stress (telephone holder, jar opener, eating utensils with built-up handles and Velcro fasteners)
- dressing sticks, reaching sticks, elevated toilet seats/chairs all facilitate mobility and independence in activities of daily living

l. reinforces proper use of mobility aids
- in addition to enabling mobility, these aids can also help to prevent flexion deformities from weight bearing
- proper fit is essential for safe use (rubber-tipped crutches, canes, walkers, braces, corrective shoes and wheelchair).

6. Instruct the patient/family/home health aide about proper/safe applications of heat and cold.

a. heat or cold can be used as separate, combined or contrast treatments usually 2 to 3 times per day depending on physician's order

b. warm baths/showers for about 15 to 20 minutes in the morning can minimize stiffness and make exercise easier

c. guidelines for safe applications of heat and cold
- do not use pack over one area for more than 20 minutes
- do not place pack between area being treated and a firm surface
- check skin during and after treatment for any signs of injury
- do not use the regimen if there is decreased/poor circulation, decreased sensation or increased sensitivity
- check with the physician if contraindications for use are evident and/or if applications intensify pain

d. heat applications (to decrease pain, relax muscles and increase motion)
- for heating packs or pads that are waterproof and designed for moist heat, follow the manufacturer's instructions
- do not use standard heating pads for wet applications
- be sure to cover the pack/pad properly before placing on joint
- after treatment, dry skin and check for injury
- for hot paraffin application, follow manufacturer's and physician's instructions

e. cold applications (to decrease pain/swelling and to increase motion) using plastic-bag ice packs

- use a double plastic bag
- wrap the pack in a slightly warm wet towel (helps the adjustment to cold pack)
- after treatment, dry skin and check for injury
  f. cold application using the ice massage
  - use a large ice cube or water frozen in a plastic cup
  - protect the hand holding the ice
  - rub ice directly on area until skin feels numb
  - stages of sensation are cooling, burning, aching (after about 3 minutes) and numbness.
7. Instruct the patient/family/home health aide about the medication plan (salicylates, nonsteroidal anti-inflammatory drugs (NSAIDs), corticosteroids, gold therapy, i.e., chrysotherapy).
   a. name, dosage, administration schedule and side effects of prescribed medications
   b. safety guidelines if the patient is taking high doses of salicylates
   - signs/symptoms of toxicity (tinnitus, decreased hearing)
   - avoid taking aspirin containing compounds, unless prescribed
   - report bleeding problems (bruising, dark stools)
   - take with food to minimize gastrointestinal irritation
   - reinforce that acetaminophen is not a substitute for aspirin
   c. with NSAIDs
   - it may take 2 to 3 weeks to feel the effects
   - administer with food to minimize gastrointestinal irritation
   d. chrysotherapy requires exacting protocols
   - patient must be under active care of the physician
   - certain laboratory tests should be performed before each injection
   - reinforce the need for immediate reporting of adverse reactions (dermatitis; stomatitis; nephrotic syndrome; blood dyscrasias; anaphylactoid effects, which may occur immediately or as long as 10 minutes after the injection and gastrointestinal reactions)
   - effects may not be felt until 3 months after onset of therapy.
8. Encourage the patient and significant other to verbalize feelings about sexual relationship.
   a. help the patient to identify positions that minimize joint stress
   b. encourage the patient to plan for sexual activity during periods of least stiffness, fatigue, pain
   c. discuss alternative ways of expressing affection.
9. Encourage the patient/family to verbalize feelings about the chronic progressive nature of the disease, changes in body image/role performance and plans/strategies to cope with long-term health care needs.
   a. encourage the patient/family to focus on the patient's strengths as a strategy to overcome limitations
   b. explain the need for the patient to achieve "emotional rest" as part of the therapeutic regimen
   c. assist the patient/family in realistic goal setting
   d. encourage the patient to participate in decision-making and to maximize independence
   e. instruct patient in stress management/relaxation techniques.
10. Identify community resources that can facilitate the patient's/family's adjustment to rheumatoid arthritis.
    a. local branch or national office Arthritis Foundation
    b. vocational rehabilitation programs

    c. counselling, psychological therapy and self-help support groups
    d. financial counselling services.
11. Coordinate additional members of the health care team such as the physical therapist, occupational therapist, social worker and registered dietician.
12. Provide progress reports and a discharge summary to the primary physician.

THERAPEUTIC ACHIEVEMENT

- The patient maintains optimal joint function, mobility and independence in activities of daily living.
- The patient /family adapts to the life style changes induced as a result of rheumatoid arthritis.

JUVENILE ARTHRITIS SUPPLEMENT

1. Rheumatoid arthritis nursing care and therapeutic achievements are applicable to the patient with juvenile arthritis.
2. Special areas of consideration include
    a. Planning exercise, rest and diversional activities directed toward
       • promoting normal growth and development
       • preventing overactivity and joint abuse
    b. Planning adequate nutritional intake when the child experiences anorexia and malaise.
       • monitoring of body weight changes is essential
       • high calorie, low volume food may be necessary
    c. Encouraging verbalizations about feelings by child and parents.
       • the child may have moderate growth retardation negatively impacting on body image
       • the child's symptoms of pain, irritability and malaise may be frightening and frustrating for both child and parents.

RELATED PATIENT INSTRUCTIONS

A Daily Food Guide—Four Basic Food Groups	Pain Medications
Arthritis	Range of Motion Exercises
Aspirin and Aspirin-like Medications	Skin Care
General Comfort Measures	Ways to Save Your Energy

UNIT
10

Joint (Hip/Knee) Replacement Care Plan

CROSS REFERENCES

Arthritis (Rheumatoid) Care Plan
Constipation Care Plan
Decubitus Care Plan
Pain Care Plan

Assistive Devices Procedure

Continuous Range of Motion Procedure
Home Safety Procedure
Range of Motion Exercises Procedure
Transcutaneous Electrical Nerve
  Stimulation (TENS) Procedure

Crutch Walking

NURSING DIAGNOSES

1. Alteration in comfort (pain) related to
   a. impaired skin integrity
   b. surgery
   c. physical rehabilitation program
   d. other.
2. Impaired skin integrity (irritation, breakdown) related to
   a. immobility
   b. brace/splint/cast irritation
   c. surgical wound
   d. other.
3. Impaired physical mobility related to
   a. pain/discomfort
   b. weakness/fatigue
   c. prescribed activity restrictions
   d. other.
4. Potential for injury (falls, infection, contractures, skin breakdown) related to
   a. weakness/fatigue
   b. impaired skin integrity
   c. inadequate compliance with therapeutic regimen
   d. inadequate transfer/ambulation techniques
   e. other.
5. Knowledge deficit (pathophysiology, underlying disease process, rehabilitation regimen, medications, exercise/activity plan, signs and symptoms to report) related to
   a. misinterpretation of information
   b. cognitive limitations
   c. lack of readiness to learn
   d. patient's request for no information
   e. other.
6. Self-care deficit (feeding, bathing/hygiene, dressing/grooming, toileting) related to
   a. fatigue/weakness
   b. discomfort/pain

   c. activity limitations

   d. other.

7. Alteration in bowel elimination related to

   a. immobility

   b. inadequate nutritional intake

   c. other.

8. Sexual dysfunction related to

   a. pain/discomfort

   b. activity/positioning restrictions

   c. other.

PROCESS INDICATORS

1. The patient /family verbalizes an understanding of joint replacement and the therapeutic regimen.

Indicators

   a. describe the underlying disease process (i.e., arthritis), therapeutic regimen and strategies to prevent complications

   b. describe proper wound care

   c. describe an activity plan that includes active/passive exercise, weight bearing/position restrictions and planned periods of rest

   d. describe medication, action, dose, administration schedule and side effects

   e. identify signs and symptoms to report to the nurse and/or physician

   f. identify appropriate community resources

   g. verbalize a plan for receiving follow-up care

   h. demonstrate proper use of assistive devices/mobility aids.

2. The patient's biopsychosocial integrity is maintained.

Indicators

   a. maintains skin integrity

   b. does not exhibit signs/symptoms of infection

   c. maintains normal healing of surgical wounds

   d. verbalizes decrease/absence of uncontrolled pain/discomfort

   e. demonstrates restoration/improvement of joint function

   f. maintains proper positioning during all activities

   g. identifies absence of falls

   h. maintains a satisfactory defecation pattern

   i. verbalizes feelings about adapting to joint replacement and rehabilitation plan

   j. expresses satisfaction with sexual relationship, if appropriate.

NURSING INTERVENTIONS

1. Assess the patient's

   a. complaints of pain/discomfort

   b. surgical wound site

   c. skin integrity (particularly around the wound site, upper back, sacrum and contact points from splints/braces)

   d. mobility

   e. replaced joint for range of motion

   f. correct use of assistive devices/mobility aids

UNIT 10

      g. position while in bed, out of bed, transferring, getting into a chair and ambulating

      h. neurovascular status of operative extremity (pulses, color, warmth, circulation, movement, sensation, capillary refill)

      i. calf edema, tenderness, swelling, pain

      j. temperature

      k. signs of bleeding.

2. Assess the patient's/family's
   a. understanding of therapeutic regimen/rehabilitation plan
   b. understanding of activity and positioning restrictions
   c. ability to correctly perform wound care
   d. understanding of signs and symptoms to report.

3. Instruct the patient/family/home health aide about joint replacement and the rehabilitation plan.
   a. correct use of assistive devices/mobility aids (crutches/walker/cane)
      - assure that straps from devices are not too tight causing excessive skin/nerve pressure
      - include use of energy saving techniques for activities of daily living
      - encourage maintaining activities within positioning restrictions
   b. performing wound care
   c. achieving/maintaining optimal body weight (to minimize stress on joints)
   d. maintaining a nutritional diet with adequate fiber/roughage to promote satisfactory bowel elimination
   e. planning to maintain the long-term rehabilitation plan (with medical follow-up)
   f. informing other health care providers about the joint replacement prior to invasive procedures/dental work (prophylactic antibiotics may be prescribed)
   g. maintaining comfort through
      - proper positioning
      - exercising
      - use of analgesics 30 to 45 minutes before exercise, if prescribed and needed
      - use of massage and other forms of relaxation
      - use of transcutaneous electrical nerve stimulation (TENS), if prescribed
   h. maintaining proper positioning within the context of the sexual relationship, if appropriate
      - encourage the patient and significant other to verbalize feelings
      - review positioning restrictions with suggestions for safe positioning
   i. using antiembolism stocking (hose) if prescribed
      - put on before getting out of bed in the morning
      - powdering the foot eases application of hose
      - apply according to instructions on package
      - remove all wrinkles
      - prevent hose from rolling down as this acts as a tourniquet
   j. advising the patient that the implant may activate metal detectors in airports.

4. Instruct the patient/family/home health aide about the prescribed activity plan and positioning restrictions for hip replacement.
   a. transferring, ambulation and gait training techniques
   b. daily exercises within prescribed parameters
      - range of motion
      - quadriceps setting and gluteal setting
      - isometric hip extension/abduction
      - flex toes and ankles

   c. maintaining operative extremity in proper alignment (trochanter rolls)

   d. maintaining activity restrictions until the physician removes restriction
- avoiding excessive hip flexion (greater than 90 degrees)
- elevating seating height (chairs with firm cushions and armrests, raised toilet seat, bed elevation to the height of the patient's mid thigh, high firm cushion for car seat)
- avoiding bending to reach objects (on the floor, bed covers, putting on socks/shoes)
- using dressing sticks/assistive devices
- avoiding rotation of hip
- keeping leg extended while riding in car, avoid driving until approved by physician
- avoiding lifting heavy objects or excessive twisting or turning
- avoiding positions during sexual activity that result in turning the knee or hip inward, flexing the hip greater than 90 degrees and moving the operative leg past the midline
- avoiding high impact activities (jogging, jumping)
- keeping knee of operated leg below hip level
- avoiding crossing of legs and standing with toes turned in
- keeping knees apart and operative extremity's foot turned out (never adduct leg past the midline)
- ascending stairs one step at a time with nonoperative leg first
- using a pillow between legs when in bed and especially when turning onto nonoperative side (avoid pillows under calf/knees)
- getting up from a chair: move to the edge first and place operative leg out in front while rising, nonoperative leg should be under the chair

   e. preventing footdrop through exercising, use of footboard/sandbags and avoiding peroneal nerve pressure

   f. preventing hip contractures by
- lying prone at least twice per day for 30 minutes
- limit sitting to 30 minutes per session, avoid sessions lasting 1 hour

   g. reporting signs and symptoms of dislocation
- severe sudden hip pain followed by continued pain and muscle spasm during hip movement
- palpable bulge over femur head
- abnormal rotation/shortening of operative leg
- impaired neurovascular status of the operative leg
- limping or inability to bear weight on operative leg.

5. Instruct the patient/family/home health aide about the prescribed activity plan and positioning restrictions for knee replacement.

   a. transferring, ambulation and gait training techniques

   b. daily exercises within prescribed parameters
- range of motion
- quadriceps setting
- active straight leg raising
- knee flexion/extension exercises to prevent flexion contractures

   c. progressive program of partial to full weight bearing

   d. use of continuous passive motion equipment, if prescribed

   e. maintaining activity restrictions until the physician removes them
- avoiding abrupt, acute flexion, of operative knee
- keeping operative knee extended while in bed
- avoiding external rotation of operative leg by use of trochanter roll

UNIT
10

- avoiding contact sports
- avoiding flexing the knee beyond the point of comfort
- avoiding heavy lifting and unusual twisting/rotation

   f. use of whirlpool baths, if allowed, to facilitate flexion/extension exercising

   g. if using a resting splint, posterior splint or knee immobilizer for ambulation
- assess tightness of knee immobilizer
- applying cornstarch under the immobilizer helps to keep skin dry

   h. if using a cast, petal the edges to minimize irritation

   i. reporting signs and symptoms of dislocation
- severe sudden knee pain followed by continued pain and muscle spasm during knee movement
- inability to move or bear weight on operative leg
- abnormal rotation/length of operative leg
- impaired neurovascular status in the operative leg.

6. Instruct the patient/family/home health aide about signs and symptoms to report.
   a. skin breakdown
   b. infection (elevated temperature, chills, redness, swelling, warmth, tenderness, unusual drainage, foul odor)
   c. falls
   d. continuous drainage of fluid from the incision
   e. sloughing or necrosis of skin in the operative area
   f. unusual/excessive bleeding
   g. loss or sensation/movement in operative leg
   h. decreasing range of motion in joint
   i. inability to flex or extend foot/toes; numbness, tingling of foot/toes
   j. thromboembolism (swelling, tenderness, redness in calf, calf pain on dorsiflexion)
   k. pain in foot during passive motion of foot/toes
   l. pallor, blanching, cyanosis, coolness and decreased or absent pulses
   m. dislocation of operative joints.

7. Instruct the patient/family/home health aide about home safety.
   a. eliminate throw rugs and slippery floors
   b. encourage uncluttered well-lit hallways/rooms
   c. allow adequate time for activities
   d. patient to wear prescribed braced supports/low-heeled shoes
   e. avoid unnecessary stair climbing.

8. Instruct the patient/family/home health aide about the medication plan.
   a. name, dosage, administration schedule and side effects
   b. safety guidelines if the patient is on anticoagulant therapy
- wear a medical identification tag
- take the medication the same time each day
- eliminate or decrease alcohol intake as directed by the physician
- avoid taking aspirin and aspirin containing compounds
- minimize/avoid tissue trauma (shave with electric razor, gently floss/brush teeth, gently blow nose and avoid straining at bowel movements)
- report excessive bleeding immediately
- apply direct pressure, if possible, if bleeding occurs.

9. Instruct the patient/family/home health aide about strategies to prevent skin breakdown.
   a. maintain schedule of position changing (at least every 1 to 2 hours) within allowed parameters of motion
   b. encourage the patient to shift weight at least every 30 minutes while awake

   c. perform range of motion exercises within prescribed parameters

   d. massage pressure points/back /elbows/heels at least twice a day

   e. keep skin clean and dry, particularly around the surgical site

   f. use pressure relief devices as needed

   g. remove antiembolism stockings at least twice a day

   h. inspect skin areas daily, especially at the contact points for splints/braces

   i. report skin breakdown immediately.

10. Identify community resources that can facilitate the patient's/family's adjustment to the long-term rehabilitation plan for joint replacement.

11. Coordinate additional members of the health-care team such as the physical therapist, occupational therapist, social worker and registered dietician.

12. Provide progress reports and a discharge summary to the primary physician.

THERAPEUTIC ACHIEVEMENT

- The patient achieves/maintains stable painless joint function with optimal motion.

RELATED PATIENT INSTRUCTIONS

A Daily Food Guide—Four Basic Food Groups	General Comfort Measures
Antibiotic Medications	Pain Medications
Arthritis	Range of Motion Exercises
Aspirin and Aspirin-like Medications	Skin Care
Changing Dressings	Ways to Save Your Energy

UNIT 10

Muscular Dystrophy Care Plan

CROSS REFERENCES

Bereavement Care Plan
Depression Care Plan
Terminal Illness Care Plan
Tracheostomy Care Plan
Ventilator Care Plan

Assistive Devices Procedure
Decubitus Care Procedure
Enteral Tube Feeding Procedure

Esophagostomy, Gastrostomy, Duodenostomy,
    Jejunostomy Tube Feeding Procedure
Home Safety Procedure
Range of Motion Exercises Procedure
Suctioning (Tracheostomy) Procedure
Tracheostomy Tube Changing Procedure

Medication Compliance Management Guidelines

NURSING DIAGNOSIS

1. Ineffective airway clearance related to
   a. neuromuscular impairment
   b. immobility
   c. other.
2. Impaired physical mobility related to
   a. muscular weakness
   b. dependence on others for care
   c. contractures
   d. other.
3. Alteration in nutrition (less than body requirements) related to
   a. immobility
   b. dependence on others for care
   c. other.
4. Potential for injury (falls, infection) related to
   a. neuromuscular impairment
   b. impaired skin integrity
   c. other.
5. Impaired skin integrity (irritation, breakdown) related to
   a. immobility
   b. brace/splint irritation
   c. other.
6. Self-care deficit (feeding, bathing/hygiene, dressing/grooming, toileting) related to
   a. muscular weakness
   b. other.
7. Fear/anxiety related to
   a. perceived powerlessness
   b. dependence on others for care
   c. loss of control
   d. other.
8. Familial fear/anxiety related to
   a. perceived powerlessness
   b. responsibility of managing the patient at home
   c. other.

9. Ineffective individual coping related to
   a. knowledge deficit
   b. progressive nature of disease with multiple life style adjustments
   c. other.
10. Impaired home maintenance management related to
    a. lack of support (family/community/financial)
    b. ineffective individual coping
    c. ineffective family coping
    d. other.
11. Disturbance in self-concept (body image, self-esteem, role performance, personal identity) related to
    a. loss of body control
    b. dependence on others for care
    c. other.
12. Knowledge deficit (pathophysiology/clinical course of muscular dystrophy, therapeutic/rehabilitation regimen, diet plan, medications, activity plan, assistive devices, signs and symptoms to report) related to
    a. misinterpretation of information
    b. cognitive limitations
    c. lack of readiness to learn
    d. patient's request for no information
    e. other.

PROCESS INDICATORS

1. The patient /family verbalizes an understanding of muscular dystrophy and the therapeutic regimen.

Indicators
   a. describes the muscular dystrophy disease process, therapeutic regimen, rehabilitation plan and strategies to prevent complications
   b. describes a diet plan that promotes adequate nutrition/caloric intake and independence in feeding
   c. describes medication's action, dose, administration schedule and side effects
   d. describes an activity plan that maintains range of motion and mobility to the fullest extent possible
   e. demonstrates appropriate safety precautions/modifications in the home
   f. identifies community resources
   g. identifies signs and symptoms to report.
2. The patient's biopsychosocial integrity is maintained.

Indicators
   a. optimal level of independence is achieved/maintained
   b. skin integrity is maintained
   c. adequate intake of food/fluid
   d. absence of contractures
   e. verbalizes feelings about adapting to muscular dystrophy
   f. maintains adequate respiration
   g. demonstrates effective coping with disease process
   h. demonstrates appropriate use of assistive devices/mobility aids
   i. expresses satisfaction with sexual relationship, if appropriate.

UNIT 10

3. The family's psychosocial integrity is maintained.
Indicators
  a. demonstrates reorganization of family roles to adjust to the patient's regimen
  b. expresses feelings that the patient's care/needs are manageable.

NURSING INTERVENTIONS

1. Assess the patient for
   a. level of activity/functioning
   b. age appropriate body weight
   c. use of assistive devices/mobility aids
   d. respiratory rate/pattern
   e. adventitious breath sounds
   f. mental/cognitive limitations
   g. understanding of the disease process
   h. range of motion/presence of contractures
   i. apical rate/rhythm.
2. Assess the family's
   a. ability to be supportive and to participate in the rehabilitation program
   b. understanding of the disease process
   c. ways of coping with the changes
   d. changes in daily pattern of living
   e. verbal/nonverbal interactions among members and the patient.
3. Instruct the patient /family/home health aide about the muscular dystrophy disease process and the therapeutic/supportive regimen.
   a. correct use of assistive devices/mobility aids
   b. use of assistive devices/mobility aids for activities of daily living and hygiene
   c. strategies to prevent respiratory infections
      • breathing exercises to minimize effects of respiratory decompensation
      • postural drainage
      • avoiding crowds during flu season
   d. strategies to prevent skin breakdown
      • keeping skin clean and dry
      • use of massage
      • use of presssure relief devices
      • repositioning schedule
   e. signs and symptoms to report
      • beginning of contracture
      • skin breakdown/irritation
      • respiratory infection
      • difficulty breathing
   f. medication's name, dosage, administration schedule and side effects.
4. Instruct the patient /family/home health aide about an activity plan that
   a. maximizes the patient's functional abilities
   b. includes range of motion exercises to prevent contractures
   c. incorporates therapy into diversional/play activities to the fullest extent possible
   d. includes return demonstration for
      • proper body alignment/positioning
      • use of assistive devices and/or mobility aids (braces/casts/wheelchair)
   e. includes planned periods of rest

    f. incorporates consultation with the physical/occupational therapists, as needed

    g. includes repositioning at least every 2 hours if the patient is confined to bed.

5. Instruct the patient/family/home health aide about a dietary plan that includes

    a. basic food groups for promotion of general nutrition and adequate caloric intake

    b. use of assistive devices/utensils to encourage independence in eating/feeding

    c. techniques for feeding the patient, as needed.

6. Instruct the patient/family/home health aide about home safety that includes

    a. wearing of prescribed braces/supports

    b. wheelchair transfers and safety, as needed

    c. use of handrails/safety rails, seat belts

    d. keeping items within easy reach

    e. encouraging uncluttered, well-lit hallways/rooms

    f. preparation for the need to adapt to the progression of the patient's weakness and muscle wasting

    g. proper technique for suctioning when needed.

7. Encourage the patient/family to verbalize their feelings about the disease and the personal and family adjustments that are required.

8. Assist children to deal with fear and grief.

9. Provide support to the family for the grieving process.

10. Encourage the patient/family to focus on the patient's strengths as a strategy to overcome limitations.

11. Assist the patient/family to establish realistic goals.

12. Identify community resources that can facilitate the patient's/family's adjustment to muscular dystrophy.

    a. local branch or the national office of the Muscular Dystrophy Association

    b. state office for handicapped children

    c. counselling, psychological therapy and self-help support groups

    d. financial counselling services

    e. resources for caretaker relief as needed.

13. Coordinate additional members of the health care team such as the social worker, occupational therapist, physical therapist and registered dietician.

14. Provide progress reports and a discharge summary to the primary physician.

THERAPEUTIC ACHIEVEMENT

UNIT
10

- The patient/family adapts to the life style changes induced as a result of muscular dystrophy.
- The patient maintains optimal functional abilities appropriate to the disease stage.

RELATED PATIENT INSTRUCTIONS

Bathing the Person in Bed	Oral Suctioning
Care of the Patient Confined to Bed	Ostomy Tube Feedings (Adult)
Comfort Measures for Dehydration	Range of Motion Exercises
Constipation	Skin Care
General Comfort Measures	Tracheostomy Care
Making the Home Environment Safe	Tube Feedings—Special Conditions
Mouth Care	Urinary Catheter Care (Female)
Nasogastric, Orogastric, Nasointestinal Tube Feedings	Urinary Catheter Care (Male)
	Ventilator Care

Multiple Sclerosis Care Plan

CROSS REFERENCES

Depression Care Plan

Assistive Devices Procedure

Home Health Aide Supervision Procedure

Home Safety Procedure

Range of Motion Exercises Procedure

Telephone Contact with Patient /Family Procedure

Medication Compliance Management Guidelines

NURSING DIAGNOSES

1. Anxiety related to
   a. lack of understanding of disease process
   b. threat to or change in socioeconomic status
   c. weakness/fatigue/unsteadiness
   d. sexual functioning and reproductive issues
   e. visual impairment (nystagmus, blurred vision, diplopia)
   f. hospitalization
   g. degenerative nature of disease
   h. other.
2. Impaired physical mobility related to
   a. weakness/fatigue/unsteadiness
   b. ataxia
   c. spasticity/contractures
   d. loss of muscle tone/paralysis
   e. impaired vision
   f. urinary incontinence
   g. other.
3. Impaired verbal communication related to
   a. weakness of facial/throat muscles
   b. dysarthria
   c. emotional lability
   d. other.
4. Impaired home maintenance management related to
   a. inadequate support systems
   b. hospitalization/complex therapy
   c. change in family roles
   d. impaired cognitive/emotional functioning (mood swings, irritability, depression, hyperexcitability)
   e. dependence on others for care
   f. impaired mobility
   g. fatigue/weakness
   h. lack of necessary equipment, aids, finances
   i. other.

5. Ineffective patient /family coping patterns related to
   a. grieving
   b. impaired cognitive/emotional functioning (mood swings)
   c. temporary family disorganization and role changes
   d. anxiety
   e. dependence on others for care
   f. inability to predict pattern of disease progression
   g. inadequate support systems
   h. other.
6. Alterations in nutrition (less than body requirements) related to
   a. nausea/vomiting
   b. difficulty feeding self/preparing foods
   c. difficulty chewing/swallowing
   d. anorexia
   e. inadequate support systems for shopping and cooking
   f. other.
7. Potential for injury related to
   a. impaired perception of pain, proprioception, temperature, tactile sensation
   b. impaired mobility
   c. weakness/fatigue/unsteadiness
   d. impaired skin integrity
   e. spasticity/muscular tremors
   f. other.
8. Self-care deficit (feeding, bathing, dressing, hygiene, toileting, self-administration of medications) related to
   a. dependence on others for care
   b. sensory impairments (visual, psychomotor, cognitive)
   c. emotional lability
   d. weakness/fatigue/unsteadiness
   e. spasticity/muscular tremors
   f. other.
9. Alteration in urinary elimination (retention, incontinence, frequency, urgency) related to
   a. inadequate fluid intake
   b. infection
   c. alteration in bladder tone
   d. decreased perception of urge to void
   e. other.
10. Alteration in bowel elimination (constipation, incontinence) related to
    a. inadequate dietary intake (bulk /fiber)
    b. decreased activity levels
    c. decreased perception of urge to defecate
    d. decreased muscle tone
    e. other.
11. Potential disturbance in self-concept (body image, self-esteem, role performance, personal identity) related to
    a. embarrassment of incontinence
    b. changes in sexual functioning
    c. dependence on others for care
    d. changes in life style/role imposed by a chronic degenerative illness
    e. impaired muscle control (ambulating, self-feeding, chewing, swallowing)
    f. emotional lability
    g. other.

UNIT
10

12. Sexual dysfunction related to
    a. altered self-concept
    b. weakness
    c. spasticity
    d. fear of incontinence
    e. decreased awareness of sensations (genital area)
    f. other.
13. Knowledge deficit related to
    a. nature of multiple sclerosis and its treatment
    b. dietary management
    c. activity program (exercise/rest)
    d. medication regimen
    e. stress management
    f. signs and symptoms to report to the physician
    g. cognitive limitations
    h. other.
14. Noncompliance with the therapeutic regimen related to
    a. cognitive limitations
    b. inadequate support (family/community/financial)
    c. difficulty integrating treatment regimen into life style
    d. dysfunctional grieving
    e. other.

PROCESS INDICATORS

1. The patient /family demonstrates an understanding of how to maintain the regimen for multiple sclerosis.

Indicators
    a. ability to describe the disease process of multiple sclerosis, the treatment regimen and strategies to prevent complications
    b. identify conditions/situations associated with precipitation of exacerbations and management strategies during exacerbations
    c. capable of describing an activity plan that promotes muscle strength and joint mobility, improves coordination and avoids overexertion
    d. develop a dietary plan that provides for adequate fiber, fluids and calories as well as the patient's ability to chew/swallow
    e. describe medication's action, side effects, administration schedule, interactions with other medications and indications for use
    f. identify signs and symptoms to report to the physician
    g. ability to develop a plan for receiving follow-up care.
2. The patient/family demonstrates effective coping patterns.

Indicators
    a. verbalization of acceptance of multiple sclerosis as a chronic disease
    d. reorganization of family roles and activities that incorporate elements of the multiple sclerosis regimen
    c. verbalization of decreased anxiety/depression/fear
    d. demonstration of satisfactory parenting skills
    e. expression of satisfactory level of sexual functioning
    f. provisions made for visual, sensory, psychomotor and cognitive impairments including use of equipment /devices

    g. creation of a plan to utilize internal/external supports such as community groups or the Multiple Sclerosis Society

    h. demonstration of effective coping with bladder dysfunction

    i. identification/implementation of appropriate safety measures

    j. demonstration of effective stress management strategies.

3. The patient establishes/maintains a satisfactory level of comfort.

Indicators

    a. undisturbed sleep

    b. successful coping with stress/anxiety

    c. maintenance of skin integrity

    d. satisfactory activity levels with ability to perform self-care activities

    e. expression of satisfaction with quality of life

    f. satisfactory defecation pattern

    g. absence of uncontrolled pain/discomfort.

NURSING INTERVENTIONS

1. Assess

    a. the patient/family's understanding of the multiple sclerosis disease process, the treatment regimen and prevention strategies for complication including but not limited to diet, activity and medication compliance

    b. the patient's current and potential level of functioning in terms of physical, cognitive, sensory and emotional capabilities

    c. the patient's complaints of weakness, fatigue and discomfort, as well as current activity level

    d. the patient's/family's development of a long-term health care plan

    e. the patient's/family's plans for safety/injury prevention.

2. Instruct the patient /family/home health about

    a. progressive nature of the disease process and the need to periodicallly reassess rehabilitation goals

    b. ways to decrease the risk of upper respiratory infection by
       • avoiding crowds during cold seasons
       • avoiding cigarette smoke and air pollution
       • practicing deep breathing

    c. effective coping strategies/stress management techniques

    d. signs and symptoms that indicate ineffective coping
       • sleep disturbances
       • increasing fatigue
       • increasing difficulty concentrating
       • irritability
       • verbalization of inability to cope
       • dysfunctional grieving
       • feelings of alienation/isolation.

3. Instruct the patient /family to report the following signs and symptoms

    a. new occurrence or increase in the intensity of
       • spasticity/weakness
       • difficulty speaking/swallowing
       • numbness/tingling
       • double/blurred/dimmed vision
       • severe mood swings

UNIT 10

- constipation/loss of bowel control
- urinary retention/incontinence
- decreased motion in any joint.
  b. inability to maintain usual nutritional status/activity level
  c. skin irritation/breakdown
  d. productive cough (purulent, green or rust-colored sputum)
  e. persistent fever/infection
  f. urinary frequency/urgency/burning or cloudy foul smelling urine
  g. signs of pregnancy (cessation of menses, tender breasts).
4. Instruct the patient /family/home health aide about an activity program that
   a. defines limitations during exacerbations
   b. is adaptable to the daily fluctuations in physical ability
   c. provides adequate periods of rest
   d. avoids overexertion
   e. incorporates diversional outlets
   f. avoids extremes in temperature (hot and cold weather/hot and cold baths).
5. Instruct the patient /family/home health aide about energy conservation techniques
   a. using a shower hose and stool in the shower/tub
   b. using a raised seat on the toilet or bedside commode
   c. using assistive devices.
6. Instruct the patient /family/home health aide about the principles/techniques of
   a. body positions
   b. body mechanics
   c. transferring
   d. gait training.
7. Instruct the patient /family/home health aide about exercises that promote muscle strengthening, mobility, balance and coordination.
   a. active or passive range of motion exercises performed every 2 hours
   b. muscle stretching exercises
      - particular emphasis on the hamstrings, gastrocnemius, hip adductors, biceps, wrist and finger flexors
      - practice stretch-hold-relax techniques (to be performed throughout the day).
8. Instruct the patient /family/home health aide about techniques to relieve spasticity.
   a. apply ice packs for 30 minutes and perform slow stretches to affected muscles (may be effective in the early stages)
   b. warm baths, warm packs and muscle relaxants (in later stages)
   c. massage spastic areas
   d. stretching exercises
   e. traction, braces, splints
   f. sleeping in the prone position.
9. Instruct the patient/family/home health aide about a dietary plan that
   a. includes foods from the basic food groups that are
      - high in fiber/bulk to promote satisfactory bowel elimination
      - low in caffeine (less diuretic effect)
      - easy to chew and swallow (custard, applesauce, puréed foods)
   b. demonstrates proper patient positioning (sitting upright) to facilitate eating
   c. reviews strategies to minimize chance of aspiration during periods of impaired swallowing
   d. incorporates use of weighted and/or broad handled eating utensils, weighted wrist cuffs and other feeding /self-help devices as advised by the occupational/physical therapist

      e. incorporates supplemental feedings after consultation with the dietician and phy-
         sician
      f. promotes adequate fluid intake (cranberry juice for greater urine acidity and prune
         . juice for constipated bowels).

10. Instruct the patient/family/home health aide about the medication regimen (anti-
    inflammatory drugs, antispasmodics, muscle relaxants, tranquilizers).
      a. names of drugs
      b. action/indications for use
      c. dosage
      d. schedule of administration
      e. possible side effects
      f. adverse effects to report to the physician.

11. Instruct the patient/family/home health aide about a plan for establishing a satisfactory
    defecation pattern.
      a. assure adequate dietary fluid, fiber and bulk
      b. teach the signs and symptoms of constipation
      c. emphasize the importance of regularity of mealtimes and evacuation times
        • strive for evacuation within 30 to 60 minutes of eating
        • use of suppositories and/or digital stimulation may be necessary
      d. provide liners for underclothes until a pattern is established.

12. Instruct the patient/family/home health aide about strategies for bladder control.
      a. establish a voiding schedule beginning with an every 2-hour interval and gradually
         increasing the time
      b. review the use of Valsalva manuever and Credé technique
      c. teach the signs and symptoms of urinary tract infection
      d. teach self-catheterization technique and/or care of an indwelling urinary catheter
        as needed
      e. keep the bedpan, urinal or commode within easy reach.

13. Instruct the patient/family/home health aide about techniques to maintain skin
    integrity.
      a. change of position every 30 minutes in a wheelchair or at least every hour in bed
      b. inspect the body, especially posterior sites every day
        • the patient can use a long-handled mirror
        • look for areas of redness or skin breakdown
      c. use pressure relief devices such as a floatation pad or sheepskin
      d. if patient uses a brace/splint
        • carefully inspect skin under the brace/splint
        • use padding over bony prominences
      e. use a sheet or bed pad over Chux waterproof pads
      f. avoid skin trauma, exposure to extreme heat/cold and prolonged pressure
      g. after bladder/bowel incontinence
        • carefully clean the skin
        • use a protective ointment or cream (Sween, Desitin)
      h. perform decubitus care as needed
      i. teach the patient to report signs and symptoms of infection.

14. Instruct the patient/family/home health aide about communication strategies.
      a. maintain a calm quiet approach, allowing adequate time for response
      b. ask questions that require short answers or nonverbal responses
      c. try to anticipate the patient's needs
      d. consult with a speech therapist as needed

UNIT 10

   e. provide materials for communication (magic-erase slate, pencil and paper, flash cards)
   f. acknowledge cognitive limitations/impaired memory
      • provide written or taped instructions
      • encourage the patient to write down questions.
15. Provide aids for visual impairment.
   a. explore use of an eye patch or a frosted lens for diplopia
   b. suggest use of corrective lenses as needed
   c. explore use of prism glasses for patients confined to bed
   d. obtain audiocassettes for patients who can't read or hold a book.
16. Review general and home safety measures.
   a. need to wear a medical identification tag
   b. keep the environment well lit and floors uncluttered
   c. keep needed items within the patient's reach
   d. provide, as needed, hand rails, cane, wheelchair, transfer belt and lap belt
   e. exercise care with use of heat or fire (matches, hot water, hot food).
17. Create opportunities for discussion with the patient/family about sexual needs.
   a. explore alternative ways of expressing caring/affection
   b. discuss use of muscle relaxants if spasticity is problematic
   c. encourage voiding/defecating before sexual activity.
18. Discuss with the physician the need for consultation with a sex therapist.
19. Identify community resources that can support the patient's/family's adjustment to multiple sclerosis.
   a. Multiple Sclerosis Society (local and national chapters)
   b. psychological therapy/self-help groups
   c. stress management/relaxation classes
   d. Division of the Blind and Physically Handicapped for audiocassettes and other aids.
20. Consult with the social worker for psychological support and financial assistance.
21. Coordinate additional members of the health care team such as the social worker, physical therapist, occupational therapist, registered dietician, speech therapist, and home health aide.
22. Provide progress reports and a discharge summary to the primary physician.

THERAPEUTIC ACHIEVEMENT

   • The patient/family adapt to the life style modifications as a result of multiple sclerosis.

RELATED PATIENT INSTRUCTIONS

A Daily Food Guide—Four Basic Food Groups	Making the Home Environment Safe
Antibiotic Medications	Muscle Relaxants
Bathing the Person in a Chair	Range of Motion Exercises
Bladder Retraining	Skin Care
Constipation	Urinary Catheter Care (Female)
General Comfort Measures	Urinary Catheter Care (Male)
Intermittent Self-Catheterization (Female)	Ways to Save Your Energy
Intermittent Self-Catheterization (Male)	

Parkinson Disease Care Plan

CROSS REFERENCES

Bladder Incontinence Care Plan   Bladder Retraining Procedure
Constipation Care Plan   Home Safety Procedure
Depression Care Plan   Telephone Contact with Patient /Family Procedure

Assistive Devices Procedure   Medication Compliance Management Guidelines

NURSING DIAGNOSES

1. Anxiety/fear related to
   a. altered body image
   b. loss of control (physical, drooling, speech)
   c. dependence on others for care
   d. lack of understanding of the process/progressive nature of the disease
   e. other.
2. Alteration in bowel elimination (constipation) related to
   a. inadequate fluid /dietary intake
   b. medication
   c. decreased activity
   d. muscle weakness
   e. other.
3. Alteration in nutrition (less than body requirements) related to
   a. difficulty in mastication/swallowing
   b. difficulty in feeding self and preparing foods
   c. anorexia
   d. muscle weakness
   e. dependence on others for care
   f. other.
4. Knowledge deficit (pathophysiology and clinical course of Parkinson disease, medications, nutrition, speech and physical therapy/rehabilitation, bowel/bladder maintenance, community resources, assistive devices) related to
   a. cognitive limitations
   b. lack of readiness to learn
   c. unfamiliarity with information resources
   d. depression
   e. other.
5. Potential for injury related to
   a. impaired mobility/tremors
   b. weakness/fatigue
   c. shuffling /unsteady gait
   d. impaired swallowing effectiveness
   e. other.

UNIT
10

6. Impaired physical mobility related to
   a. muscle weakness/fatigue
   b. tremors
   c. bradykinesia
   d. muscular rigidity of upper/lower extremities (particularly large joints)
   e. other.
7. Impaired home maintenance management related to
   a. inadequate support system
   b. insufficient finances
   c. ineffective individual coping
   d. change in family roles
   e. impaired mobility
   f. fatigue/weakness
   g. lack of necessary equipment /aids
   h. other.
8. Impaired verbal communication related to
   a. excessive saliva buildup/drooling
   b. weakness of muscles controlling respiration, phonation and articulation
   c. depression
   d. other.
9. Depression related to
   a. social withdrawal
   b. drooling
   c. dysfunction from progression of disease
   d. other.
10. Self-care deficit (feeding /bathing /grooming /hygiene/toileting) related to
    a. dependence on others for care
    b. weakness/fatigue/unsteadiness
    c. muscular tremors
    d. impaired mobility
    e. rigidity of upper/lower extremities
    f. other.
11. Sleep pattern disturbance related to
    a. tremors
    b. anxiety
    c. other.

PROCESS INDICATORS

1. The patient's biopsychosocial integrity is maintained.
Indicators
   a. no skin irritation or breakdown
   b. weight is maintained
   c. absence of dehydration (fluid intake is minimally 1200 ml/day)
   d. patient performs self-care/activities of daily living as appropriate with his or her capabilities; uses assistive devices as needed
   e. personal hygiene is adequate
   f. bowel /bladder patterns are regular and continent
   g. patient /family validates balance among patient's rest, exercise and nutrition
   h. patient /family maintains a satisfactory level of social-community interaction.

2. The patient/family adapts to the Parkinson disease treatment regimen in terms of medication, physical therapy/rehabilitation and nutrition.

Indicators
   a. the patient maintains satisfactory nutritional status, eats slowly without choking, maintains acceptable weight and takes supplemental feedings as needed
   b. explains the purpose, administration schedule and adverse reactions of medications
   c. identifies signs of parkinsonian crisis to report to the physician/nurse
   d. patient exercises daily and maintains an activity plan that preserves functional capabilities and prevents severe disabilities
   e. develops a plan for long-term care.
3. The patient's psychological health is supported.

Indicators
   a. patient expresses satisfaction with his or her life experiences
   b. patient exhibits a reduction of anxiety-induced thoughts, feelings and behaviors
   c. patient spontaneously shares his or her thoughts and feelings about his or her condition, changing life style and functional losses
   d. patient/family utilizes community supports/resources that facilitate adaptation to biopsychosocial/sensory-motor losses.

NURSING INTERVENTIONS

1. Assess
   a. patient's/family's understanding of the Parkinson disease process and the treatment regimen (diet, activity, medication)
   b. patient's current level of functioning in terms of physical capabilities, activities of daily living and communicative abilities
   c. patient's complaints of weakness, fatigue and discomfort
   d. patient's/family's plans for safety/injury protection
   e. patient's bowel/bladder elimination pattern
   f. patient's nutritional status
   g. availability/reliability of support systems.
2. Instruct the patient/family/home health aide about
   a. progressive nature of the disease process and the need to periodically reassess rehabilitation goals
   b. the need for skin care and personal hygiene
   c. the need for weekly weight monitoring
   d. the signs and symptoms of parkinsonian crisis
      • sudden and severe increase in bradykinesia, rigidity and tremors
      • potential for impaired airway, tachycardia and hyperpnea
   e. signs and symptoms to report to the nurse/physician
      • change in mentation (confusion, agitation)
      • blurred vision
      • difficulty in urination
      • fever
      • rash.
3. Instruct the patient/family/home health aide about a daily activity program that includes principles/techniques of physical therapy/rehabilitation.
   a. perform active/passive range of motion exercise of each joint daily
   b. perform stretch/hold/relax exercises to loosen joints
   c. relieve spasticity by warm baths/packs, massage and stretching exercises

UNIT
10

    d. schedule periods of rest to avoid fatigue and feelings of being hurried

    e. consult with a physical/occupational therapist for exercises that increase muscle strength, improve coordination, treat muscle rigidity and prevent contractures

    f. use assistive devices as needed (raised toilet seat, trapeze over bed, shower chair, wheelchair, cane, walker)

    g. use proper body positioning
- use straight backed arm chair and firm mattress
- teach proper body alignment while patient is in bed, chair and when walking
- use side-lying positions or elevate the head of bed to prevent choking
- change position every hour

    h. use gait training techniques
- explore patient's feelings of fear of falling
- approach the patient in a calm, unhurried manner (allow ample time for any activity)
- have the patient use a broad-based gait (feet wide apart)
- encourage the patient to swing arms while walking, to lengthen strides and to use a heel-toe gait

    i. to begin forward motion when the patient feels "frozen" or "glued" to the floor, instruct the patient to
- raise his or her head and toes
- take a small step backward and then start forward *or*
- step sideways and then start forward *or*
- rock from one foot to the other with knees slightly bent and then start forward
- do not try to pull the patient.

4. Instruct the patient/family/home health aide about a dietary plan that

    a. includes foods from the basic food groups which are
- high in fiber/bulk to promote satisfactory bowel elimination
- easy for the patient to chew and swallow

    b. reviews strategies to minimize aspiration due to impaired swallowing
- demonstrate proper patient positioning (sitting upright) to facilitate eating/swallowing
- review swallowing technique of placing food on tongue, closing lips/teeth, lifting the tongue up, then back and swallowing
- instruct the patient to consciously chew food thoroughly

    c. maintains weight within an acceptable range

    d. incorporates supplemental feedings after consultation with the dietician/physician

    e. allows small feedings, 4 to 5 times a day

    f. incorporates feeding/self-help devices as advised by the occupational/physical therapist such as weighted and/or broad handled eating utensils, nonspill cup, lipped plate and warming tray

    g. permits fluid intake (at least 1200 ml/day) to compensate for excess salivation/perspiration.

5. Instruct the patient/family/home health aide about the medication regimen (antiviral and anticholinergic agents, tricyclic antidepressants, dopamine replacement).

    a. names, action, dosage, administration schedule, side and adverse effects and drug interactions

    b. need to discuss the introduction of any new medications with the physician prior to initiation

    c. strategies to assist the patient who has an impaired concept of time with adhering to the administration schedule

      d. scheduling medication times with meals as appropriate

      e. reinforcing with the patient /family that the medications decrease symptoms but do not stop disease progression.

6. Instruct the patient /family/home health aide about a plan for establishing a satisfactory defecation pattern.

      a. assure adequate dietary fluid, fiber and bulk

      b. teach the signs and symptoms of constipation

      c. emphasize the importance of regularity of mealtime and evacuation time.

7. Instruct the patient /family/home health aide about communication strategies.

      a. maintain a calm quiet approach, allowing adequate time for response

      b. ask questions that require short answers or nonverbal responses

      c. consult with a speech/language pathologist for assessment and therapy as needed

      d. amplification devices help a weak voice

      e. have the patient face the listener and speak in short sentences

      f. have the patient practice reading in front of a mirror and/or into a tape recorder while he or she exaggerates pronunciations
- read aloud 15 minutes twice daily
- singing is also an acceptable exercise

      g. have the patient practice facial muscle exercises
- make faces in front of a mirror
- grimace, smile, frown and so forth

      h. have the patient practice tongue exercises (extend tongue and try to touch chin, nose, cheek)

      i. encourage the patient to control saliva buildup by planning to swallow frequently and to hold the head upright
- provide tissues for expectoration
- instruct the patient to cough and deep breathe periodically.

8. Discuss strategies with the patient /family/home health aide to prevent depression and social isolation.

      a. encourage the patient to participate in social and recreational events, particularly those that require the use of voice, hands, arms or legs

      b. plan a program of activities to engage in throughout the day

      c. discuss allowing extra time for activities (a hurried/tense situation will result in increased patient dysfunction)

      d. encourage the patient /family to discuss fears and anxieties (such as feelings of dependency; embarrassment due to speech, drooling, body movements, facial expressions; loss of control)

      e. explore community resources to support the patient and family

      f. because of the mask-like facial expression of Parkinson disease, encourage the patient to share his or her feelings since nonverbal communication may not be effective.

9. Instruct the patient /family/home health aide about general and home safety measures.

      a. need for the patient to wear medical identification tag

      b. keep the environment well lit with uncluttered/nonskid floors

      c. keep items within the patient's reach

      d. provide hand rails, cane, walkers, wheelchairs as needed

      e. encourage the patient to wear firm soled shoes instead of slippers

      f. encourage the patient to change positions slowly and wear elastic stockings to prevent postural hypotension

UNIT
10

    g. avoid overexertion on hot, humid days
- overheating in hot weather is possible because of the effects of certain drugs in reducing the excessive diaphoresis common in Parkinson disease
- avoid chilling by fans and air conditioners

    h. encourage independence by wearing shoes that do not have laces and loose fitting clothes that close with Velcro.

10. Coordinate referrals, as necessary to
    a. social worker
    b. physical therapist
    c. occupational therapist
    d. speech therapist
    e. self-help groups
    f. financial counselling service
    g. dietician
    h. The American Parkinson's Disease Association.
11. Obtain blood work as ordered.
12. Provide progress reports and a discharge summary to the primary physician.

THERAPEUTIC ACHIEVEMENT

- The patient/family adapts to life style changes induced as a result of a progressive neurological disease.
- The patient's sense of self-esteem is maintained.

RELATED PATIENT INSTRUCTIONS

A Daily Food Guide—Four Basic Food Groups
Constipation
Making the Home Environment Safe

Mouth Care
Range of Motion Exercises
Skin Care

Seizure Disorder Care Plan

CROSS REFERENCES

Bereavement Care Plan
Depression Care Plan

Home Safety Procedure
Seizure Precaution/Management Procedure

Medication Compliance Management Guidelines

NURSING DIAGNOSES

1. Potential for injury related to
   a. lack of knowledge about seizure precautions
   b. safety hazards in the home
   c. failure to follow medication regimen
   d. oral/musculo-skeletal/airway vulnerability after seizure activity
   e. other.
2. Knowledge deficit (medication regimen, seizure precautions, seizure process, treatment plan) related to
   a. sociocultural differences
   b. low readiness for acceptance of information
   c. language barrier
   d. cognitive limitations
   e. severe anxiety
   f. other.
3. Anxiety/fear of the patient /family related to
   a. lack of understanding about the clinical process of seizure activity
   b. uncontrolled seizure activity
   c. fear of rejection by significant others/community
   d. threat of long-term disability/life style changes/limitations
   e. sociocultural beliefs
   f. ineffective airway clearance during seizure activity
   g. other.
4. Noncompliance with treatment plan related to
   a. denial
   b. sociocultural conflict
   c. knowledge deficit
   d. lack of belief in therapeutic effectiveness
   e. nonsupportive family/environment
   f. side effects of medication/prescribed therapy
   g. other.
5. Sleep pattern disturbance related to
   a. seizure activity
   b. anxiety/depression/fear
   c. environmental changes
   d. other.
6. Disturbance in self-concept related to
   a. seizure disorder

UNIT
10

    b. situational/occupational role changes
    c. perceived sense of powerlessness
    d. uncontrollable bowel / bladder incontinence during seizure activity
    e. other.
7. Social isolation related to
    a. embarrassment about seizure activity/precautions
    b. alteration in self-concept
    c. fear of environmental hazards
    d. fear of rejection by significant others/community
    e. other.
8. Potential alteration in health maintenance related to
    a. knowledge deficit
    b. lack of perceived threat to health
    c. sociocultural beliefs
    d. alteration in self-concept
    e. depression/anxiety
    f. other.
9. Alteration in family process related to
    a. ambivalent patient /family relationships
    b. knowledge deficit
    c. exhausted supportive capacity among family members
    d. changes in family roles
    e. altered financial circumstances
    f. sociocultural conflicts with treatment plan
    g. other.
10. Grieving related to altered body function.
11. Impaired verbal communication related to
    a. impaired articulation
    b. post-seizure disorientation
    c. other.

PROCESS INDICATORS

1. The patient is protected from seizure-related injury.
Indicators
    a. rearrangement of the home environment to eliminate known safety hazards
    b. family/home health aide demonstrates recall of management actions during seizure activity
    c. patient /family/home health aide feedback reflects an adequate understanding of the seizure process
    d. patient /family identifies actions to be taken when an aura occurs
    e. patient /family/home health aide feedback reflects an accurate awareness of activities and environmental factors that can be life-threatening in the presence of a seizure.
2. The patient /family alters their previous pattern of daily living to incorporate seizure management /precautionary techniques.
Indicators
    a. patient /family/home health aide feedback reflects an adequate understanding of the treatment plan

b. patient /family/home health aide recalls the purpose, side effects and precautions for prescribed medications
c. patient /family/home health aide administers anticonvulsant medications as pre-scribed
d. patient accepts wearing of an emergency medical identification tag or bracelet
e. patient /family demonstrates ability to appropriately participate in daily living even in presence of anxiety
f. patient /family maintains satisfactory level of social-community interaction
g. patient /family accurately verbalizes state laws relative to the seizure disorder and activities of daily living.

NURSING INTERVENTIONS

1. Assess
   a. level /causes of patient/family anxiety
   b. patient / family support systems
   c. sociocultural beliefs about seizure disorders
   d. patient /family perceptions about personal vulnerability to the seizure disorder and its sequelae
   e. sensorimotor deficits during seizure activity.
2. Provide instruction to the patient /family/home health aide about
   a. clinical process of the specific seizure disorder (grand mal, petit mal, myoclonic, status epilepticus)
   b. seizure precautions
   c. seizure management
   d. modification of diet, exercise, rest, environment
   e. stress-management techniques
   f. medications (purpose, side effects, administration, precautions)
   g. importance of wearing an emergency medical identification tag or bracelet
   h. auras and preseizure management
   i. importance of avoiding environmental stimuli that might precipitate seizure activity
   j. post-seizure symptoms and appropriate care
   k. importance of physician and laboratory follow-up
   l. how to record seizure activity
   m. state laws regarding the seizure disorder and activities of daily living (check with division of motor vehicles).
3. Involve the patient /family/home health aide in
   a. problem solving
   b. care planning
   c. determination of which behaviors indicate satisfactory compliance.
4. Consult with the attending physician about changes in the medical regimen in order to encourage patient /family compliance.
5. Coordinate/facilitate referrals to
   a. Epilepsy Foundation of America
   b. community social service
   c. self-help groups
   d. pastoral care/spiritual adviser
   e. psychiatric liaison nurse
   f. legal counsel (relative to state laws).

UNIT
10

THERAPEUTIC ACHIEVEMENT

- The patient/family adapts to the life style changes induced as a result of the seizure disorder.

RELATED PATIENT INSTRUCTIONS

Anticonvulsant Medications
Guidelines for Describing Seizure Activity
Making the Home Environment Safe

Management of Seizure Activity
Medication Compliance
Seizure Precautions

Procedures

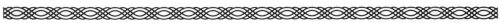

Continuous Passive Motion (CPM) Equipment Procedure

PURPOSE

- To provide continuous passive motion to the leg.
- To maintain joint function.

EQUIPMENT

- continuous passive motion unit with patient control switch
- sheepskin cover with Velcro closures
- adhesive tape

Steps

1. Confirm physician's order for therapy and coordinate with the physical therapist.

2. If compatible with agency policy, a piece of adhesive tape can be placed above the control knobs to record the current prescribed settings.

3. Wash hands.
4. Reinforce patient/family understanding of the procedure.
5. Assure that the patient is comfortably positioned.
6. Plug CPM unit into the power outlet and activate the power switch on the panel.
7. Place the CPM unit on or near the bed on the side of the patient's affected extremity.
8. Place the patient's affected extremity carefully on the CPM unit frame.

Key Points

1. The physician order must specify the CPM unit's settings for speed and degree of flexion and extension. Initial application and frame adjustment are made by the physical therapist. Maintenance of the therapy can be supervised by the nurse.

2. To assure the accuracy of this method, the tape should be dated and signed by the health care professional who sets the control knobs.

4. Review skin care safety and indications for calling the nurse/physician.

UNIT
10

9. Recheck the control knobs for *current* prescribed settings.
10. Start the CPM unit in motion by pushing the patient control button.
11. Reinforce with the patient/family that the unit may be stopped at any time by pushing the patient control button.
12. Push the patient control button to stop the CPM unit.
13. Turn off the power switch on the panel.
14. Carefully lift the patient's affected extremity from the unit.
15. Remove the CPM unit.

9. Check the flexion, extension and speed settings.

DOCUMENTATION

1. The time the CPM unit was applied as well as the settings for flexion, extension and speed.
2. Patient tolerance of procedure and progress in increased length of time using the unit.
3. Patient/family understanding of procedure and indications for calling the nurse/physician.
4. The time the CPM unit was removed as well as the schedule of reapplication times with proper settings of controls.
5. Any significant information concerning surgical site, dressings and neurovascular status.
6. Consultation with the physical therapist as appropriate.
7. Report to the primary physician.

Seizure Precaution/ Management Procedure

PURPOSE

- To teach the patient/family how to manage a seizure disorder at home.
- To teach the family how to observe and record seizure activity.

EQUIPMENT

- padded tongue blade/oral airway/mouth gag

Steps	**Key Points**
1. Assess patient/family level of knowledge.	1. A baseline of what the patient/family knows will facilitate teaching.
2. Teach the patient/family about seizure precautions.	2. Useful materials/information can be obtained from the Epilepsy Foundation of America.
a. compliance with medication regimen	
b. use of an emergency medical bracelet or tag	
c. diet modification (no caffeine/alcohol)	
d. use of axillary/rectal temperatures	
e. quick access to mouth gag/oral airway/padded tongue blade	
f. no swimming alone	
g. no smoking	
h. no tub bathing until seizure free	
i. no operating heavy equipment until seizure free	i. Refer to legal counsel/local law enforcement agencies regarding the operation of heavy machinery/equipment/cars/trucks.
j. no driving until seizure free	
k. avoidance of environmental stimuli (flashing lights, screeching noises) that may precipitate seizure activity.	
3. Teach the family about seizure management.	3. It is important for the family to express confidence regarding seizure management.

UNIT 10

a. lower patient to the floor
b. clear the area around the patient
c. place something soft under the patient's head
d. insert mouth gag /oral airway/padded tongue blade if the patient's jaws are not clenched
e. loosen constrictive clothing around the patient's head, neck and chest
f. do not restrain /interfere with the patient's movements
g. give artificial respiration, if needed
h. turn the patient on his or her side after the seizure
i. remain with the patient during and after the seizure

j. reorient the patient after the seizure.

4. Teach the family about observations to be made/recorded about the patient's seizure activity:
a. precipitating factors
b. aura
c. what part of the body the seizure starts in
d. generalized or focal seizure
e. changes in the eyes
f. incontinence (bowel/bladder)
g. respiratory pattern
h. loss of consciousness
i. postictal status
j. frequency and duration.

i. Familial calmness and acceptance comforts the patient and decreases the possibility of a fear reaction.

4. A written outline of items to observe during seizure activity may be helpful if given to the family.

DOCUMENTATION

1. Assessment of patient's/family's level of knowledge.
2. Assessment of patient's/family's capability to learn.
3. Instructions given about seizure precautions, seizure management and observation of seizure activity.
4. Patient /family response to information.
5. Patient /family validation of learning (e.g., reiteration and explaining how they understand the material).

Resources

Crutch-Walking

FOUR-POINT GAIT PATTERN

Crutch Walking
Four-point gait pattern

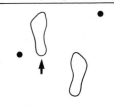

(5) Advance opposite leg.

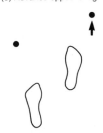

(4) Advance right crutch.

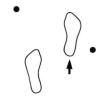

(3) Advance opposite leg.

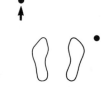

(2) Advance left crutch.

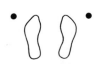

(1) Begin with weight on both legs and both crutches.

THREE-POINT GAIT PATTERN

Crutch Walking
Three-point gait pattern

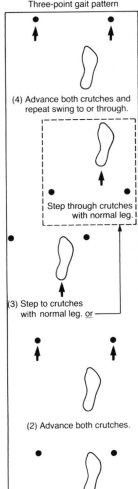

(4) Advance both crutches and repeat swing to or through.

Step through crutches with normal leg.

(3) Step to crutches with normal leg. or

(2) Advance both crutches.

(1) Begin with weight on normal leg and both crutches.

TWO-POINT GAIT PATTERN

Crutch Walking
Two-point gait pattern

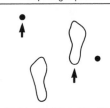

(3) Advance left crutch with the opposite leg.

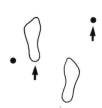

(2) Advance right crutch with the opposite leg.

(1) Begin with weight on both legs and both crutches.

UNIT 10

Beebe, W. and Gomez, K. Amyotrophic Lateral Sclerosis. Home Healthcare Nurse, 3(3): 1985, pp. 8–17.

Caroscio, J. T. (ed.). Amyotrophic Lateral Sclerosis: A Guide to Patient Care. New York: Thieme Medical Publishers, Inc., 1986.

Dickinson, G. A Home Care Program for Patients with Rheumatoid Arthritis. Nursing Clinics of North America, 15(2): June 1980, pp. 403–418.

Maloney, F. P., Burkes, J. S. and Rengel, S. P. (eds.). Interdisciplinary Rehabilitation of Multiple Sclerosis and Neuromuscular Disorders. Philadelphia: J. B. Lippincott Co., 1985.

McCarthy, D. J. (ed.). Arthritis and Allied Conditions: A Textbook of Rheumatology, 10th ed. Philadelphia: Lea & Febiger, 1985.

Moskowitz, R. W. and Haug, M. R. (eds.). Arthritis and the Elderly. New York: Springer, 1986.

Porter, S. F. Arthritis Care: A Guide for Patient Education. Norwalk, Connecticut: Appleton-Century Crofts, 1984.

Rabin, David. Practical Tips for Patients with A.L.S. Nursing 86, February 1986, pp. 47–49.

Rich, J. Action Stat: Generalized Motor Seizure. Nursing, 6(4): 1986, p. 33.

Scott, S., Carol F. I. and Williams, B. O. Communication in Parkinson's Disease. Rockville, Maryland: Aspen Systems, 1985.

Souliere, C. Home Administration of Gold Therapy for Rheumatoid Arthritis. Home Healthcare Nurse, 3(4): 1985, pp. 28–32.

Yanko, J. What Your Patient Should Know About Parkinson's Disease. Nursing 88, 18(1): February 1988, pp. 32p–32s.

Elimination Alterations

UNIT
11

Care Plans

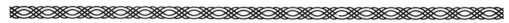

Bladder Incontinence Care Plan

CROSS REFERENCES

Bladder Retraining Procedure
Home Health Aide Supervision Procedure
Infection Control Procedure
Intermittent Self-Catheterization Procedure

Medication Compliance Management Guidelines
Mental Health Assessment /Intervention Guide

NURSING DIAGNOSES

1. Alteration in pattern of urinary elimination (incontinence) related to
   a. sphincter dysfunction (traumatic injury, surgery, childbirth)
   b. urgency (urinary tract infection, brain tumor, traumatic brain injury, meningitis)
   c. neuromuscular impairment (spinal cord injury/lesion, compression of the spinal cord, obstructive bladder disorder)
   d. sensorimotor impairment (elderly, coma, no definite cerebral pathology)
   e. intra-abdominal pressure (elderly, childbirth, coughing, sneezing, physical strain)
   f. urinary catheter drainage
   g. other.
2. Potential /actual impairment of skin integrity related to
   a. frequent contact with urinary irritants
   b. poor personal hygiene
   c. caking of excessive talc after showering or bathing
   d. hypersensitivity to perineal deodorant spray
   e. other.
3. Disturbance of body image related to
   a. urinary odor
   b. physical discomfort
   c. lack of control over basic function of elimination
   d. other.
4. Disturbance in self-esteem related to
   a. dependence on others
   b. feelings of powerlessness
   c. other.
5. Social isolation related to
   a. uncontrolled bladder function
   b. embarrassment
   c. urinary odor
   d. other.
6. Sleep pattern disturbance related to nocturnal enuresis.
7. Knowledge deficit (bladder retraining, personal hygiene, urinary catheter care, protective devices for incontinence, skin care, fluid intake modifications) related to

a. cognitive limitation
b. unfamiliarity with information resources
c. misinterpretation of information
d. lack of exposure to information
e. other.

PROCESS INDICATORS

1. The patient establishes control over his or her pattern of urinary elimination.
Indicators
    a. no suprapubic distention
    b. residual urine of less than 50 ml
    c. voiding _____ ml at each continent episode
    d. indwelling urinary catheter does not leak
    e. patient/family demonstrates appropriate use of urine collection devices
    f. patient/family validates adherence to the bladder management program.
2. The patient's physical integrity is maintained.
Indicators
    a. absence of perineal/anogenital skin irritation
    b. absence of foul urinary odor
    c. clear, yellow urine
    d. patient/family adequately describes the relationship between hygiene and skin integrity
    e. patient/family validates a balanced food and fluid intake that facilitates bowel and bladder training.
3. The patient's/family's psychological equilibrium is maintained.
Indicators
    a. patient verbalizes/expresses feelings of social acceptability
    b. patient/family participates in social activities in and out of the home
    c. patient/family verbalizes their frustrations and feelings regarding incontinence
    d. patient/family identifies where and when to seek help, if problems are encountered.

NURSING INTERVENTIONS

1. Assess
    a. patient's health conditions associated with incontinence
    b. times, amounts and frequency of incontinent episodes
    c. patient's pattern of fluid intake
    d. patient's pattern of bowel elimination
    e. patient's awareness of the need to void
    f. medications that may induce incontinence (fast-acting diuretics, hypnotics, diazepam, phenothiazines)
    g. environmental impediments to continence (patient's clothing, obstructed pathways, location of toilet, etc.)
    h. patient's skin for irritation/breakdown
    i. patient's urine (color, clarity, odor)
    j. method(s) used by the patient/family to control/cope with the incontinence
    k. patient's/family's feelings about the incontinence
    l. patient's/family's ability to learn.

UNIT
11

2. Identify a program of bladder management that is consistent with the patient's/family's capabilities and the etiology of the incontinence.
3. Consult with the attending physician regarding treatment approach, intermittent/retention catheter orders and prescribed medications.
4. Coordinate, as necessary, referrals to the enterostomal therapist and dietician.
5. Monitor the therapeutic/nontherapeutic effects of the prescribed medications.
6. Teach the patient/family/home health aide about
   a. physiology of micturition
   b. physiology/etiology of the patient's incontinence
   c. methods to increase sphincter/perineal muscle tone (Kegel exercises, no smoking, diet that facilitates bowel elimination, stopping and starting urine flow)
   d. how to measure intake and output
   e. modification of fluid intake to prevent incontinence (establish a consistent fluid intake schedule, avoid large fluid intakes in short periods of time, limit fluid intake before leaving the house, do not drink fluids after 7:00 pm, avoid coffee, tea and citrus juices)
   f. modification of fluid intake to prevent urinary tract infection (increase fluid intake to at least 3000 ml per day, drink cranberry juice, add 2 gm ascorbic acid to daily intake)
   g. signs/symptoms of urinary tract infection (fever, pain, cloudy urine, foul odor)
   h. how to take/administer diuretics at times that prevent/diminish nocturnal enuresis
   i. how to respond quickly to the patient's urge to void
   j. methods to reduce impediments to voiding (use of Velcro closures on clothing, dresses/skirts for women, easy accessibility to toilet/commode/bedpan/urinal)
   k. skin and perineal care (avoid excess powder/cornstarch, wash with soap and water after each incontinent episode, dry the skin thoroughly, use protective sprays/wipes/zinc oxide, maintain personal hygiene, change wet bed linens/clothes as soon as possible)
   l. noninvasive devices for urine collection (bedpan, urinal, external catheter, leg bag, adult diapers)
   m. care of indwelling urinary catheters (change drainage bags, empty urine, positioning of the patient, physical activity for the patient, fluid intake, hygiene, catheter irrigation technique)
   n. intermittent (self) catheterization
   o. methods to control odor (good hygiene, frequent change of bed linens and underclothes, use and frequent change of absorbent pads, deodorant sprays)
   p. methods to protect furniture (rubber/plastic sheets, absorbent pads, use of commode seat on a favorite chair, use of commode wheelchairs)
   q. noninvasive methods of urine collection for the chronically bedridden patient (Bradford frame; use of padding to build up around a depressed area in which to place a drainage receptacle; cut a hole in the mattress, pad the edges and place a funnel/collection bottle beneath the opening)
   r. methods to facilitate socialization (good grooming, dressing in street clothes, coordinating social activities and pattern of incontinence)
   s. purposes, side effects and administration of prescribed medications.
7. Create situations that encourage the patient/family to express their thoughts and feelings.
8. Provide progress reports and a discharge summary to the attending physician.

THERAPEUTIC ACHIEVEMENT

- The patient/family identifies a reduction in the number of episodes of urinary incontinence.
- The patient/family identifies restoration of urinary continence.

RELATED PATIENT INSTRUCTIONS

Antibiotic Medications
Bladder Retraining
Infection Control for the Home
Intermittent Self-Catheterization (Female)
Intermittent Self-Catheterization (Male)

Measuring Liquid Intake and Output
Medication Compliance
Skin Care
Urinary Catheter Care (Female)
Urinary Catheter Care (Male)

UNIT
11

Chronic Renal Failure Care Plan

CROSS REFERENCES

Bereavement Care Plan
Congestive Heart Failure Care Plan
Constipation Care Plan
Depression Care Plan
Home Peritoneal Dialysis Care Plan
Hypertension Care Plan
Pain Care Plan
Seizure Disorder Care Plan

Terminal Illness Care Plan

Assistive Devices Procedure
Decubitus Care Procedure
Home Safety Procedure

Range of Motion Exercises
Medication Compliance Management Guidelines
Mental Health Assessment/Intervention Guide

NURSING DIAGNOSES

1. Alteration in fluid volume (excess) related to
   a. excess fluid intake
   b. excess sodium intake
   c. fluid retention
   d. impaired urinary output
   e. other.
2. Alteration in fluid volume (deficit) related to
   a. increased fluid loss
   b. decreased fluid intake
   c. other.
3. Anxiety related to
   a. lack of understanding of the disease, prognosis, therapeutic regimen
   b. repeated hospitalizations/invasive procedures
   c. life style changes resulting from disease/treatments
   d. failure to achieve normal growth patterns
   e. fear of death
   f. powerlessness/hopelessness
   g. financial demands of treatment
   h. other.
4. Alteration in urinary elimination related to
   a. disturbance of renal function
   b. decreased urine output
   c. other.
5. Ineffective breathing pattern related to
   a. decreased energy/fatigue
   b. fluid volume overload
   c. anxiety
   d. other.
6. Alteration in comfort (stomatitis, nausea/vomiting, muscle cramps, paresthesias/ burning /numbness/tingling, pruritus) related to
   a. irritation of oral mucous membranes

   b. electrolyte imbalance
   c. peripheral nerve irritation
   d. skin irritation (dryness/uremic frost)
   e. other.
7. Ineffective individual coping related to
   a. dependence on others for care
   b. denial
   c. multiple life changes
   d. failure to achieve normal growth
   e. other.
8. Alteration in bowel elimination (constipation) related to
   a. medications
   b. fluid restrictions
   c. dietary restrictions
   d. lack of physical activity
   e. other.
9. Alteration in bowel elimination (diarrhea) related to
   a. fear/anxiety
   b. medications
   c. gastrointestinal irritation
   d. other.
10. Self-care deficit (feeding, bathing, hygiene, dressing, grooming, toileting) related to
   a. fatigue/weakness
   b. discomfort /pain
   c. activity restrictions
   d. depression
   e. other.
11. Activity intolerance related to
   a. fatigue/weakness
   b. neuromuscular impairment
   c. muscle cramps
   d. other.
12. Alteration in nutrition (less than body requirements) related to
   a. anorexia /decreased appetite
   b. nausea /vomiting
   c. stomatitis
   d. altered taste sensation
   e. inadequate support systems (cooking, shopping)
   f. personal /cultural /religious barriers
   g. other.
13. Impairment of skin integrity (irritation and breakdown) related to
   a. itching /pruritus
   b. deposits of waste products on the skin
   c. other.
14. Alteration in oral mucous membrane (dryness, stomatitis) related to
   a. ineffective oral hygiene
   b. infection /irritation
   c. inadequate nutrition
   d. other.
15. Potential for injury (falls, bleeding, infection, thermal injury) related to
   a. impaired skin integrity

UNIT 11

   b. paresthesias
   c. inadequate compliance with regimen
   d. other.
16. Sleep pattern disturbance related to
   a. muscle cramps
   b. pruritus
   c. anxiety /fear
   d. other.
17. Alteration in thought process (memory deficit, confusion, altered attention span, impaired reasoning) related to
   a. partial /total loss of hearing /vision
   b. sensory overload
   c. other.
18. Sexual dysfunction (impotence, decreased libido) related to
   a. altered body function /image
   b. medication side effects
   c. other.
19. Disturbance in self-concept (body image, self-esteem, role performance, personal identity) related to
   a. loss of body function /control
   b. repeated hospitalizations /invasive procedures
   c. change in role/job/life style
   d. dependence on others for care
   e. other.
20. Impaired home maintenance management related to
   a. lack of support (family/community/financial)
   b. lack of knowledge
   c. health /cultural beliefs /values
   d. ineffective individual coping
   e. other.
21. Knowledge deficit (nature of disease process/therapeutic regimen, follow-up care, signs and symptoms to report) related to
   a. cognitive limitations
   b. lack of readiness to learn
   c. patient's request for no information
   d. misinterpretation of information
   e. other.
22. Noncompliance with the therapeutic regimen related to
   a. knowledge deficit
   b. lack of support (family/community/financial)
   c. difficulty integrating regimen into life styles
   d. dysfunctional relationship with health care providers
   e. expressed feelings of hopelessness
   f. other.

PROCESS INDICATORS

1. The patient /family verbalizes an understanding of chronic renal failure and the therapeutic regimen.

Indicators

    a. describes renal failure disease process, therapeutic regimen and strategies to prevent complications

    b. verbalizes a diet plan that includes parameters for maintaining fluid and electrolyte balance, protein /basic nutrition and promotion of bowel evacuation

    c. describes medication's action, dose, administration schedule and side effects

    d. maintains an activity plan that provides for periods of activity, planned rest periods and diversional activities (taking into consideration age and specific growth and development, as appropriate).

2. The patient's biopsychosocial integrity is maintained.

Indicators

    a. maintains blood pressure and pulse within the patient's normal range

    b. maintains an optimal urine output

    c. maintains skin /mucous membrane integrity

    d. does not exhibit signs of infection

    e. maintains an appropriate fluid balance

    f. maintains an adequate nutrition level

    g. maintains weight within the acceptable range for the patient based upon age and body structure

    h. maintains a satisfactory defecation pattern

    i. verbalizes feelings about adapting to renal failure

    j. expresses satisfaction with sexual relationship, as appropriate.

3. The patient establishes/maintains a satisfactory level of comfort.

    a. verbalizes /exhibits an absence of uncontrolled pain /discomfort /itching

    b. verbalizes /exhibits successful coping with anxiety

    c. expresses satisfaction with the quality of life

    d. reports undisturbed sleep.

NURSING INTERVENTIONS

1. Assess the patient for

    a. urinary output
- any signs of obstruction or infection
- usual daily output (reports of anuria, oliguria, polyuria)

    b. general nutritional status
- measurement of triceps skin folds
- usual daily intake.

2. Assess the patient for signs and symptoms of fluid and electrolyte disturbances including

    a. history of body weight changes and patterns of increases or decreases in weight

    b. hyponatremia /hypernatremia

    c. hyperkalemia

    d. hyperphosphatemia

    f. thirst (although not a reliable indicator)

    g. dehydration (which can lead to a crisis).

3. Assess the patient for signs and symptoms of metabolic and endocrine disturbances including

    a. glucose intolerance

    b. sex hormone disturbance (particularly during puberty)

    c. metabolic acidosis.

UNIT
11

4. Assess the patient for signs and symptoms of dermatological disturbances including
   a. nails—brittleness, red bands on nails (Muercke lines) or proximal half of nails appear white and distal half appear brown
   b. hair—brittle with loss
   c. skin—turgor, dryness, color (pallor, grey-yellow, hyperpigmentation, purpura, petechiae, ecchymoses), uremic frost, pruritus.
5. Assess the patient for signs and symptoms of hematological disturbances including
   a. color of oral mucous membranes (for pallor)
   b. bleeding tendencies/bruising
   c. fatigue and cold intolerance (resulting from anemia).
6. Assess the patient's cardiovascular status including
   a. blood pressure measurements (sitting, standing, supine in both arms)
   b. peripheral edema (palpate tibia, ankles, sacrum, back; assess for puffiness of face and eyelids, assess for demarcation patterns from shoes and clothing on the body)
   c. signs of neck vein distension
   d. evidence of electrocardiogram (ECG) changes (peaked and elevated T waves with widened QRS and flattened or absent P waves indicate hyperkalemia that requires emergency treatment)
   e. auscultation of heart sounds (rate, rhythm, S_3 and /or S_4 gallop rhythms, arrhythmias, pericardial rub)
   f. assessment of peripheral pulses and circulation.
7. Assess the patient's respiratory status including
   a. auscultation of breath sounds (rate, rhythm, depth, adventitious sounds, Kussmaul respiration, Cheyne-Stokes respiration)
   b. signs of orthopnea, paroxysmal nocturnal dyspnea, dyspnea.
8. Assess the patient's gastrointestinal status including
   a. symptoms of anorexia, nausea, vomiting
   b. signs of blood in vomitus, urine, stool
   c. assessment of oral mucous membrane and gingiva moistness and integrity (indicators of stomatitis-inflammation, ulcers, leukoplakia, pain, dysphagia, viscous saliva)
   d. complaints of constant bitter metallic or salty taste in mouth, hiccoughs
   e. signs of fetid, fishy or ammonia-like breath.
9. Assess the patient's neuromuscular status including
   a. complaints of fatigue, weakness, lethargy, paresthesias (burning, tingling, numbness), dysarthria
   b. signs of muscle cramps, twitching seizures, sleep disorders, drowsiness
   c. signs of irritability, headache, difficulty concentrating
   d. evidence of growth retardation in children.
10. Assess the patient for personality changes including
    a. increased lability
    b. depression
    c. changes in mentation.
11. Assess the patient's/family's understanding of the disease process and treatment regimen.
12. Monitor, record and review the patient's/family's records of
    a. intake and output
    b. specified vital signs
    c. body weight.
13. Instruct the patient/family/home health aide about chronic renal failure and/or end stage renal failure disease process and the treatment regimen.

    a. preparing the patient/family for treatment protocols, as appropriate (i.e., dialysis or kidney transplant)

    b. properly performing and recording
- intake and output
- specified vital signs
- body weight

    c. understanding the relationship of
- daily weight changes
- fluid and dietary sodium intake
- fluid loss (including urinary output, vomiting, diarrhea, diaphoresis)

    d. preventing complications and fluid and electrolyte imbalances.

14. Instruct the patient/family/home health aide about a dietary plan that complies with the prescribed parameters.

    a. dietary restrictions/adjustments according to the patient's status (particularly fluid weight gain and blood pressure)
- sodium restriction to _____/day (avoid monosodium glutamate, pickled foods, processed meats, salty snacks, added salts)
- fluid restriction to _____/day
- distribution of food/fluid allowances throughout the day
- potassium restriction to _____/day (limitations on salt substitutes containing potassium, citrus fruits, bananas, dried fruits)
- phosphorus restrictions (limitations on meat, milk, legumes, carbonated beverages)

    b. maintenance of adequate caloric intake to prevent wasting syndrome (loss of body weight, muscle mass and adipose tissue)
- carbohydrate powders/supplements may be necessary
- carbohydrate intolerance may require adjustment of insulin dosages in patients with diabetes mellitus
- protein intake _____/day (if amino acid–rich foods such as meats, eggs and dairy products cannot be consumed; amino acid and vitamin supplements may be needed on protein-restricted diets)
- using extra sweeteners, spices and seasonings to increase consumption

    c. relief of nausea
- encourage patient to eat dry foods (toast) and avoid liquids with meals when nauseated
- encourage the patient/family to maintain a relaxed pleasant environment at mealtime (eliminate noxious odors and sights)
- instruct the patient to change positions slowly
- encourage oral hygiene before and after meals (and after each emesis)
- instruct the patient to avoid foods/fluids irritating to the gastrointestinal tract (i.e., spicy foods, citrus fruits/juices, chocolate, coffee, tea, colas)
- obtain a prescription for antiemetics (if needed) and assess for effectiveness

    d. incorporation of cultural/religious/personal preferences

    e. written instructions/recipes for reference

    f. plan for smaller more frequent meals

    g. plan for rest before and after meals (elevate head after meals)

    h. instruct the patient to eat/drink slowly (use of a warming tray can keep food warm)

    i. a complete 72 hour food log, if needed for nutritional assessment

    j. consultation with the dietician and/or physician for dietary adjustments and/or for alternative methods for providing nutrition (tube feedings) as needed.

UNIT 11

15. Instruct the patient /family/home health aide about the prescribed medications.
   a. minimizing the risk for medication toxicity
      • toxic reactions for all medications must be carefully explained
      • usual published dosage ranges may be altered
   b. taking medications with applesauce or other foods (i.e., mashed potatoes), if permitted, rather than liquids for those on fluid-restricted diets
   c. consulting with the nurse /physician before taking any medication, particularly over-the-counter and nephrotoxic medications.
16. Instruct the patient /family/home health aide about an activity plan including
   a. strategies to compensate for fatigue, weakness, joint pain and bone demineralization (increased incidence of fractures)
   b. use of assistive devices/mobility aids to assist with activities of daily living, to save energy and to provide for safety
   c. use of range of motion exercises, as needed
   d. diversional activities appropriate for the patient's energy level, age and growth and development
   e. planned periods of uninterrupted rest
   f. planned periods of minimal environmental stimulation and activity prior to sleep
   g. instructions to stop activities that result in signs and symptoms of overactivity
      • pulse rate increase greater than 20 beats/minute above the resting rate
      • marked increase in blood pressure (40 mmHg systolic and/or 20 mmHg diastolic)
      • chest pain
      • dyspnea
      • excessive fatigue/weakness
      • diaphoresis.
17. Instruct the patient /family/home health aide about signs and symptoms to report.
   a. appearance of irregular heart rate, palpitations, chest pain
   b. increased dizziness, headache, drowsiness, restlessness, confusion, hallucinations
   c. seizures
   d. dyspnea, orthopnea, paroxysmal nocturnal dyspnea, rapid /shallow respirations
   e. appearance of poor skin turgor, skin breakdown, oral mucous membrane ulceration, tan-bronze or yellow skin color
   f. urine output of less than _____ /day
   g. weight gain or weight loss of greater than 1 lb. (0.45 kg)/day
   h. increasing or decreasing blood pressure
   i. appearance of peripheral edema
   j. increased weakness/fatigue
   k. increase in severity of nausea, vomiting, itching, muscle cramps, twitching, tremors, paresthesias, metallic taste in mouth, diarrhea
   l. unusual bleeding (petechiae, multiple ecchymotic areas, bleeding gums, frequent or uncontrolled epistaxis, unusual joint pain or swelling, hematemesis, melena, red or smoke-colored urine, excessive menses, increase in abdominal girth)
   m. signs and symptoms of infection (elevated temperature, cloudy or foul-smelling urine, burning /pain /urgency /increased frequency of urination, skin breakdown with redness/swelling /tenderness/warmth /drainage).
18. Instruct the patient/family/home health aide about measures to maintain skin integrity including
   a. nutrition, mobility, hygiene, early recognition and treatment of skin breakdown
   b. identification and elimination of irritants
   c. promotion of vasoconstriction with a cool (not cold) environment, loose/nonconstrictive light clothing and avoidance of excessive bedding

   d. inspection of skin for redness and breakdown particularly at bony prominences, pressure points, dependent areas, edematous areas (including scrotum) and perineal area
   e. avoidance of direct skin contact with waterproof underpads
   f. thorough cleaning and drying of the perineal area after voiding and after each bowel movement (apply protective ointment/cream if needed)
   g. performance of decubitus care if skin breakdown occurs
   h. for immobile patients
      • performing range of motion exercises _____ /day
      • repositioning the patient at least every 2 hours
   i. for edematous patients
      • elevating affected extremities when possible
      • using a scrotal support for scrotal edema
      • handling edematous areas carefully
      • instructing in proper application of elastic wraps/hose for lower extremities if ordered
   j. trimmed nails and/or mittens
   k. treatment of pruritus
      • instruct in use of prescribed emollients/lotions, cool/moist compresses, and/or antihistamines
      • for bathing use tepid/cool baths with moisturizing oils to relieve dry skin
      • keep skin clean using a mild soap
      • rinse skin thoroughly to remove all soap residue and pat skin dry
      • use of cutaneous stimulation techniques to avoid scratching (firm pressure, massage, vibration) at the site of itching or acupressure points.
19. Instruct the patient/family/home health aide about strategies to promote comfort including
   a. relief of muscle cramps and paresthesis
      • provide a footboard to keep bed linens off the feet and for the patient to push against with his or her feet for foot and/or leg cramps
      • instruct the patient to change positions slowly
      • instruct the patient in relaxation techniques and use of diversional activity
      • consult with the physician concerning use of warm packs, analgesics, and/or muscle relaxants
   b. assistance of the patient with cold intolerance to identify the most comfortable environmental temperature in combination with layers of loose clothing (thermal clothing is an option for some patients)
   c. relief of shortness of breath
      • avoid overactivity and adhere to periods of planned rest
      • maintain a semi-Fowler position after meals
      • discontinue smoking.
20. Instruct the patient/family/home health aide about mouth care.
   a. perform oral hygiene before meals, after meals, after emesis and when ever necessary
   b. avoid foods (such as hot, acidic, spicy foods or fluids) that irritate the oral mucous membranes
   c. use a soft bristle brush; review proper brushing and flossing techniques
   d. maintain the prescribed fluid intake
   e. discontinue mouth breathing (when possible) and smoking
   f. follow prescribed routines/medications for mouth care
      • rinsing the mouth with 25% acetic acid and cool water

UNIT 11

- use of topical anesthestics, oral protective pastes, antifungal /antibacterial agents and artificial saliva
- avoid lemon-glycerine swabs and mouthwashes containing alcohol

g. for relief of dry mouth
- perform prescribed mouth care routine
- lubricate lips
- use a spray bottle and /or ice chips (fluid intake needs to be part of prescribed total)
- use hard candy

h. if mouth discomfort continues, increase frequency of oral hygiene (for patients with dentures, remove dentures and replace only for meals).

21. Instruct the patient /family/home health aide about promoting a satisfactory defecation pattern including

a. a plan based on the patient's previously successful defecation pattern and within the prescribed parameters for fluid intake/restrictions, high fiber food (restrictions due to potassium and phosphorus), exercise (intolerance) and medication side effects (constipation from aluminum hydroxide)

b. strategies to prevent /treat constipation (consult with the physician for use of)
- intermittent antacids that have a laxative effect
- emollient stool softeners
- bulk, stimulant, lubricant laxatives (compounds containing magnesium or phosphorus can cause electrolyte imbalance)
- small volume, gentle stimulant enemas (avoid large volume saline or water enemas)

c. strategies to relieve diarrhea
- avoid foods irritating to the gastrointestinal tract (foods that are extremely hot / cold, spicy, high in fat, high in caffeine or gas producing)
- eat small frequent meals
- discontinue smoking (stimulates the gastrointestinal tract)
- consult with the physician for use of antacids that have a constipating effect and /or the use of medication to decrease motility.

22. Instruct the patient /family/home health aide about a plan to promote patient safety including

a. protection against falls due to neuro-musculo-skeletal changes (susceptibility to fractures, gait changes, seizures)
- keep bed in the low position
- use padded side rails and review seizure precautions (if the patient has experienced seizures)
- keep needed items within easy reach
- instruct the patient to wear low-heeled shoes with nonskid soles
- encourage uncluttered well-lit hallways/rooms and removal of hazards that cause tripping
- use mobility aids (walkers, hand rails) as needed
- allow time for ambulation /activity, avoid rushing the patient

b. protection against thermal injuries
- let foods cool slightly to decrease risk of burns from spills
- assess bath water or warm pack temperature before and during use
- avoid use of cold applications in areas of decreased sensation

c. minimization of bleeding risks
- avoid taking aspirin, aspirin-containing compounds and alcohol
- use care when shaving (use an electric razor), cutting nails, brushing and flossing teeth

- avoid situations, (i.e., contact sports) where injury/trauma could result
- avoid straining to have a bowel movement
- blow nose gently
- if bleeding occurs apply firm prolonged pressure to the area (for epistaxis apply ice packs and pressure to the nasal area as well as the Fowler position)

d. avoidance of nephrotoxic exposure such as chemical fumes (antifreeze, insecticides, carbon tetrachloride, mercuric chloride, lead, arsenic and creosote)

e. protection from infection due to impairment of the immunological system
  - use of good handwashing technique
  - maintaining aseptic technique when needed (procedures/treatments)
  - avoiding others who have infections and especially crowds during the flu season
  - using good perineal care (remind female patients to clean from the front to the back).

23. Instruct the patient/family/home health aide about strategies to cope with the patient's cognitive limitations (forgetfulness, impaired judgment, inability to concentrate).
    a. assess the patient's mentation status prior to involvement in decision-making or teaching
    b. speak clearly using short simple sentences
    c. repeat instructions/directions
    d. provide simple written or tape recorded directions/schedules for reference
    e. keep routines simple and consistent
    f. reorient patient and correct distortions when necessary
    g. attempt to ask the patient to participate in decisions when he or she is feeling alert and well; assist with problem-solving as needed
    h. allow adequate time for communication
    i. keep environmental stimulation/distraction to a minimum during communications
    j. assist family with plans for telephone visitation, homebound communications and constant patient supervision, if necessary
    k. appearance of delusions or increasing psychological impairment indicates the need for referral.

24. Promote the patient's sense of self-esteem and sense of control.
    a. use of makeup and colorful clothing to minimize the skin's appearance
    b. use of a wig/scarf for hair loss
    c. use of assistive devices to minimize dependence on others for care
    d. for impotence (males) and decreased libido
       - allow for rest before and after sexual activity
       - explore ways of expressing affection
       - discuss underlying issues to identify reversible factors (anxiety, fatigue, medications).

25. Encourage the patient/family to verbalize feelings about personality changes, increased lability and depression.
    a. assist the patient/family with the grieving process as end stage renal disease approaches
    b. discuss strategies for patient/family communication and coping
    c. refer the patient/family to support groups or counselling (dysfunctional grieving, hysteria and suicidal behavior require immediate assistance).

26. Identify community resources that can facilitate the patient's/family's adjustment to chronic and/or end stage renal failure.
    a. state or local Kidney Disease Foundation
    b. American Kidney Fund
    c. counselling, psychological therapy and self-help support groups
    d. financial counselling services.

UNIT
11

27. Coordinate additional members of the health care team such as the social worker, occupational therapist and registered dietician.
28. Obtain orders for blood work (chemistry and hematology) and culture/sensitivity tests (skin and mucous membranes).
29. Provide progress reports and a discharge summary to the primary physician.

PEDIATRIC CONSIDERATIONS

1. Assessment of signs and symptoms.
   a. age appropriate growth and development (growth retardation)
   b. age appropriate endocrine disturbances (secondary amenorrhea in girls past puberty, delayed or absent sexual maturation)
   c. bone or joint pain
   d. bed wetting
   e. pattern of intercurrent infections
   f. decreased interest in usual activities.
2. Encourage the patient/family to verbalize feelings about the
   a. impact of growth retardation and socialization
   b. impact of fatigue on school/socialization
   c. child's fear of death
   d. need for urinary manipulation ("good touch, bad touch" may need further explanation/reinforcement)
   e. need for repeated hospitalizations/procedures, particularly for dialysis and/or renal transplant.

THERAPEUTIC ACHIEVEMENT

- The patient/family adapt to the life-style changes induced as a result of chronic and/or end stage renal failure.
- For children, the patient's developmental findings are appropriate for gestational age.

RELATED PATIENT INSTRUCTIONS

Clinical Signs of Imminent Death
Constipation
Continuous Ambulatory Peritoneal Dialysis
Continuous Ambulatory Peritoneal Dialysis: Special Conditions
Diuretic Medications

General Comfort Measures
High Blood Pressure Medications
Restricted Protein Diet
Seasonings for Sodium Restricted Diets
Skin Care
Ways to Save Your Energy

Constipation Care Plan

CROSS REFERENCES

Pain Care Plan

Fecal Disimpaction Procedure
Home Health Aide Supervision Procedure

Range of Motion Exercises

NURSING DIAGNOSES

1. Alteration in bowel elimination (constipation) related to
   a. immobility
   b. painful defecation
   c. inadequate fiber/bulk in diet
   d. inadequate fluid intake
   e. inadequate exercise
   f. medication
   g. use of laxatives
   h. lack of privacy
   i. emotional status
   j. stressful life style
   k. neuromuscular impairment
   l. altered environment
   m. other.
2. Anxiety/fear related to
   a. change in normal bowel function
   b. interference with daily living
   c. other.
3. Alteration in comfort (back pain, abdominal pain, headache) related to
   a. hard stools
   b. hemorrhoids
   c. fecal impaction
   d. irritated perianal area
   e. other.
4. Knowledge deficit (modifications to restore normal bowel function) related to
   a. cognitive limitations
   b. sociocultural differences
   c. communication disorder
   d. information misinterpretation
   e. other.

UNIT 11

PROCESS INDICATORS

1. The patient establishes a satisfactory pattern of defecation.
Indicators
   a. soft formed stool
   b. easy passage of feces without straining

    c. patient's verbalization that the defecation problem has abated
    d. defecation more than 3 times/week
    e. soft abdomen and bowel sounds.
2. The patient /family/home health aide demonstrates an understanding of how to maintain a normal pattern of defecation.

Indicators

    a. ability to describe the factors contributing to the defecation problem
    b. ability to identify methods to counteract, reduce and eliminate the contributing factors.

NURSING INTERVENTIONS

1. Assess the magnitude of the defecation problem based on patient's
    a. type and duration of symptoms
    b. eating, activity and bowel habits
    c. own perception of normal bowel pattern
    d. drug usage (laxatives, anticholinergics, antidepressants, antacids, narcotics, iron preparations)
    e. age and weight.
2. Determine if the patient is impacted.
    a. rectal examination
    b. changes in vital signs (tachycardia, hyperventilation, elevated temperature, elevated blood pressure)
    c. related symptoms (oozing of stool, abdominal cramping, malaise, anorexia, urinary retention)
    d. abdominal assessment.
3. Manually disimpact if indicated (see Fecal Disimpaction Procedure).
4. Provide instruction to the patient /family/home health aide about
    a. increasing fluid intake to between 960 ml and 1200 ml per day
    b. increasing daily crude fiber (bran, whole, and cracked wheat cereals, fresh fruits, fresh vegetables, prunes and prune juice)
    c. bowel training (defecate when the urge is first felt, establish a regular time for defecation, avoid straining, drink decaffeinated coffee or tea 1 hour before scheduled defecation time, spend at least 15 minutes on the bedpan or toilet, sit so that the thighs can be flexed against the abdomen)
    d. importance of privacy
    e. increasing daily activity (brisk walk, ambulation, active/passive range of motion exercises)
    f. stress management techniques
    g. comfort measures for perianal irritation (sitz baths, protective emollients, cool compresses)
    h. long-term effects of laxative use
    i. maintaining a bowel elimination record.
5. Obtain prescriptions (stool softeners, enemas, suppositories) from the physician, as necessary.
6. Consult with the physician regarding medication changes, laxatives, antiseptic agents, local anesthetics.

THERAPEUTIC ACHIEVEMENT

- The patient identifies the restoration of a satisfactory pattern of defecation.

Home Peritoneal Dialysis Care Plan

CROSS REFERENCES

Constipation Care Plan
Depression Care Plan
Hypertension Care Plan

Chronic Renal Failure Care Plan
Infection Control Procedure

NURSING DIAGNOSES

1. Alteration in fluid volume (excess) related to
   a. inadequate compliance with dialysis regimen
   b. excess fluid intake
   c. excess sodium intake
   d. other.
2. Alteration in comfort (low back pain, leg cramping, abdominal/rectal pain, referred shoulder blade pain, constipation, shortness of breath) related to
   a. adequate performance of dialysis procedure (side effects)
   b. inadequate compliance with dialysis regimen
   c. other.
3. Impaired home maintenance management related to
   a. ineffective individual coping
   b. ineffective family coping
   c. lack of support (family/community/financial)
   d. lack of knowledge
   e. other.
4. Sleep pattern disturbance related to
   a. pain/discomfort
   b. anxiety
   c. dialysis regimen
   d. other.
5. Ineffective breathing pattern (shortness of breath) related to
   a. fluid excess (dialysate pressure on the diaphragm)
   b. anxiety
   c. other.
6. Potential for injury related to
   a. inadequate compliance with dialysis regimen
   b. impaired skin integrity
   c. other.
7. Knowledge deficit (nature of disease process and dialysis regimen including procedure, medication, diet, follow-up care, skin care, signs and symptoms to report) related to
   a. cognitive limitations
   b. lack of readiness to learn
   c. patient's request for no information
   d. misinterpretation of information
   e. other.

UNIT
11

8. Alteration in nutrition related to
    a. insufficient financial resources
    b. anorexia /nausea
    c. altered sense of taste
    d. inadequate support systems (shopping, cooking)
    e. personal /cultural /religious barriers
    f. inadequate compliance with prescribed diet
    g. other.
9. Disturbance in self-concept (body image, self-esteem, role performance, personal identity) related to
    a. change in role/job/life style
    b. dependence on others for care
    c. verbalizations of hopelessness/powerlessnes
    d. loss of body function /control
    e. other.
10. Noncompliance with the therapeutic regimen related to
    a. knowledge deficit
    b. lack of support (family/community/financial)
    c. difficulty integrating regimen into life style
    d. other.
11. Anxiety related to
    a. uncertainty of future, disease process, treatment plan
    b. changes in life style/role functioning /socioeconomic status
    c. performance of dialysis procedure
    d. pain /discomfort
    e. disturbances in sleep-rest patterns
    f. other.
12. Alteration in bowel elimination (constipation) related to
    a. medication (side effects)
    b. dietary restrictions
    c. other.

PROCESS INDICATORS

1. The patient /family verbalizes an understanding of home peritoneal dialysis management.

Indicators
    a. describes the disease process, dialysis regimen and strategies to prevent complications
    b. performs dialysis procedure accurately
    c. describes the diet plan that includes parameters for fluid, sodium, potassium and protein intake as well as foods to promote bowel elimination
    d. identifies medication action, dose, administration schedule and side effects for both oral intake and for dialysis instillation
    e. identifies signs and symptoms to report to the physician
    f. describes a plan for receiving follow-up care
    g. identifies community/financial resources.
2. The patient's biopsychosocial integrity is maintained.

Indicators
    a. maintains an adequate nutrition level
    b. maintains an appropriate fluid balance

c. does not exhibit signs of infection (peritoneum, skin)

d. maintains a satisfactory defecation pattern.

3. The patient establishes/maintains a satisfactory level of comfort.

Indicators

a. reports undisturbed sleep

b. verbalizes successful coping with anxiety

c. verbalizes absence of uncontrolled pain /discomfort

d. expresses satisfaction with quality of life.

NURSING INTERVENTIONS

1. Assess the patient for
   a. skin integrity (catheter exit site, subcutaneous tunnel)
   b. signs of fluid overload (increasing abdominal girth, shortness of breath, gallop rhythm on cardiac auscultation, pitting edema)
   c. symptoms of infection (cloudy dialysate, low grade fever, malaise, abdominal pain, rebound tenderness)
   d. nutritional status
   e. minor complications (asymptomatic hernia, low back pain, bladder pressure, rectal pressure, epigastric pressure, inflow pain, outflow failure)
   f. signs of electrolyte imbalance (particularly hypernatremia when using dialysate with dextrose concentrations of 4.25%).

2. Assess
   a. type of dialysis regimen prescribed—continuous ambulatory peritoneal dialysis (CAPD) or continuous cycled peritoneal dialysis (CCPD)
   b. patient's/family's abilities/limitations in terms of performance of the dialysis procedure, maintenance of aseptic technique, trouble-shooting the equipment (if used) and prevention of complications
   c. patient's/family's understanding of the dialysis regimen and the relationship among blood pressure, weight, fluid intake and diet
   d. home environment for routine sanitary practices, for space needed to store supplies/equipment and area to perform the dialysis procedure
   e. current durable medical equipment (DME) vendor and availability/acceptability of the service (particularly emergency repairs)
   f. patient's/family's financial /insurance needs
   g. patient's/family's record keeping system.

3. Monitor and record the patient's
   a. vital signs
      - be alert for low grade temperature
      - blood pressure readings should be taken in both arms with the patient in standing, sitting and lying positions
   b. body weight
   c. monthly tubing changes performed by the nurse, if ordered by the physician.

4. Instruct the patient /family about aseptic technique and infection control.
   a. review the need for handwashing, use of masks and gloves and maintaining sterility
   b. points to review in the dialysis procedure for potential breaks in techniques
      - connecting and disconnecting the tubing
      - changing the bottles (transferring the spike without contaminating it)
      - adding medication to the dialysate solution
      - caring for the catheter between exchanges
   c. skin and dressing care at the exit site following physician's order (iodophor and a dry sterile occlusive or transparent dressing).

UNIT 11

5. Instruct the patient/family about the
   a. disease process and therapeutic regimen
   b. principles of dialysis (osmosis and diffusion)
   c. setup/purging of the tubing and the equipment; checking each container for correct concentrations, leaks or particles; allow for return demonstrations
   d. maintenance and trouble-shooting
   e. use of an automatic cycler, if appropriate
      • review the manufacturer's instructions for problems that set off alarms (such as catheter kinking during sleep, inadequate amount of drainage during outflow and catheter lodging against the peritoneum)
      • changing positions typically alleviates problems
   f. promotion of sleep pattern by learning to position patient during sleep to prevent lying on and kinking the catheter
   g. need to call the nurse/physician when experiencing problems with dialysis
   h. emergency action plan including a 24-hour telephone access number
   i. need for a plan for achieving follow-up care.
6. Instruct the patient/family about minor complications that need to be reported to the nurse/physician. Physician consultations/orders are required for select interventions.
   a. low back pain due to pressure and weight of dialysate in abdomen may require prescriptions for analgesics and/or exercises to improve muscle tone
   b. asymptomatic hernia due to increased abdominal pressure may require a patient to avoid overexertion or a prescription to alleviate nausea, vomiting and constipation
   c. pressure in the bladder and rectal or epigastric areas is related to catheter placement (if pressure persists the physician may need to correct the catheter's placement)
   d. inflow pain/cramping usually decreases in the first 2 weeks and can result from intraperitoneal irritation (if due to infection the physician must be notified); cold dialysate (warm dialysate to body temperature using heating pads, heater component in the cycler or a microwave oven—check the temperature carefully); acid dialysate (dialysate concentration may need to be adjusted); stretching and irritation of the diaphragm or referred shoulder blade pain (decrease the infusion or drainage rate; strive for complete drainage of solution, the amount of dialysate used at exchanges may need adjustment; clamp off dialysate tubing with fluid remaining in the tubing to prevent air from entering the abdomen)
   e. outflow failure can result from a full colon (bowel evacuation is needed), catheter obstruction (changing position or ambulation may help), peritonitis signs and symptoms (requires immediate notification of the physician), bed or chair height not high enough for gravity flow (raise bed or chair height), dislodged catheter or kinked catheter (due to subcutaneous scarring) requires medical attention
   f. dialysate leaking around catheter can result from excessive instillation of dialysate (amount of dialysate at each exchange may need adjustment), catheter obstruction (the physician may order sterile normal saline irrigation), catheter position problems (require medical intervention).
7. Instruct the patient and family about signs and symptoms (particularly peritonitis) to report to the nurse/physician.
   a. fever (patients with end stage renal disease typically have subnormal temperatures; therefore, a slightly elevated temperature can be clinically significant)
   b. persistent abdominal pain
   c. abdominal fullness
   d. cloudy outflow (contains shreds of fibrin/mucus)
   e. bright yellow outflow (bladder perforation)

    f. feces in outflow (bladder perforation)

    g. little or sporadic outflow

    h. general malaise

    i. redness, swelling and tenderness around catheter and /or over subcutaneous tunnel

    j. inflow difficulties (kinking of catheter)

    k. scrotal edema (may result from subcutaneous leakage of dialysate in male patients)

    l. dialysate leakage around the catheter.

8. Instruct the patient /family about a dietary plan that complies with the prescribed parameters including

    a. dietary restriction of sodium and fluids as related to the patient's fluid weight gains and blood pressure
   - dietary sodium intake restriction to _____ /day (avoid monosodium glutamate, pickled foods, processed meats, salty snacks, added salt)
   - fluid restriction to _____ /day
   - potassium may not be restricted

    b. strategies to relieve dry mouth
   - hard candy, ice chips and ¼ cup mouth wash diluted with ¼ cup ice water (take into consideration the patient's age and calorie intake and oral mucous membrane pH, e.g., the alcohol content of mouth wash and the danger of aspirating on candy)

    c. protein intake
   - protein loss across the peritoneal membrane can be 40 gm/day when an infection is present
   - patient with chronic renal disease may develop an aversion to meat
   - identify protein sources acceptable to the patient
   - depending upon patient's age/condition, he or she may need to consume a minimum of 1 gm/kg of body weight

    d. caloric intake
   - dextrose in the dialysate is absorbed by the body resulting in an increase in blood glucose level and calories
   - certain patients may require caloric restrictions and monitoring of blood glucose levels

    e. foods to promote satisfactory bowel elimination
   - bran, fresh fruits and vegetables are high in potassium and phosphorus and may be permitted only in limited quantities for select patients
   - patient's plan will require careful adjustment

    f. written instructions/recipes for reference

    g. incorporation of cultural/religious parameters and personal preferences

    h. consultation with the dietician.

9. Instruct the patient/family about the medication plan (through the oral route and through dialysis instillation) including

    a. names, actions, dosages, administration schedule, side and adverse effects and drug interactions

    b. need to discuss the introduction of any new medications with the physician prior to initiation

    c. addition of medications (antibiotics, heparin) to the dialysate using aseptic technique

    d. multi-vitamins and folic acid–supplements may be prescribed

    e. analgesics may be prescribed for lower back pain

    f. stool softeners or mild laxatives may be necessary on a routine basis to prevent colonic distension which interferes with effective dialysis.

UNIT 11

10. Instruct the patient/family about promoting a satisfactory defecation pattern.
    a. design a plan based on the patient's previously successful defecation pattern, keeping in mind that fluids, exercise and high fiber foods may not be advisable for renal disease patients who require dialysis
    b. end stage renal disease patients whose hyperphosphatemia conditions are treated with aluminum hydroxide compounds are more likely to suffer from constipation
    c. fluid intake must be carefully planned within the patient's dialysis regimen
    d. patients with end stage renal disease tend to experience chronic anemia resulting in fatigue (exercise may not be feasible)
    e. high fiber foods may be limited for select patients owing to high potassium and phosphorus contents
    f. preventative bowel management requires close collaboration with the physician for inclusion of one or more of the following
       • emollient/stool softeners for constipation prevention and treatment
       • bulk, stimulant or lubricant laxatives (cathartics containing magnesium or phosphorus can cause electrolyte imbalances)
       • small volume, gentle stimulant enemas (large volume saline or water enemas must be avoided).
11. Instruct the patient/family about record keeping to include the following suggested elements
    a. weight (before and after dialysis)
    b. temperature (before and after dialysis and whenever fever or symptoms are present)
    c. pulse (before and after dialysis), check for irregularities
    d. blood pressure (before and after dialysis)
    e. respiratory rate and quality (before and after dialysis)
    f. type of dialysate
    g. medications (added to dialysate or taken orally)
    h. dialysis details (total number of exchanges, length of inflow/dwell/outflow periods, percentage/type of dialysate, amount of dialysate infused and recovered)
    i. quality of outflow—color, clarity and presence of other particles such as fibrin, mucus and feces
    j. any unusual events before, during and after dialysis
       • swelling, redness, tenderness or drainage at the exit site
       • signs and symptoms of peritonitis (fever, persistent abdominal fullness and cloudy outflow drainage)
       • shortness of breath
       • dialysate flow problems (catheter related)
       • discontinuation of dialysis for any reason (including reason and length of time).
12. Encourage the patient/family to verbalize feelings/fears/anxieties.
    a. identify stressors and foster coping strategies
    b. promote the patient's/family's sense of control
    c. create opportunities for the patient and partner to discuss their feelings/concerns about their sexual relationship
    d. involve siblings when the patient is a child
    e. create opportunities for the patient to discuss self-concept.
13. Identify community resources that can facilitate the patient's/family's adjustment to the life style modifications of the dialysis regimen.
    a. state or local Kidney Disease Fund
    b. counselling, psychological therapy and self-help groups for support
    c. financial counselling service
    d. consultation with the physician and initiation of referrals as needed.

14. Coordinate additional members of the health care team such as the social worker, registered dietician and DME vendor.
15. Obtain orders for blood work (electrolyte values) and for peritoneal fluid analysis (culture/sensitivity tests, Gram stain and cell count).
16. Provide progress reports and a discharge summary to the primary physician.

THERAPEUTIC ACHIEVEMENT

- The patient /family adapts to the life style changes induced as a result of long-term peritoneal dialysis.
- The patient /family performs peritoneal dialysis safely in the home.
- For children, the patient's developmental findings are appropriate for gestational age.

RELATED PATIENT INSTRUCTIONS

Antibiotic Medications
Changing Dressings
Continuous Ambulatory Peritoneal Dialysis
Continuous Ambulatory Peritoneal Dialysis:
  Special Conditions

Infection Control for the Home
Restricted Protein Diet
Seasonings for Sodium Restricted Diets

UNIT 11

Ostomy Care Plan

CROSS REFERENCES

Chemotherapy Care Plan
Depression Care Plan

Infection Control Procedure

NURSING DIAGNOSES

1. Anxiety related to
   a. lack of emotional support
   b. alteration in body image
   c. disease process/prognosis
   d. insufficient financial resources
   e. dependence on others for care
   f. lack of adequate information
   g. disruption of regular routines
   h. change in social involvement/fear of rejection or reaction by others
   i. other.
2. Grieving related to
   a. loss of body organ
   b. change in life style
   c. loss of bodily function/control
   d. other.
3. Noncompliance with treatment regimen related to
   a. patient's health care value system
   b. cultural/spiritual beliefs
   c. cognitive limitations/lack of interest in learning
   d. difficulty integrating treatment regimen into life style
   e. insufficient financial resources
   f. dysfunctional grieving
   g. depression/anxiety/anger
   h. repulsion of stoma/pouching
   i. denial
   j. fatigue
   k. other.
4. Knowledge deficit (colostomy/ileostomy/urostomy care, skin care, colostomy irrigation, diet, medication, odor control, obtaining supplies) related to
   a. cognitive limitations
   b. denial
   c. patient's request for no information
   d. misinterpretation of information
   e. lack of interest in learning
   f. other.
5. Social isolation related to
   a. alteration in physical appearance
   b. anxiety

    c. embarrassment
    d. fear of rejection
    e. other.
6. Self-care deficit (toileting, hygiene, grooming) related to
    a. dependence on others for care
    b. depression /anxiety
    c. fatigue
    d. repulsion of stoma /pouching
    e. cognitive limitations
    f. psychomotor limitations
    g. other.
7. Ineffective patient /family coping patterns related to
    a. grieving
    b. depression /anxiety
    c. sociocultural implications
    d. other.
8. Sleep pattern disturbance
    a. depression /anxiety
    b. physical /discomfort
    c. leakage /fear of leakage
    d. other.
9. Alteration in fluid and electrolyte balance related to
    a. fistula drainage
    b. inadequate sodium intake
    c. inadequate fluid intake
    d. other.
10. Alteration in comfort related to
    a. abdominal /perineal incisional pain
    b. flatulence
    c. skin irritation
    d. other.
11. Alteration in skin integrity related to
    a. faulty pouching system
    b. wound drainage
    c. frequent pouch removal /skin stripping
    d. irritation from soap /cleanser residue
    e. dermatological conditions (from radiation, allergy, fungal /bacterial contamination)
    f. other.
12. Potential disturbance in self-concept (body image, self-esteem, role performance, personal identity) related to
    a. dependence on others for care
    b. change in social involvement /fear of rejection or reaction by others
    c. fear of body odor /leakage
    d. embarrassment
    e. loss of bodily function /control
    f. other.
13. Alteration in sexual function related to
    a. fear of rejection
    b. fear of body odor /leakage
    c. change in body image
    d. loss of bodily function /control
    e. other.

UNIT 11

PROCESS INDICATORS

1. The patient's biopsychosocial integrity is maintained.
Indicators
    a. maintains skin integrity
    b. maintains a dietary plan that incorporates the basic food groups and eliminates foods that result in patient discomfort
    c. establishes satisfactory management of elimination.
2. The patient/family demonstrates effective coping patterns.
Indicators
    a. patient shares his or her feelings regarding the change in his or her body image
    b. patient looks at and touches the stoma
    c. patient resumes presurgical social interactions and relationships
    d. patient/family states the disease process and the surgical creation of the ostomy using appropriate terminology
    e. patient/family verbalizes decreased anxiety/depression/fear
    f. patient/family verbalizes acceptance of the ostomy
    g. patient expresses satisfactory level of sexual functioning
    h. patient/family utilizes resources such as community groups and United Ostomy Association, as appropriate
    i. patient/family verbalizes the indications for contacting the nurse/physician/enterostomal therapist/DME supplier.

NURSING INTERVENTIONS

1. Assess
    a. the patient's/family's understanding of the surgical procedure, reason for creation of the ostomy
    b. the patient's/family's abilities to learn/perform care/manage the ostomy as assessed at the start and at the conclusion of the visit
    c. the patient's/family's ability to make adjustments within the regimen (e.g., alter diet, adjust to stoma size changes)
    d. patient's emotional status and process of grieving/adjustment
    e. patient's previous coping mechanisms
    f. family's/support system's ability to cope
    g. patient's dietary intake.
2. Inspect
    a. stoma for color, moistness, size, protrusion
    b. mucosal-cutaneous junction for abnormalities such as separation, scar tissue formation
    c. peristomal skin for abnormalities such as maceration, denudation with or without weeping, allergic reaction, fungal rash.
3. Instruct the patient/family about ostomy care (refer to the appropriate ostomy instructions).
    a. Colostomy
    b. Ileostomy
    c. Urostomy.
4. Create situations for the patient/family to verbalize feelings, fears, and concerns.
5. Counsel the patient/family for coping strategies/sexual functioning.
    a. the stoma is not harmed by physical contact
    b. an empty pouch and ostomy deodorizer, if needed, foster a sense of well-being

c. refer to the United Ostomy Association, counselling services, sex therapist as needed

d. promote an environment that allows sufficient time, privacy, and support during the adjustment period

e. allow the patient to proceed at a negotiated pace.

6. Coordinate additional members of the health care team such as the social worker, enterostomal therapist, occupational therapist, registered dietician, and home health aide.

7. Provide the patient/family with a list of local ostomy suppliers.

8. Assist the patient/family with the use of community resources, educational resources, and organization support.

a. United Ostomy Association

b. ostomy supply manufacturers provide many helpful pamphlets at no cost.

9. Obtain orders from the primary physician as necessary for medications, laboratory tests, aids/equipment.

10. Provide progress reports and a discharge summary to the primary physician.

THERAPEUTIC ACHIEVEMENT

- The patient completes the rehabilitation process.
- The patient identifies the restoration of a satisfactory quality of life and level of independence.

RELATED PATIENT INSTRUCTIONS

Changing Dressings	Ileostomy Care
Colostomy Care	Urostomy Care
Colostomy Irrigation	Skin Care

COLOSTOMY CARE

1. Instruct the patient/family about the pouching system.

a. patients with right-sided colostomies (i.e., ascending and transverse colostomies) generally should use a drainable (open-ended) pouching system owing to the often unpredictable and frequent liquid-like to soft fecal output

b. patients with left-sided colostomies (such as sigmoid) should use either an open-ended or a closed-end pouch. If a closed-end pouch requires changing more than once or twice a day, the patient should switch to a drainable pouch.

c. the stoma size should be measured initially once per week
- stoma size decreases over time with the most substantial shrinkage occurring in the first 12 weeks postoperatively
- weekly measurements should continue for 8 weeks or so
- measurements can be reduced to once every other week for weeks 8 through 12; thereafter, measurement is recommended on a monthly basis.

2. Instruct the patient/family about a dietary plan.

a. follow a well-balanced diet

b. take note if any particular foods seem to upset the regular bowel pattern; reduce or eliminate these foods from the diet accordingly

UNIT
11

3. Instruct the patient/family about odor control.
   a. good hygiene and regular pouch emptying and rinsing is essential
   b. natural foods assisting to reduce fecal odor are parsley, buttermilk, and yogurt
   c. avoid foods thought to increase fecal odor such as fish, eggs, onions, peas, cabbage, broccoli
   d. commercial liquid deodorizers are available
   e. discourage putting aspirin in the pouch, as it can irritate the stoma and cause bleeding.
4. Instruct the patient/family about flatus control.
   a. gas can usually be controlled by diet
   b. avoid foods and beverages thought to increase flatus (mushrooms, beer, carbonated beverages, onions, eggs, cabbage, beans, milk)
   c. most closed-end pouches are manufactured with built-in gas/odor filters.
5. Instruct the patient/family about colostomy irrigation if appropriate.
   a. patient with a sigmoid colostomy may be instructed in colostomy irrigation as an alternative in colostomy management
   b. careful, professional evaluation combined with patient/family participation discussions about advantages, disadvantages, and contraindications are prerequisite to this procedure.

   Special Note. Ascending and transverse colostomies have a liquid-like output and are not appropriate for irrigation, as they are generally temporary and cannot usually be regulated owing to the nature of the liquid-like output.

6. Provide the patient/family with a list of ostomy suppliers in the geographical area he or she resides in.
7. Inform the patient/family of the availability of support groups such as the local United Ostomy Association.
8. Provide the patient with related literature to review. Many pamphlets are available at no cost from manufacturers of ostomy supplies.

ILEOSTOMY CARE

1. Instruct the patient/family about the pouching system.
   a. pouches should be emptied every 2 to 3 hours
   b. if using reusable pouches, remove only the pouch leaving the skin barrier in place every morning
   c. the entire system should be changed every 7 days
   d. the stoma size should be measured initially once per week
      • stoma size decreases over time with the most substantial shrinkage occurring in the first 12 weeks postoperatively
      • weekly measurements should continue for 8 weeks or so
      • measurement can be reduced to once every other week for weeks 8 through 12; thereafter, measurement is recommended on a monthly basis.
   e. meticulous skin care is essential as the small bowel contains high levels of enzymes that can quickly damage the peristomal skin
   f. attention should be given to proper size, application, and adherence of the skin barrier and pouch
   g. a leaky pouch should never be allowed to remain on the skin.
2. Instruct the patient/family about a dietary plan.
   a. follow a well-balanced diet
   b. note if any particular food seems to upset the regular bowel pattern; reduce or eliminate those foods from the diet accordingly

    c. strategies to prevent a bolus food blockage such as eating slowly; chewing foods very well; avoiding foods such as cheese, lima beans, nuts, corn, orange pulp, celery, pineapple; drinking plenty of fluids with meals

    d. patient should contact nurse/physician immediately if a food blockage occurs

    e. a gentle ileostomy lavage procedure may be necessary to release the bolus.

3. Instruct the patient/family about odor control.

    a. good hygiene and regular pouch emptying and rinsing are essential

    b. natural foods assisting to reduce fecal odor are parsley, buttermilk, and yogurt

    c. avoid foods thought to increase fecal odor such as fish, eggs, onions, peas, cabbage, broccoli

    d. commercial liquid deodorizers are available

    e. discourage putting aspirin in the pouch as it can irritate the stoma and cause bleeding.

4. Instruct the patient/family about avoiding dehydration.

    a. increase daily fluid intake

    b. recognize precipitating factors such as fever, vomiting, diarrhea, excessive perspiration, decreased environmental humidity, and increased environmental temperature

    c. if diarrhea/vomiting is present it is particularly important to act quickly to prevent dehydration and electrolyte imbalance

    d. examples of replacement fluids are tea, chicken broth, carbonated beverages, and Gatorade.

5. Instruct the patient/family about medications.

    a. advise the patient to alert any health care provider of his or her ileostomy before taking medications

    b. oral medications that do not dissolve in the mouth, esophagus, stomach, or small bowel will not benefit the patient; they may not dissolve properly before reaching the stoma and may fall into the pouch whole; examples include enteric-coated tablets, time-released spansules/tablets

    c. caution against the use of laxatives; diarrhea and dehydration may ensue and can be life-threatening.

6. Instruct the patient/family that neither rectal temperature measurements nor enemas should be attempted.

7. Provide the patient/family with a list of ostomy suppliers in the geographical area he or she resides in.

8. Inform the patient/family of the availability of support groups such as the local United Ostomy Association.

9. Provide the patient with related literature to review. Many pamphlets are available at no cost from manufacturers of ostomy suppliers.

10. Confirm with the physician if a restrictive fat diet and/or vitamin B_{12} injections are needed when the patient has had more than 100 cm of the terminal portion of the ileum removed.

UNIT 11

UROSTOMY CARE

1. Instruct the patient/family about the pouching system.

    a. patient should empty his or her pouch every 2 hours. Urine that stagnates in the pouch develops a high pH. This alkaline urine has a stronger odor and can deposit crystals around the stoma, skin, and pouch lining.

    b. encourage the patient to wear a belted urostomy system to provide support to the pouch and prevent loosening of the seal due to constant pulling as urine constantly flows into the pouch

c. encourage the use of an antirefluxing pouch to prevent urine from "bathing" the stoma area and refluxing into the kidneys especially when lying down; refluxing alkaline urine increases danger of kidney infection; most pouches developed in the last 10 years are designed with an antireflux mechanism.

d. if the patient is using an older urostomy system without an antireflux valve the following procedure may be advised to reduce urine alkalinity and stoma crystalization
   • fill the pouch from the spout with a vinegar and warm water solution (1 part vinegar to 2 or 3 parts water);
   • have the patient lie down and bathe the stoma for a few minutes. This should be done one or two times a day.

e. inform the patient that urine flows almost continuously from the stoma and contains mucus
   • to diminish urine output to facilitate easier pouch change, the patient may limit fluid intake 2 to 3 hours prior to the scheduled change
   • often the best time for pouch change is prior to breakfast

f. advise the patient to utilize a large, straight bedside drainage bag at night or while in bed; this will reduce stagnation of urine in the pouch thus reducing weight, odor, and backflow of urine into the stoma

g. The stoma size should be measured initially once per week
   • stoma size decreases over time with the most substantial shrinkage occurring in the first 12 weeks postoperatively
   • weekly measurements should continue for 8 weeks or so
   • measurement can be reduced to once every other week for weeks 8 through 12; thereafter, measurement is recommended on a monthly basis.

2. Instruct the patient/family about a dietary plan.
   a. follow a well-balanced diet
   b. take note if any particular food seems to upset the regular bowel pattern; reduce or eliminate those foods from the diet accordingly.

3. Instruct the patient/family about odor control.
   a. good hygiene and regular pouch emptying and rinsing are essential
   b. vinegar to rinse and/or soak pouches will aid in odor reduction
   c. asparagus particularly increases urine odor and should be avoided
   d. when using commercial liquid deodorizers, follow label directions
   e. discourage putting aspirin in the pouch as it can irritate the stoma and cause bleeding.

4. Instruct the patient/family about signs and symptoms to report
   a. fungal rashes (especially *Candida albicans*) can develop on the peristomal skin owing to the warm moist environment provided by urine
      • the risk increases during oral antibiotic therapy as the normal floras are reduced
      • the rash appears as red and/or white papules with an erythematous, irregular bordered blush of the skin
      • the itch may be intense
   b. urinary tract infection symptoms are fever, hematuria, increasingly cloudy or foul-smelling urine, flank pain.

5. Provide the patient/family with a list of ostomy suppliers in the geographical area he or she resides in.

6. Inform the patient/family of the availability of support groups such as the local United Ostomy Association.

7. Provide the patient with related literature to review. Many pamphlets are available at no cost from manufacturers of ostomy suppliers.

Procedures

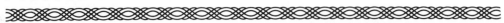

Bladder Retraining Procedures

PURPOSE

- To train the patient's bladder to empty at regular and predictable times.
- To teach the patient how to achieve/maintain urinary continence.

EQUIPMENT

- pencil
- paper

Special Note. If the patient has an indwelling urinary catheter, instruct the patient/family to clamp it for intervals of 2 to 3 hours during the 48 hours preceding its removal. This procedure will strengthen the bladder's muscle tone prior to initiating the retraining program. Reinforce that close monitoring is necessary to avoid bladder overdistension.

Steps	Key Points
1. Assess the patient's mental capacity to learn and adhere to a bladder retraining program.	1. If the patient lacks the mental capacity, identify someone who will be able to make sure that the patient strictly adheres to the retraining schedule until bladder control is relearned.

2. Identify the patient's usual pattern of voiding
  a. time
  b. amount
  c. voluntary/involuntary
  d. physically sensing the need to void
  e. behavior/feelings/activities preceding micturition.
	2. A reliable pattern can usually be obtained in 48 to 72 hours. Common times for voiding are
	  a. first thing in the morning
	  b. after naps
	  c. 30 minutes after drinking
	  d. before retiring for the night.

3. Determine a schedule for voiding based on the patient's usual pattern.	3. Give the patient/family a written copy of the schedule.
4. If, after several days, the schedule based on the patient's usual pattern is not successful, develop a schedule of toileting every 1 to 2 hours on a 24 hour basis.	4. As the patient achieves success with the toileting schedule, gradually lengthen the times between voiding.
5. Teach the patient/family a. how to measure and record intake and output	

UNIT 11

b. the physiology of micturition

c. how to recognize the physical sensations indicative of a full bladder (restlessness, diaphoresis, chills, headache, feeling of fullness in the lower abdomen)

d. void as soon as the urge is felt

e. assume as natural a position as possible (females sitting; men standing)

f. to increase the fluid intake to at least 3000 ml daily (if no contraindications)

g. to limit fluid intake when away from home and increase it upon return

h. to schedule fluid intake so that little is taken after 7:00 pm in order to prevent incontinence at night

i. to do toileting in the bathroom or in surroundings that will remind the patient of the toileting function

j. skin and perineal care

k. methods of external urinary protection (rubber sheets, waterproof pants, adult diapers, absorbent pads).

b. Gear discussion to the patient/family's level of understanding to increase compliance with the retraining program.

f. An adequate amount of fluid is necessary to produce enough urine to stimulate the voiding reflex.

g and h. Fluid intake should be on a regular schedule to facilitate establishment of a predictable voiding routine.

6. Teach the patient/family methods to stimulate urination

a. digital pressure at the side of the urinary meatus

b. rocking back and forth

c. running water in the sink

d. stroking the abdomen and thighs

e. application of cold to the abdomen

f. hot water bottle applied to the abdomen

g. sitz bath

h. pouring warm water over the perineum

i. pressure in a circular motion over the bladder

j. Credé maneuver (if not contraindicated)

k. inhaling oil of peppermint

l. placing a cottonball saturated with ammonia in the urine receptacle

m. putting the patient's hands in warm water

n. thinking about water in motion (rain, rivers).

6. The success of each method is dependent upon the patient's susceptibility to it.

7. Teach the patient Kegel exercises to strengthen bladder tone (tense perineal muscles by pressing buttocks together; hold for 3 seconds; relax; repeat 15 to 20 times/hour).
8. Teach the patient to learn voluntary control of micturition by stopping the urinary flow, holding back a few seconds, and starting the stream again.
9. Discuss with the patient/family
   a. normal expectation of accidents during the training period
   b. that it may take weeks to months to regain bladder control
   c. importance of consistency in successful bladder training
   d. feelings about dependency
   e. feelings about being unable to control a basic body function
   f. criteria to define when acceptable and realistic success of the bladder training program has been achieved.

DOCUMENTATION

1. The patient's/family's capacity to learn and adhere to the bladder retraining program.
2. The patient's usual pattern of voiding.
3. The toileting schedule.
4. The criteria to define success of the retraining program.
5. Patient progress in achieving bladder control.

Colostomy Irrigation Procedure

PURPOSE

- To stimulate the large intestine to expel stool at a selected time of day, thereby establishing a regular bowel movement via colostomy.

EQUIPMENT

- irrigation kit
- irrigation fluid container
- tubing with regulator clamp
- catheter or cone-tip attachment
- drainable irrigation sleeve
- belt (optional)
- pouch closure clip (optional)
- lukewarm tap water (100 to 105°F)
- water-soluble lubricant
- paper towels

Special Note. Manufacturers of colostomy supplies provide all-inclusive irrigation kits. It may be easiest to select the appropriate kit in accordance with the brand of colostomy pouch being used.

Steps	Key Points
1. Gather and prepare all equipment as related to company instructions.	1. Explain all equipment to the patient using proper terminology.
2. Fill irrigation fluid container with designated amount of lukewarm water. Between 250 and 500 ml maximum of water should be used on the first irrigation to assess tolerance. Increase by 250 ml for each successive irrigation until a maximum of 1000 to 1500 ml is reached.	2. Water that is too cool may cause cramps. Water that is too warm may burn the mucosa of the bowel. Most patients require between 750 and 1000 ml.
3. Unclamp regulator to allow water to run completely through the tubing to clear out all the air. Reclamp the regulator when the water flows readily through the tip of the tube.	3. Clearing the tube of air prior to commencing procedure will prevent air from entering the bowel thus minimizing abdominal cramping.

4. Lubricate the tip of the cone/catheter tip.

5. The irrigation container may be hand held; however, it is preferable to hang it on a hook on the wall at a height that aligns the bottom of the fluid container with the patient's shoulder.

6. Before beginning actual procedure
   a. Ensure patient comfort. Have the patient seated comfortably either on the toilet or on an adjacent chair.

   b. Assess integrity of the irrigation sleeve where attached to the body and as it enters the toilet.

7. Gently insert catheter/cone into the stoma. Never force.

8. Holding the cone/catheter in place, open the regulator clamp and allow water to flow in slowly over a period of 10 to 15 minutes. Apply gentle pressure against the cone to prevent water from backing out.

9. Once the desired amount of fluid is instilled, clamp regulator to Off and remove the cone/catheter. Close the top of irrigator sleeve securely.

10. Allow approximately 40 minutes for complete evacuation to occur.

11. After completion of procedure, all parts should be washed in lukewarm water and mild liquid soap. Rinse and dry well. Hang equipment to dry.

4. Always use water-soluble jelly. The cone tip is preferred to the catheter tip to reduce the danger of bowel perforation.

   a. Pillows may be necessary to support the back. Many postoperative patients with anteroposterior resections find sitting on toilets uncomfortable and prefer chairs.

   b. Depending on brand and style of the system, the sleeve may attach to the body by a faceplate, belt, or adhesive. It is critical to obtain a complete seal or the evacuating fluid will leak. Be sure that the sleeve hangs freely and far enough into the toilet.

7. If using a cone, fit tip snugly into stoma. If using a catheter, maximum insertion is 2 to 3 in. If resistance is met, encourage a few deep breaths to relax abdominal muscles.

8. Slow instillation will minimize cramping. If cramps occur, the flow should be slowed or shut off via the regulator clamp until cramps subside.

10. The bulk of the returns will be expelled in the first 15 to 20 minutes. After this time, the sleeve may be rinsed, folded, and clamped at the bottom to allow the patient to ambulate. This step may also stimulate additional evacuation.

UNIT 11

12. Wash and dry the peristomal area. Apply desired colostomy pouching system.

12. Refer to Colostomy Care Procedure.

DOCUMENTATION

1. The date and time of the procedure.
2. The indicators that prompted the procedure.
3. The amount of fluid used.
4. The amount and characteristics of the returns.
5. The patient's response to the procedure.
6. The patient/family teaching done.
7. The name and relationship of the person taught, if other than the patient.
8. The quality of the return demonstration.
9. The plans for follow-up.

Fecal Disimpaction Procedure

PURPOSE

- To relieve the patient's discomfort.
- To prepare the patient for initiation of a bowel regimen.
- To remove a fecal impaction.

EQUIPMENT

- gloves (nonsterile)
- absorbent pads
- water-soluble lubricant
- topical anesthesia (lidocaine ointment, 5%)*
- mineral oil–enema or full-strength hydrogen peroxide*
- bedpan
- packaged enema of sodium phosphate and sodium biphosphate (Fleet) or bisacodyl suppository (Dulcolax)*

Special Note. This procedure may be contraindicated in patients with cardiac alterations.

Steps	Key Points
1. Explain the procedure to the patient.	1. Anxiety may cause the patient to misunderstand or forget the explanation.
2. Provide for the patient's comfort and privacy.	2. The presence of a significant other is sometimes reassuring.
3. Place the absorbent pads under the patient's buttocks and put the bedpan in an easily accessible spot.	
4. Soften the intestinal contents a. instill 30 to 60 ml full strength hydrogen peroxide *or* b. give 115 ml warm mineral oil enema, have patient retain for 20 to 30 minutes.	4. The manipulation of hardened fecal material may erode the rectum and result in bleeding.
5. Apply a topical anesthetic to the perianal area 5 to 10 minutes before disimpaction.	
6. Position the patient on the left side, with his or her knees flexed.	

UNIT 11

*Physician's order may be required.

7. Instruct the patient to take slow deep breaths.

8. Gently insert a gloved lubricated index finger into the rectum and gently massage around the stool to loosen it.

9. Pause frequently to allow the patient to rest.

10. Observe the client for facial pallor, diaphoresis, change in pulse rate, and complaints of severe cramps, dizziness, and chest pain.

11. Complete the disimpaction.

12. Allow patient to rest.

13. Stimulate evacuation
    a. administer a packaged enema of sodium phosphate and sodium biphosphate or
    b. administer a bisacodyl suppository if the stool is soft.

14. Advise patient that the bowel pattern may be irregular for 2 to 3 days.

15. Instruct the client /family/home health aide
    a. to be safety conscious as patient may be weak or dizzy
    b. to provide a fluid replacement
    c. to administer a mild laxative in the late evening.*

7. Controlled breathing provides distraction and relaxation and discourages Valsalva maneuver.

8. Be very cautious if the client has rectal, perineal, or prostatic cancer.

9. Removal of a large amount of stool can lower intrabdominal pressure.

10. Stop the procedure if severe pain or rectal bleeding occurs. Notify the physician.

11. Consider three consecutive daily visits if the disimpaction is difficult and the patient is frail /elderly.

13. Avoid large enemas as sudden distention may cause mild shock in the elderly.

15. Be particularly attentive in follow up to the mentally impaired, those with severe cardiac problems, those with decreased mobility, and the depressed.

DOCUMENTATION

1. The indicators that prompted the procedure.
2. Activities of fecal disimpaction.
3. The amount and characteristics of the fecal material.
4. The patient's response to the procedure.
5. Instructions to client /family/home health aide.
6. Plans for bowel regimen follow-up.

---

*Physician's order may be necessary.

Incontinence Rash Procedure

PURPOSE

- To protect skin that is excoriated or shows a rash as a result of exposure to urine and/or feces.

EQUIPMENT

- nystatin (Mycostatin) powder (requires a physician's prescription)
- liquid antacid
- nonsterile gloves
- nonsterile 4 × 4 gauze pad
- washcloth
- towel
- hair dryer with a cool setting
- warm water in a basin

Steps

1. Explain the procedure to the patient/family.
2. Wash your own hands.
3. Put on nonsterile gloves.
4. Gently cleanse the affected area with warm water.
5. Pat the area dry.
6. Sprinkle Mycostatin powder on the affected area, spreading it evenly.
8. Dry the area with the cool setting of the hair dryer.
9. Teach the family to repeat steps 1 to 8 after every incontinent episode.

Key Points

1. Knowing what to expect increases patient/family compliance.

4. Do not use soap as it may cause further irritation.

8. The area can also air dry.

9. Reinforce the importance of cleaning the patient as soon as possible after an incontinent episode.

UNIT
11

DOCUMENTATION

1. The date and time of the procedure.
2. The condition of the affected skin.
3. Patient/family teaching done.
4. The family members to whom the procedure was taught.
5. Quality of return demonstration.
6. Patient/family response to the procedure.
7. Plans for follow-up.

Intermittent Self-Catheterization Procedure

PURPOSE

- To enable the patient who has no bladder control to independently maintain urinary continence.

EQUIPMENT

- #14 to #16 straight catheter (rubber or plastic)
- soap, water, and towel or moist disposable towelettes
- water-soluble lubricant (males only)
- plastic bag/glass jar for used catheter
- container for collecting urine (if toilet isn't available or if urine has to be measured)
- mirror (females only)

Special Note. Clean technique is used in the home, as it is easier and less expensive for the patient and has not been shown to increase the incidence of urinary tract infection (UTI).

Steps	Key Points
1. Review the procedure with the patient.	1. Knowing what to expect increases patient compliance.
2. Have the patient try to void prior to the procedure.	
3. Have the patient wash his or her hands.	3. Good handwashing is an essential component of clean technique.
4. Help the patient organize the supplies within his or her reach.	
5. Have the patient assume as normal a position as possible.	5. Men may either stand or sit. Women may sit on the edge of a chair or stand with one leg elevated on a stool.
6. Have the male patient	
a. wash his penis (being sure to retract the foreskin if not circumcised)	a. remind the patient to keep the foreskin retracted during the procedure
b. lubricate the catheter tip and the adjacent 2 in with the water-soluble lubricant	b. lubrication is necessary because the male urethra is susceptible to traumatic urethritis
c. hold his penis erect and slowly insert the catheter until urine starts to flow (about 7 in)	c. place the draining end of the catheter so that the urine flows into the toilet or container
d. advance the catheter another 2 in	d. further advancement ensures placement in the bladder

e. change position, Credé maneuver (if not contraindicated), or strain the abdominal muscles when the urine flow stops.
7. Have the female patient
   a. wash her perineal area with downward strokes
   b. hold the catheter about ½ in from the tip (as though holding a pen)
   c. seprate the labia with her other hand

   d. slowly insert the catheter into the urethra until the urine starts to flow (about 2 in)
   e. advance the catheter another 1 in

   f. Credé maneuver (if not contrain-dicated) or strain the abdominal muscles when the urine flow stops.
8. When the urine stops draining, in-struct the patient to slowly withdraw the catheter.
9. Have the patient wash his or her hands and redress.
10. Have the patient
    a. wash the catheter with warm water and soap
    b. rinse the catheter (inside and out) with clear water
    c. dry the catheter thoroughly with the towel
    d. store the catheter in the plastic bag /glass jar
    e. wash his or her hands.
11. Instruct the patient
    a. to use each catheter once *then*
    b. to boil used catheters for 20 min-utes in water
    c. to store boiled catheters in fresh bags, jars, or freshly laundered towels
    d. to replace cracked or hard cathe-ters.

e. this step ensures complete empty-ing of the bladder.

b. Lubrication is not necessary be-cause of the female's natural ure-thral lubrication.
c. A mirror may be propped be-tween the legs to locate the mea-tus. Advise the patient not to be-come dependent upon the mirror because she may not always have one available.
d. Place the draining end of the catheter so that the urine flows into the toilet or container.
e. Further advancement ensures placement in the bladder.
f. This step ensures complete emp-tying of the bladder.

8. Remind the patient to keep the cath-eter tip up to avoid dribbling urine.

a. If soap and water aren't available, use a moist towelette until the cleaning can be done with soap and water.

11. Remind the patient to keep used and clean catheters separate.

UNIT 11

12. Review the catheterization schedule with the patient (most schedules begin with catheterization every 2 hours, with half hour increments after each 24 hours dry, until dryness is achieved with a 4-hour schedule).

12. The schedule is tailored to the individual patient. If wetness/incontinence continues, reevaluate the catheterization technique to be sure the bladder is being completely emptied.

13. Teach the patient to
    a. adjust fluid intake
    b. avoid caffeine-containing beverages
    c. avoid calcium-rich and phosphorus-rich foods

    c. This will reduce the chance of kidney stone formation.

    d. monitor intake and output
    e. monitor pertinent data about his or her urine (color, odor, clarity)
    f. recognize the signs of UTI (fever, pain, cloudy urine, foul odor)

    f. Patients with spinal cord injuries may not feel pain.

    g. adhere to the prescribed medication regimen.

14. Discuss regimen with the patient
    a. his or her feelings regarding this procedure/incontinence
    b. the importance of planning his or her day to include regular self-catheterization

    b. Overdistention of the bladder can lead to infection.

    c. the use of external collection devices between catheterizations.

15. Teach the procedure to at least one other responsible family member.

15. It is important for another family member to know the procedure in the event that the patient is unable to do the catheterization.

DOCUMENTATION

1. The teaching, the procedure, the quality of the return demonstration, and the name and relationship of the person taught, if other than the patient.
2. The appearance (color, clarity), odor, and amount of drained urine.
3. The patient's/family's response to the procedure.
4. Plans for follow-up.
5. Patient's progress in achieving bladder control.

Bibliography

Bradshaw, T. Making Male Catheterization Easier for Both of You. RN, December 1983, pp. 43–45.
Bradwell, D. C. and Jackson, B. Principles of Ostomy Care. St. Louis: C. V. Mosby Co., 1982.
Binkley, L. Keeping Up with Peritoneal Dialysis. American Journal of Nursing, June 1984, pp. 729–733.
Brundage, D. J. Nursing Management of Renal Problems, 2nd ed. St. Louis: C. V. Mosby Co., 1980.
Chambers, J. Bowel Management in Dialysis Patients. American Journal of Nursing, July 1983, pp. 1051–1052.
Implementing Urologic Procedures. Nursing Photobook Nursing 84 Books, Springhouse Corp., Springhouse, Pa.
Lancaster, L. E. (ed.). The Patient with End Stage Renal Disease, 2nd ed. New York: John Wiley & Sons, 1984.

Lewis, B. Streamlining the Process of Elimination. American Journal of Nursing, 85(7): 1985, pp. 774.

Mager-O'Connor, E. How to Identify and Remove Fecal Impactions. Geriatric Nursing, May/June 1984, pp. 158–161.

Mahoney, J. M. Guide to Ostomy and Nursing Care. Boston: Little, Brown & Co., 1976.

Mc Connell, E. A. and Zimmerman, M. F. Care of Patients with Urologic Problems. Philadelphia: J. B. Lippincott Co., 1983.

Miller, J. Helping the Aged Manage Bowel Function. Journal of Gerontological Nursing, 11(2): pp. 37–41.

Mullen, B. D. and McGinn, K. A. The Ostomy Book. Palo Alto: Bill Publishing Co., 1980.

Murphy, L. M. and Cole, M. J. Renal Disease: Nutritional Implications. Nursing Clinics of North America, March 1983, pp. 57–70.

Performing GI Procedures. Nursing Photobook Nursing 84 Books, Springhouse Corp., Springhouse, Pa.

Shefts, D., et al. Bowel Management Protocol. Home Healthcare Nurse, 2(5): 1984, pp. 17–20.

Simons, J. Does Incontinence Affect Your Client's Self Concept? Journal of Gerontological Nursing, 11(6): 1985, pp. 37–42.

Sohn, N. and Lenneberg, E. T. Modern Concepts in the Management of Patients with Intestinal and Urinary Stomas. Clinical Obstetrics and Gynecology, 15(2): June 1972.

Stark, J. and Hunt, V. Helping Your Patient with Chronic Renal Failure. Nursing 83, September 1983, pp. 54–63.

Strangio, L. Believe It or Not. Peritoneal Dialysis Made Easy. Nursing 88, January 1988, pp. 43–46.

Van Stone, J. C. Dialysis and the Treatment of Renal Insufficiency. New York: Grune & Stratton, 1983.

Whitman, S. and Kursh, E. Curbing Incontinence. Journal of Gerontological Nursing, 13(4): 1987, pp. 35–40.

Wilde, M. Living with a Foley. American Journal of Nursing, 86(10): 1986, pp. 1121–1123.

Zappacosta, A. R. and Perras, S. T. Continuous Ambulatory Peritoneal Dialysis. Philadelphia: J. B. Lippincott Co., 1984.

Ziemann, L., et al. Incidence of Leakage from Indwelling Urinary Catheter in Homebound Patients. Home Healthcare Nurse, 2(5): 1984, pp. 22–26.

Digestive Alterations

Care Plans

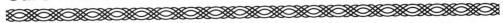

Eating Disorders Care Plan

CROSS REFERENCES

Alcohol Abuse Care Plan
Depression Care Plan

Suicidal Patient: Indications for Requesting Hospitalization

NURSING DIAGNOSES

1. Anxiety related to
   a. situational/maturational crises
   b. threat to self-concept/distorted body image
   c. fear of obesity/loss of control of eating
   d. weight gain
   e. amenorrhea
   f. other.
2. Ineffective individual coping related to
   a. situational/maturational crises
   b. inadequate support systems
   c. inadequate relaxation skills
   d. poor nutrition
   e. substance abuse
   f. unrealistic perceptions
   g. disturbed sleep patterns
   h. other.
3. Potential fluid volume deficit related to
   a. excessive losses through oral/rectal routes
   b. inadequate intake
   c. medications (diuretics)
   d. other.
4. Alteration in health maintenance related to
   a. perceptual or cognitive impairment
   b. ineffective individual coping
   c. ineffective family coping
   d. weakness/fatigue
   e. other.
5. Ineffective family coping (compromised) related to
   a. situational/maturational crises
   b. chronically unexpressed feelings of anxiety/guilt/despair

UNIT 12

    c. prolonged treatment regimen/therapy that impacts upon the entire family

    d. anxiety about eating behaviors/weight gain

    e. other.

6. Alteration in bowel elimination (constipation) related to
   a. inadequate dietary intake (food, fluid, bulk)
   b. chronic use of medication and enemas
   c. emotional status/anxiety
   d. vomiting after eating
   e. other.

7. Knowledge deficit (dynamics of eating disorder, medications, healthful nutrition, limit setting, stress management techniques, identification of suicidal risk, community resources) related to
   a. cognitive limitations
   b. lack of interest in learning
   c. patient's request for no information
   d. other.

8. Noncompliance with therapeutic regimen related to
   a. health-care beliefs about susceptibility to disease (denial, consequences of disease, value of treatment)
   b. cognitive limitations/lack of interest in learning
   c. dysfunctional patient-health care provider relationship
   d. substance abuse
   e. lack of financial resources
   f. distorted body image
   g. depression/suicidal ideas
   h. other.

9. Alteration in nutrition (less than body requirements) related to
   a. body weight about 20% under the ideal weight for height and frame
   b. reported/evidence of inadequate food intake
   c. anxiety/lack of interest in food
   d. abdominal pain
   e. decreased appetite due to medication
   f. vomiting meals
   g. difficulty eating (oral mucosa/dental conditions)
   h. other.

10. Alteration in oral mucous membrane related to
    a. dehydration
    b. malnutriton
    c. chemical trauma (vomiting)
    d. other.

11. Disturbance in self-concept (body image, self-esteem, role performance, personal identity) related to
    a. verbalization of feelings of hopelessness/powerlessness
    b. change in body appearance/function (weight loss, amenorrhea)
    c. impaired ability to perceive/acknowledge body appearance/changes
    d. withdrawal (social)
    e. other.

12. Sensory-perceptual alterations related to
    a. altered sensory reception and/or interpretation of body stimulus (hunger)
    b. sleep pattern disturbances
    c. chemical alterations/electrolyte imbalance

    d. anxiety/psychological stress
    e. impaired ability to concentrate
    f. other.
13. Sleep pattern disturbance related to
    a. anxiety/psychological stress
    b. other.
14. Potential for violence (self-directed) related to
    a. substance abuse
    b. self-destructive behavior and/or suicidal acts
    c. depression/distorted body image
    d. metabolic imbalance
    e. other.
15. Potential for injury related to
    a. bingeing followed by purging (vomiting, laxatives/enemas)
    b. hypovolemia
    c. electrolyte/metabolic imbalance
    d. malnutrition
    e. suicidal ideas or feelings
    f. other.
16. Alteration in thought processes related to
    a. electrolyte/metabolic imbalance
    b. inability to concentrate
    c. distorted body image
    d. preoccupation with food/dieting
    e. sleep pattern disturbance
    f. other.

PROCESS INDICATORS

1. The patient's biopsychosocial integrity is maintained.
Indicators
    a. patient maintains prescribed weight gain/attains targeted body weight
    b. patient does not demonstrate dysfunctional behaviors (lack of eating, bingeing/purging)
    c. patient/family validates a balance among the patient's nutrition, activity, and rest as prescribed in the therapeutic regimen
    d. patient identifies nonfood-related strategies for dealing with stress
    e. patient establishes adequate nutrition, hydration, and elimination patterns
    f. patient/family describes the therapeutic regimen/goals for diet, activity, and medication
    g. patient/family identifies signs and symptoms to report to the physician/nurse
    h. patient/family participates in follow-up care/counselling as appropriate
    i. patient does not exhibit self-directed injury and complications of malnutrition
    j. patient develops more effective/satisfying interpersonal relationships with family and others.
2. The patient/family demonstrate effective coping patterns.
Indicators
    a. patient verbalizes decreased feelings of anxiety/depression/fear
    b. patient/family identifies community resources/self-help groups
    c. patient/family identifies strategies to cope with stress

UNIT 12

  d. patient expresses feelings of positive self-esteem/satisfaction with quality of life
  e. patient verbalizes feeling of increased control over eating behaviors.
3. The patient achieves a satisfactory level of comfort.

Indicators
  a. satisfactory pattern of bowel elimination (without laxatives)
  b. satisfactory sleep patterns
  c. intact oral mucous membrane.

NURSING INTERVENTIONS

1. Assess the patient's
   a. eating patterns/diet (compliance with regimen)
   b. current weight and progress on weight goals
   c. sleeping patterns (early morning waking, difficulty falling asleep)
   d. activity levels
   e. use/abuse of medications/substances (antidepressants, laxatives, diuretics, amphetamines, alcohol/drugs, ipecac)
   f. elimination color, amount, consistency, frequency (a history of laxative/enema abuse requires careful monitoring of bowel function)
   g. verbalizations of feelings of self-esteem, depression, suicidal ideas, body image, and abilities to cope with stress/interpersonal relationships
   h. attitudes toward food ("bad" foods and "soothing" foods) and weight
   i. complaints of and signs of impaired ability to concentrate, amenorrhea, abdominal pain, vomiting, esophagitis, constipation, pale dry skin, poor skin turgor, brittle nails, hair loss, poor oral/dental hygiene-note decay and caries, feeling cold, signs of electrolyte imbalance (hypokalemia with cardiac arrhythmias).
2. Assess the patient's/family's
   a. interactions/communication patterns/coping abilities (include assessment for physical/sexual and/or alcohol abuse)
   b. participation in follow-up care/counselling
   c. understanding of the therapeutic regimen concerning target weight, diet, activity, and medication parameters
   d. use of food in the family as punishment and/or reward.
3. Instruct the patient/family/home health aide about consultation with a recreational/occupational therapist who may provide nonfood ways for the patient to relax/spend leisure time.
   a. nonfood strategies for coping with stress and relaxation techniques
      • reinforce instructions patient may have received during therapy
      • exercise, as a relaxation technique, may be used only as approved within the prescribed activity parameters.
   b. strategies for satisfactory sleep pattern
      • avoiding stimulants (caffeine, activity, stress) before bedtime
      • relaxation techniques that can be performed in bed (imagery, controlled breathing)
   c. activity/exercise parameters
   d. medications (name of drugs, action, dosage, schedule of administration, possible side effects, adverse effects to report to the physician)
   e. good oral hygiene practices including a dental examination.

4. Instruct the patient/family/home health aid about a dietary plan that
   a. complies with the prescribed parameters including foods that
      - form the basic food groups to foster good nutrition/to prevent malnutrition
      - are high in fiber/bulk (bran, vegetables, fruit, whole grains, fruit juices) to promote satisfactory bowel elimination and maintenance of targeted weight
      - are low in caffeine (coffee, tea, colas, chocolate) to decrease sympathetic nervous system stimulation prior to bedtime
   b. includes a 3-day diet recall completed by the patient
   c. incorporates cultural, religious, and personal preferences
   d. includes a consultation with the dietician as appropriate
   e. encourages the patient to eat 3 to 4 meals daily within the prescribed parameters
      - avoiding large meals and overeating/bingeing (which could lead to vomiting/purging)
      - incorporating nutritional supplements as appropriate
      - keeping "binge" foods out of the home
   f. incorporates weight control/behavior modification strategies as described by the therapeutic regimen
      - encouraging a pleasant relaxing environment for eating (relaxation techniques may be needed before and after meals)
      - remaining in the presence of others for 30 to 60 minutes after eating
      - maintaining a food/weight log
      - drinking adequate amounts of water (6 to 8 glasses/day)
   g. incorporates administration of tube feedings if appropriate.
5. Instruct the patient/family/home health aide about signs and symptoms to report to the physician/nurse.
   a. extreme weight loss (loss of 20 to 25% of predicted body weight)
   b. compulsive/excessive exercise
   c. unusual/change in eating habits (including fasting, bingeing/purging)
   d. substance abuse (alcohol/drugs)
   e. destructive behavior toward self and sense of desperation
      - suicidal intent may develop as eating-disordered symptoms decrease
      - recognition of suicidal intent requires immediate reporting
   f. withdrawal (social) from others
   g. obsession (dysfunctional with regard to body weight, dieting, and calorie counting)
   h. failure to adhere to therapeutic regimen with exacerbation of symptoms.
6. Encourage the patient/family to verbalize fears, anxieties, and feelings of helplessness/hopelessness.
7. Identify community resources that can facilitate the patient's/family's recovery from eating disorder.
   a. American Anorexia and Bulimia Association, Inc.
   b. National Anorexic Aid Society, Inc.
   c. Anorexia Nervosa and Associated Eating Disorders
   d. local self-help groups.
8. Support/participate in patient contract for regimen compliance
   a. reinforce self-control and positive self-esteem
   b. reinforce coping and stress management/relaxation strategies.
9. Monitor and record patient's weight, vital signs, and any signs and symptoms of noncompliance, dehydration, bowel dysfunction, malnutrition, electrolyte imbalance (cardiac arrhythmias), and esophagitis.
10. Obtain blood for electrolytes, acid-base balance, and so forth as ordered.

UNIT
12

11. Insert nasogastric tube and instruct patient/family about nasogastric tube care and feeding directions if appropriate.
12. Coordinate and consult with additional members of the health care team such as the recreational/occupational therapist, social worker, registered dietician, dentist, and mental health provider.
13. Provide progress report and discharge summary to the primary physician.

THERAPEUTIC ACHIEVEMENTS

- The patient maintains targeted body weight.
- The patient maintains regular, adequate patterns for nutrition, hydration, elimination, and activity.

Special Note. The eating disorders care plan should be used selectively in meeting the individualized needs of the patient and family members. Although eating disorders, in general, focus on an intense preoccupation with food/eating/dieting, each type of disorder demands a different focus.

Depending upon the patient's diagnosis (anorexia nervosa/bulimia), level of nutritional compromise, type/length of treatment, and therapeutic regimen/goals, the care plan requires a combination of different approaches for the patient and family. Nursing interventions can assist patients and their support systems (family/peers) to create environments in which the eating disorder behaviors are not needed.

Hepatic Cirrhosis Care Plan

CROSS REFERENCES

Alcohol Abuse Care Plan
Hypertension Care Plan

NURSING DIAGNOSES

1. Alterations in nutrition (less than body requirements) related to
   a. anorexia
   b. nausea/vomiting
   c. chronic dyspepsia/gastric distress
   d. dependence on others for cooking/shopping
   e. hematemesis
   f. other.
2. Alterations in bowel elimination (constipation, diarrhea, melena) related to
   a. inadequate dietary intake
   b. inadequate medication compliance
   c. impaired mobility
   d. other.
3. Knowledge deficit (prevention and treatment of cirrhosis, signs and symptoms to report to physician/nurse, medication/dietary/activity regimen, programs for alcohol rehabilitation) related to
   a. cognitive limitation
   b. lack of interest in learning
   c. unfamiliarity with information resources
   d. other.
4. Potential for injury related to
   a. weakness/fatigue
   b. increased abdominal distension (ascites)
   c. dyspnea
   d. increased bleeding tendencies (epistaxis, ecchymosis, petechiae, bleeding gums)
   e. hematemesis
   f. weight loss
   g. change in mentation (depression, confusion)
   h. other.
5. Anxiety/fear related to
   a. unemployment
   b. chronic nature of disease
   c. other.
6. Impaired skin integrity related to
   a. edema
   b. impaired mobility
   c. altered metabolic state resulting in skin itchiness
   d. altered immune response
   e. impaired nutritional state (anorexia)
   f. increased risk of bleeding

**UNIT
12**

    g. inadequate hygiene/skin care

    h. other.

7. Activity intolerance related to

    a. ascites

    b. nausea/vomiting

    c. dyspnea

    d. edema

    e. diarrhea

    f. fever

    g. weakness

    h. other.

8. Self-care deficit (feeding, bathing, grooming, hygiene, toileting) related to

    a. immobility/activity intolerance

    b. dyspnea

    c. changes in mentation

    d. dependence on others for care

    e. malaise/anorexia

    f. other.

9. Noncompliance with therapy related to

    a. denial

    b. substance abuse

    c. dependence on others for care/inadequate support systems

    d. changes in mentation

    e. other.

10. Sleep pattern disturbance related to

    a. dyspnea

    b. nausea/vomiting

    c. changes in mentation

    d. diarrhea

    e. restlessness

    f. other.

11. Ineffective individual/family coping related to

    a. fatigue/weakness

    b. unemployment

    c. change in family roles/responsibilities

    d. dependence on others for care

    e. substance abuse

    f. other.

12. Alteration in thought process related to

    a. changes in mentation

    b. coma

    c. substance abuse

    d. other.

PROCESS INDICATORS

1. The patient's biopsychosocial integrity is maintained.

Indicators

    a. no skin irritation or breakdown

    b. patient performs self-care/activities of daily living as appropriate with his or her capability/activity tolerance

    c. patient/family validates balance among the patient's rest, activity, and nutrition
    d. patient/family utilizes community resources/substance abuse rehabilitation programs
       (Alcoholics Anonymous, Alanon, Alateen)
2. The patient/family adapts to the cirrhosis regimen for convalescence and prevention of
   disease progression.

Indicators

    a. patient maintains satisfactory nutritional status, maintains acceptable body weight,
       eats small frequent meals, and takes vitamin supplements as prescribed
    b. patient/family explains the purpose, administration schedule, and adverse effects of
       prescribed medications
    c. patient/family identifies the need to avoid taking any medication, including over-
       the-counter medication, without prior physician approval
    d. patient maintains an activity plan that includes rest periods
    e. patient/family identifies signs and symptoms to report to the nurse/physician
    f. patients/family verbalizes factors that can aggravate or precipitate cirrhosis
    g. patient/family verbalizes decreased feelings of anxiety/depression.

NURSING INTERVENTIONS

1. Assess the patient
    a. skin integrity, color of skin and sclera, presence of pruritus, jaundice
    b. nutritional status/appetite (nausea, vomiting, weight loss, anorexia), frequency of
       meals
    c. evidence of bleeding tendencies (ecchymosis, petechiae, epistaxis, melena, hem-
       atemesis, bleeding gums)
    d. level of comfort/discomfort (dyspnea, dyspepsia, epigastric discomfort)
    e. bowel/bladder patterns, change in habits, color of stool/urine, presence of frank/
       occult blood
    f. activity level/tolerance (weakness, lassitude, muscle twitching, asterixis)
    g. psychological state (changing mentation, depression, substance abuse)
    h. presence of peripheral edema, ascites, hemorrhoids.
2. Assess
    a. availability/reliability of support systems
    b. patient's/family's understanding of causes of cirrhosis and treatment
    c. patient's/family's awareness of community resources (alcohol/drug rehabilitation
       programs as appropriate)
    d. patient's/family's understanding of the cirrhosis regimen (nutrition, activity, medi-
       cation, and elimination of alcohol intake)
    e. patient's/family's ability to effectively cope.
3. Instruct the patient/family/home health aide about the medication regimen (diuretics,
   antibiotics, hematenics, blood coagulants, laxatives and stool softeners, antacids,
   antiemetics, antidiarrheals, antipruritics, supplemental vitamins and minerals)
    a. names of drugs
    b. action/indication for use
    c. dosage
    d. schedule of administration
    e. possible side effects
    f. adverse effects to report to the physician
    g. avoiding any medications without prior approval of the physician
       • includes over-the-counter medications, such as acetylsalicylic acid (ASA) and
        birth control pills and
       • many drugs that are hepatotoxic.

UNIT 12

4. Instruct the patient/family/home health aide about skin care.
   a. clean the skin daily, avoiding alkaline soap
   b. apply emollient lotions as necessary (prn)
   c. treat skin breakdown immediately to prevent infection
   d. prevent skin trauma by using an electric razor and soft bristled toothbrush
   e. keep nails clean, short, and trimmed
   f. change position at least every 2 hours if on bed rest.
5. Discuss strategies with the patient/family/home health aide to promote patient self-esteem and successful patient/family coping.
   a. encourage the patient/family to verbalize feelings/concerns
   b. encourage the patient to perform daily grooming
   c. refer to Alcoholics Anonymous, Alanon, and Alateen.
6. Instruct the patient/family/home health aide to report the following signs and symptoms to their nurse/physician:
   a. evidence of bleeding tendencies (epistaxis, petechiae, ecchymosis, bleeding gums, hematemesis, melena)
   b. changes in mentation (depression, euphoria, inappropriate behavior, fatigue, irritability, loss of judgment)
   c. weight change
      • weight gains with edema, increasing ascites
      • weight loss with anorexia, vomiting
   d. skin breakdown, increasing skin itchiness/pruritus
   e. signs of impending hepatic coma (nausea, vomiting, low grade fever, abdominal pain)
   f. changes in gastrointestinal status (nausea, anorexia, vomiting, diarrhea, constipation).
7. Instruct the patient/family/home health aide about a plan that promotes rest and balanced activities.
   a. restricted activity during acute episodes and when fatigued
   b. avoiding activities that increase the risk of bleeding due to trauma (avoid straining at stools, forceful nose blowing, coughing, sneezing, trauma due to falls)
   c. position the patient in semi-Fowler or high-Fowler position to relieve dyspnea/orthopnea related to ascites.
8. Instruct the patient/family/home health aide about a dietary plan that
   a. incorporates sodium and fluid restrictions, if the patient has fluid retention and ascites (avoid table salt, salty foods, canned and frozen foods)
   b. incorporates a balanced diet within the prescribed parameters for percentages of protein, carbohydrate, and fat
      • protein may be restricted if ammonia levels rise
      • reinforce that the diet may change as blood levels vary
      • supplemental feedings
   c. encourages the patient to assume a semi-Fowler or high-Fowler position for meals, particularly if ascites is present
   d. allows small frequent meals (4 to 5 times/day)
   e. provides a list of foods that are permitted and restricted
      • avoid foods that are mechanically or chemically irritating or high in ammonia (gelatin, strong cheeses)
      • include foods that promote bowel evacuation
   f. includes supplemental feedings that may be needed to maintain adequate caloric intake (enteral feedings may need to be instituted).

9. Instruct the patient/family about
   a. need to eliminate patient's alcohol intake
   b. recording intake and output as appropriate
   c. need to record weekly weight
   d. testing of stool for blood as ordered.
10. Request/obtain orders, as necessary for blood work, medications, vitamin K.
11. Test urine/feces for blood as ordered.
12. Measure/monitor abdominal girth as ordered.
13. Coordinate/refer to as necessary
    a. social worker
    b. occupational therapist
    c. self-help/community resources
    d. substance abuse rehabilitation programs
    e. financial counselling services
    f. dietician.
14. Provide progress reports and a discharge summary to the primary physician.

THERAPEUTIC ACHIEVEMENT

- The patient/family adapts to the life style changes as a result of cirrhosis.

RELATED PATIENT INSTRUCTIONS

A Daily Food Guide—Four Basic Food Groups
Constipation
Diuretic Medications
General Comfort Measures

Infection Control for the Home
Measuring Liquid Intake and Output
Medication Compliance
Skin Care

UNIT
12

Procedures

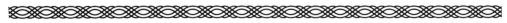

Enteral Tube Feeding Procedure

PURPOSE

- To administer feedings directly to the duodenum or jejunum through a feeding tube.

EQUIPMENT

- feeding solutions/medications
- large volume container
- stethoscope
- tap water
- clamp
- gauze sponges
- nonallergic tape
- for syringe feeding
  - bulb or plunger syringe (at least 50 cc)
- for gravity drip and pump feeding
  - enteral therapy administration set
  - piston syringe
  - IV pole or wall hook
  - pump, if used
- Optional
  - water-soluble lubricant
  - cotton-tipped applicators
  - feeding tube/administration set tube adapter
  - feeding tube cap/plug
  - ice bag/pouch.

Special Note
1. Check the expiration date on commercially prepared feeding formulas.
2. Check the date and time of home prepared feeding solution
   a. discard if it has not been refrigerated or if it is more than 48 hours old
   b. do not hold the formula at room temperature for longer than 10 hours.
3. Always label prepared solutions with time, date, contents, and volume.
4. If the patient is permitted solid food, mix it in a blender. The residue and fiber promote bowel function.
5. Warm the solution to room temperature to prevent cramps and reduce gas formation.

Steps

1. Explain the procedure to the patient/family.
2. Gather supplies.
3. Wash hands.
4. Measure the feeding solution and water in graduated containers.
5. Prepare the administration set equipment.
   a. *Gravity drip and pump method.* Pour the feeding solution into the administration set. Hang the feeding container about 2 ft above an adult's head (6 to 8 in above an infant's head). Fill the drip chamber about ½ full. Flush the tubing to remove excess air.
   b. *Syringe method.* Remove the bulb/plunger. Flush the tubing to remove excess air.
6. Place the patient in semi-Fowler or high-Fowler position unless contraindicated. Position infants supine or lying on the right side with head and chest slightly elevated.
7. Administer the feeding.
   a. *Gravity drip and pump method.* Connect the feeding set to the tube.
   b. *For gravity feeding,* open and adjust the flow regulator clamp for the prescribed rate
   c. *For pump feeding,* open the flow regulator clamp, turn on the pump, and set the flow rate. When the feeding solution has infused, close the flow regulator clamp before the drip chamber is empty; if using a pump, turn it off. Flush the tubing with the prescribed amount of water. Flushing can be done by using a gravity drip, pump, or syringe. After flushing is completed, close the flow regulator clamp and detach the administration set.

Key Points

1. Knowing what to expect increases patient/family compliance.

4. As the patient's tolerance grows, the volume can be increased.
5. Follow the instructions for the pump and/or administration set. If the administration set contains an ice pouch, fill the pouch with ice. The formula may be diluted initially to ½ or ¾ strength.

6. Do not allow the patient to lie flat because of regurgitation/aspiration. During the feeding, the infant should be held and given a pacifier, if possible.

c. Follow manufacturer's instructions for operation/rate setting. Avoid allowing the feeding container to empty, some pumps will pump air. Flushing is critical to maintain tube patency.

UNIT 12

d. *Syringe method.* Attach the syringe to the feeding tube. Pour the feeding solution into the syringe. Add more solution when the syringe is ¼ full. Regulate the flow rate by adjusting the height of the syringe. When the feeding solution has infused, pour the prescribed amount of water into the syringe. After flushing is completed, close the clamp. Detach the syringe.

d. Holding the tube upright with a slight tilt will allow air bubbles to escape. Adding more solution before the syringe empties prevents air from entering the tube. The feeding should last about 15 to 20 minutes for an adult and 20 to 45 minutes for an infant. Periodically interrupt the feeding to allow infants to burp. Flushing is critical to maintain tube patency.

8. Instruct the patient to remain sitting upright for about 30 minutes after the feeding. Position an infant on the abdomen or right side for at least 1 hour after the feeding.

8. If not contraindicated, walking can aid digestion. Instruct the ambulatory patient to hold the pole securely while walking. Be sure the pump converts to battery power after unplugging it.

9. Clean the administration set.
   a. Wash the feeding administration set (container and tubing) and/or syringe in hot soapy water
   b. Rinse thoroughly and dry
   c. Store the equipment in a clean covered container.

10. Change the administration sets.
    a. When changing administration sets, follow the steps for Preparation of Administration Set Equipment at step 5.
    b. Close the flow clamp on the current administration set.

    b. If using a pump, turn it off.

    c. Clamp/pinch the feeding tube to prevent air from entering the intestine.
    d. Disconnect the current administration set from the feeding tube
    e. Connect the new administration set
    f. Open the flow clamp to adjust the rate

    f. If using a pump, turn it on.

    g. If reusing the administration sets be sure to thoroughly wash, rinse, and dry before storing.

11. Instruct the patient/family about mouth care.

11. A schedule of mouth care 3 to 4 times daily is important for an unconscious patient.

12. Instruct the patient/family about nostril care.

12. Nostril cleaning and lubrication, as well as assessing the skin for signs of breakdown should be performed daily.

13. Instruct the patient/family about maintaining hydration and administering medications, if ordered.

13. If ordered antidiarrheal agents and other medications can be administered through the tube, except for enteric-coated drugs. Tablets must be crushed and capsules opened and diluted in water. Scheduled water supplements may be necessary for the patient's hydration (in addition to flushing the tube with water after feedings/medication administration).

14. Monitor/record intake, output, and weight. Periodic measurements of abdominal girth may also be necessary.

14. Assist the patient/family to keep accurate records.

15. Monitor the patient's tolerance to feedings.

15. Assess for patient's complaints of feeling too full or regurgitation after a feeding.
    a. Smaller, more frequent feedings may be needed.
    b. Maintaining a constant flow rate will decrease complications such as hyperglycemia, glycosuria, and diarrhea.
    c. Ausculate for bowel sounds as needed.
    d. Assess for signs of the dumping syndrome (nausea, vomiting, diarrhea, cramps, pallor, sweating, and fainting) in patients with a duodenostomy or jejunostomy.

16. Monitor
    a. blood and urine glucose levels
    b. serum electrolytes
    c. other blood studies as ordered/ needed.

DOCUMENTATION

1. Record the date, time, amount, and type of each feeding. Assist the family to develop a log book for recording intake, output, and weight.

2. Record the administration of any medications.

3. Record the volume of water used.

4. Record the patient's tolerance to feedings as well as any complaints of regurgitation/ intolerance to feedings, dumping syndrome, diarrhea, and the like. Include the condition of the skin around the tube as well as tube placement checks.

5. Document the patient's/family's progress in mouth/nostril care, administration of feedings, administration set changes, and recording in the log book.

6. Notify the physician of any deviations from expected outcomes; document the date, time, and details of the consultation.

UNIT
12

Esophagostomy, Gastrostomy, Duodenostomy, Jejunostomy Tube Feeding Procedure

PURPOSE

- To administer feedings directly to the esophagus, stomach, duodenum, or jejunum through a surgical opening.

EQUIPMENT

- feeding solutions/medications
- large volume container
- stethoscope
- tap water
- clamp
- gauze sponges
- nonallergic tape
- for syringe feeding
  - 50 cc bulb or plunger syringe
- for gravity drip and pump feeding
  - administration set
  - piston syringe
  - IV pole or wall hook
  - pump, if used
- Optional
  - water soluble lubricant
  - skin protectant ointment
  - drain sponges
  - abdominal pads
  - abdominal binder
  - cotton-tipped applicators
  - hydrogen peroxide
  - normal saline
  - baby-bottle nipple
  - gastrostomy tube/urinary catheter with appropriate size balloon

Special Note
1. Check the expiration date on commercially prepared feeding formulas.
2. Check the date and time of home prepared feeding solution
   a. discard if it has not been refrigerated or if it is more than 48 hours old
   b. do not store the formula at room temperature for longer than 10 hours.

3. Always label home prepared solutions with time, date, contents, and volume.
4. If the patient is permitted solid food, mix it in a blender. The residue and fiber promote bowel function.
5. Warm the solution to room temperature to prevent cramps and reduce gas formation.
6. Prior to age 1 year, infant formula and breast milk are used; after age 1 year, home prepared or commercially prepared products may be used.

Steps	**Key Points**
1. Explain the procedure to the patient/family.	1. Knowing what to expect increases patient/family compliance.
2. Gather supplies.	
3. Wash hands.	
4. Measure the feeding solution and water in graduated containers.	4. As the patient's tolerance grows, the volume can be increased.
5. Prepare the administration set equipment	
a. *Gravity drip and pump method*	a. Follow the instructions for the pump and/or administration set.
• pour the feeding solution into the administration set	
• hang the feeding container about 2 ft above the patient's head	
• fill the drip chamber about ½ full	
• flush the tubing to remove excess air	
b. *Syringe method*	
• remove the bulb/plunger	
• flush the tubing to remove excess air.	
6. Place the patient in semi-Fowler or high-Fowler position unless contraindicated. Position an infant supine or lying on the right side with the head and chest slightly elevated.	6. Do not allow the patient to lie flat because of regurgitation/aspiration. During the feeding, the infant should be held and given a pacifier, if possible.
7. Prepare the ostomy tube	
a. *For tube insertion*	a. Do not cut the dressing off; you may cut sutures, if any are present.
• remove the ostomy dressing and dispose of properly	
• if the patient has a prosthesis, remove the cap	• a patient with an esophagostomy usually will remove the tube between meals.
• lubricate the distal end of the tube with water-soluble lubricant or water	
• insert the tube into the ostomy opening.	• this measurement is about 4 to 6 in for an adult and 2 to 3 in for an infant.

UNIT 12

b. *For a tube that is already in place*
- remove the dressing to expose the tube; dispose of the dressing properly.

c. *For changing a gastrostomy tube* (urinary catheter type)
- remove the dressing if present
- deflate the urinary catheter balloon
- instill water into the ballon of the new catheter
- check for leaks, then remove the water
- *(for infants only)* cut three to four small air vents in the wide part of the nipple. Pull the catheter tip (using a clamp or tweezers) through the opening in the top of the nipple
- lubricate the distal end of the tube with water or water soluble lubricant
- insert the catheter into the stomach
- instill water to inflate the balloon of the catheter
- gently pull back on the catheter until resistance is met
- slide the nipple down until it rests against the skin (for infants only).

9. If ordered, aspirate for gastric residual contents prior to the feeding.

10. Administer the feeding
a. Connect the feeding set/syringe tubing to the ostomy tube
b. *For gravity feeding,* open and adjust the flow regulator clamp for the prescribed rate
c. *For pump feeding,* open flow regulator clamp, turn on the pump, and set the flow rate

d. *For syringe feeding,* attach the syringe to the feeding tube
- pour the feeding solution into the syringe

b. Do not cut the dressing off; you may cut the tube or sutures.

c. Plan tube changing prior to a feeding so that the stomach is empty.

- Do not cut off the top of the nipple.

9. Residual contents can be returned to the stomach or discarded, depending upon physician's orders.

c. Follow manufacturer's instructions for operation/rate setting. Avoid allowing the feeding container to empty. Some pumps will pump air.

- holding the tube upright with a slight tilt will allow air bubbles to escape

- add more solution when the syringe is ¼ full

- regulate the flow rate by adjusting the height of the syringe

e. When the feeding solution has infused, close the flow regulator clamp
  - do not allow the tubing to empty
  - if using a pump, turn it off.
11. Flush the tubing/syringe with the prescribed amount of water.
12. After flushing is completed, close the flow regulator clamp. Close the clamp on the ostomy tube.
13. Detach the administration set from the ostomy tube.
14. Instruct the patient to remain sitting upright for about 30 minutes after the feeding.

15. Wash the feeding administration set (container and tubing) and/or syringe in warm soapy water. Rinse thoroughly and dry. Store the equipment in a clean covered container.
16. If the ostomy tube is removable and will be reused for each feeding, wash it in hot soapy water. Rinse thoroughly and dry.
17. Instruct the patient/family to wash the peristomal skin with soap and water at least daily.

18. Instruct the patient/family about proper dressing procedure if appropriate.

- adding more solution before the syringe empties prevents air from entering the tube
- the feeding should last about 15 to 20 minutes for an adult and 20 to 45 minutes for an infant
- for an infant elevate the syringe 4 in above the abdominal wall
- interrupt the feeding periodically to allow infants to burp.

11. Flushing is critical to maintain tube patency.

14. If not contraindicated, walking can aid digestion. Infants should be positioned upright or lying on the right side for at least 1 hour after the feeding.

16. Check the tube carefully for any damage, hardening, or cracks.

17. Encrusted secretions can be removed from the skin or tube with cotton-tipped applicators or a clean cloth soaked in a mixture of half hydrogen peroxide and half water (or saline). Rinse the area and dry the skin carefully. A skin protectant may also be prescribed.

UNIT
12

19. Instruct the patient/family about maintaining hydration and administering medications if ordered.

19. If ordered, antidiarrheal agents and other medications can be administered through the tube. Scheduled water supplements may be necessary for patient hydration (in addition to flushing the tube with water after feeding/medication administration). Medications should be mixed well with water, strained fruit, or pudding.

20. Monitor/record intake, output, and weight. Periodic measurements of abdominal girth may also be necessary.

20. Teach the patient/family to keep accurate records.

21. Monitor the patient's tolerance to feedings.

21. Assess for the patient's complaints of feeling too full or regurgitating after a feeding. Smaller, more frequent feedings may be needed. Auscultate for bowel sounds as needed. Assess for signs of the dumping syndrome (nausea, vomiting, diarrhea, cramps, pallor, sweating, and fainting) in patients with a duodenostomy or jejunostomy.

22. Monitor blood/urine glucose levels, serum electrolytes, and other blood studies as ordered/needed.

DOCUMENTATION

1. Record the date, time, amount, and type of each feeding. Assist the family to develop a log book for recording intake, output, and weight.

2. Record the administration of any medications.

3. Record the volume of water used.

4. Record the patient's tolerance to feedings as well as any complaints of regurgitation or intolerance to feedings, dumping syndrome, diarrhea, and so forth. Include the condition of the peristomal skin and the stoma.

5. Document the patient's/family's progress in stoma care, administration of feedings, dressing procedure, and recording in the log book.

6. Notify the physician of any deviations from expected outcomes. Document the date, time, and the details of the consultation.

Gastric Tube Feeding Procedure

PURPOSE

- To administer feedings/medications directly into the stomach.

EQUIPMENT

- feeding solution/medication
- large volume containers
- stethoscope
- tap water
- clamp
- nonallergic tape
- for syringe feeding
  - bulb or plunger syringe (almost 50 ml)
- for gravity drip or pump feeding
  - administration set
  - piston syringe
  - IV pole or wall hook
  - pump, if used
- optional
  - water soluble lubricant
  - cotton-tipped applicators
  - adaptor

Contraindication
- absence of bowel sounds/possible intestinal obstruction

Special Note
1. Check the expiration date on commercially prepared feeding formulas.
2. Check the date and time of home prepared feeding solutions.
   a. discard if they have not been refrigerated or if they are more than 48 hours old
   b. do not hold the formula at room temperature for longer than 10 hours.
3. Always label prepared solutions with time, date, contents and volume. Follow package instructions or defined dietary parameters to prepare the feeding solution.
4. If the patient is permitted solid food, mix it in a blender. The residue and fiber promote bowel function.
5. Warm the solution to room temperature to prevent cramps and reduce gas formation. If the solution has been refrigerated remove the amount needed for the feeding. Warm the container with the solution in a basin of hot water or let it stand until it reaches room temperature. Do not heat the solution over direct heat as the solution may curdle or chemically decompose. The solution's temperature may become too warm and cause injury to the patient.

UNIT 12

Steps	*Key Points*

1. Explain the procedure to the patient/family.

   1. Knowing what to expect increases patient/family compliance.

2. Gather supplies.
3. Wash your hands.
4. Measure the feeding solution into the graduated container.

   4. As the patient's tolerance grows, the volume can be increased.

5. Prepare the administration set equipment.

   5. Follow the instructions for the pump and/or administration set. If the administration set contains an ice pouch, fill the pouch with ice. The formula may be diluted initially to ½ or ¾ strength.

   a. *Gravity drip and pump method.* Pour the feeding solution into the administration set. Hang the feeding container about 2 ft above an adult's head (6 to 8 in above an infant's head). Fill the drip chamber about ½ full. Flush the tubing to remove excess air.

   b. *Syringe method.* Remove the bulb/plunger. Flush the tubing to remove excess air.

6. Place the patient in semi-Fowler or high-Fowler position. Infants should be positioned supine or lying on their right side with head and chest slightly elevated.

   6. This position aids digestion and decreases the risk of aspiration due to gastroesophageal reflux.

7. Place the towel or absorbent pad over the patient's chest.
8. Remove the cap or plug from the feeding tube.
9. Check for tube patency and proper placement by injecting 5 to 10 cc of air through the tube for an adult (½ to 5 cc for an infant). Simultaneously auscultate the patient's stomach with the stethoscope.

   9. Proper placement is confirmed if a whooshing sound is heard and if gastric contents can be aspirated. Never give a tube feeding until proper placement is confirmed. Aspiration for gastric residual contents can be performed at this point if indicated.

10. Administer the feeding.

    a. *Gravity drip and pump method.* Connect the feeding tube to the gavage tubing.

       a. An adapter may be needed to connect the tubings.

    b. *For gravity feeding,* open and adjust the flow regulator clamp for the prescribed rate.

c. *For pump feeding*, open the flow regulator clamp, turn on the pump, and set the flow rate. When the feeding solution has infused, close the flow regulator clamp before the drip chamber is empty; if using a pump, turn it off. Flush the tubing with the prescribed amount of water. Flushing can be done using a gravity drip, pump or syringe. After flushing is completed, close the flow regulator clamp and detach the administration set.

d. *Syringe method*. Attach the syringe to the feeding tube. Pour the feeding solution into the syringe. Add more solution when the syringe is ¼ full. Regulate the flow rate by adjusting the height of the syringe. When the feeding solution has infused, pour the prescribed amount of water into the syringe. After the flushing is completed, close the clamp. Detach the syringe

11. Monitor the administration.

12. During continuous feedings assess the patient for abdominal distension/vomiting. Infants should be held and given pacifiers if possible.

13. Cap/plug the end of the feeding tube. *Option:* Bend the tube in half near the proximal opening, wrap a piece of gauze over the opening, and secure it with a rubber band.

14. Instruct the patient to remain in the semi-Fowler or high-Fowler position for at least 30 minutes. Position infants on their right side or abdomen for at least 1 hour after the feeding.

c. Follow the manufacturer's instructions for operation/rate setting. Avoid allowing the feeding container to empty; some pumps will pump air. Flushing is critical to maintain tube patency.

d. Holding the tube upright with a slight tilt will allow air bubbles to escape. Adding more solution before the syringe empties prevents air from entering the tube. The feeding should last about 15 to 20 minutes for an adult and 20 to 45 minutes for an infant. Periodically interrupt the feeding to allow infants to burp. Flushing is critical to maintain tube patency.

11. Periodically squeeze the bag to agitate the solution and to prevent clogging.

12. Reverse peristalsis can obstruct the flow of solution. If you suspect this problem, change the patient's position to assess if the solution will flow more freely. Burp the infant during the feeding.

14. If not contraindicated, walking aids in digestion. Instruct the patient to securely hold the pole while walking.

UNIT 12

15. *Clean the administration set.* Wash all reusable equipment in warm soapy water. Rinse thoroughly and dry. Store the equipment in a clean closed container.
16. Aspirate stomach contents about 2 to 3 hours after the patient's first feeding and before all subsequent feedings to verify adequate gastric emptying.
17. *Change the administration set.*
    a. When changing the administration sets, follow the steps for preparation of administration set equipment at *step 5.*
    b. Close the flow clamp on the current administration set.
    c. Clamp/pinch the feeding tube to prevent air from entering the intestine.
    d. Disconnect the current administration set from the feeding tube.
    e. Connect the new administration set.
    f. Open the flow clamp to adjust the rate.
    g. If reusing the administration sets be sure to thoroughly wash, rinse and dry before storing.

    b. If using a pump, turn it off.

    f. If using a pump, turn it on.

18. Instruct the patient/family in oral/nasal care.

18. A schedule of mouth care 3 to 4 times daily is important for an unconscious patient. Nostril cleaning and lubrication, as well as assessing the skin for signs of breakdown, should be performed daily.

19. Instruct the patient/family about maintaining hydration and administering medications, if ordered.

19. If ordered antidiarrheal agents and other medications can be administered through the tube except for enteric-coated drugs. Tablets must be crushed and capsules opened and diluted in water. Scheduled water supplements may be necessary for the patient's hydration (in addition to flushing the tube with water after feeding/medication administration).

20. Establish a diary for the patient/family to record date, time the feeding began and ended, type and amount of formula administered, amount of water given, other foods or fluids given, weight, stool frequency and consistency.

20. If constipation occurs
    a. the fruit, vegetable or sugar content of the feeding must be increased by the physician
    b. assess the patient's hydration status to be sure dehydration is not the cause
    c. increase the fluid intake, as necessary
    d. request orders for enemas/laxatives/stool softeners from the physician.
    If diarrhea occurs
    a. administer small, frequent, less concentrated feedings
    b. assess storage and preparation procedures
    c. request antidiarrheal medication from the physician
    d. ensure good perineal and skin care.

21. Monitor blood/urine glucose levels, serum electrolyte values and other blood studies as ordered/needed.

DOCUMENTATION

1. Record the date, time, amount and type of each feeding. Assist the family to develop a log book for recording intake, output and weight.

2. Record the administration of any medications.

3. Record the volume of water used.

4. Record the patient's tolerance to feedings as well as any complaints of regurgitation/intolerance to feedings, constipation, diarrhea and the like. Include the condition of the skin around the tube as well as tube placement checks.

5. Document the patient's/family's progress in mouth/nostril care, administration of feedings, administration set changes and recordings in the log book.

6. Notify the physician of any deviations from expected outcomes; document the date, time and details of the consultation.

UNIT
12

Nasogastric Tube Insertion Procedure

PURPOSE

- To remove gastric contents.
- To administer feedings (gavage) and medication directly into the gastrointestinal (GI) tract.

EQUIPMENT

- nasogastric tube or feeding tube with or without guide (sizes range from 6 to 18 French; 12 French is typical)
- towel or absorbent pad
- tissues
- emesis basin
- water-soluble lubricant
- ice chips or glass of water with straw
- penlight
- tongue blade
- ½- to 1-in nonallergic tape
- 50 ml syringe
- stethoscope
- rubber band
- safety pin
- optional
  - metal clamp
  - tincture of benzoin
  - ice
  - warm water
  - suction equipment

Special Note

1. Exercise caution during the insertion procedure in pregnant patients and patients who may have aortic aneurysms, myocardial infarctions, gastrointestinal hemorrhages, or esophageal varices.

2. Inserting the tube nasally is preferred unless certain conditions exist, such as impaired patency of the nostrils.

3. Newer nasogastric feeding tubes made of silicone, polyvinyl chloride, rubber, and polyurethane are more comfortable and less irritating than traditional plastic tubes.

4. Feeding tubes weighted with mercury require special handling for disposal.

Steps	*Key Points*
1. Explain the procedure to the patient/ family.	1. Knowing what to expect increases patient/family compliance.

2. Provide privacy.
3. Gather supplies.
4. Wash hands.
5. Prepare the equipment
   a. inspect the tube for defects; run water through the tube to assure patency
       a. For eash of insertion place a limp rubber tube in ice; place a stiff tube in warm water.
   b. follow the instructions on the package.
6. Place the patient in semi-Fowler or high-Fowler position.
7. Stand at the patient's right side if you are right handed. Stand on the patient's left side if you are left handed.
8. Drape the patient's chest with an absorbent pad.
9. Measure the tube length
   a. place the distal end of the tube at the tip of the patient's nose; extend the tube to the earlobe (Fig. 12–1A)
       a. Keep this portion (about 3 to 4 in in an adult) coiled until insertion
   b. extend the uncoiled portion from the earlobe to the xiphoid process (Fig. 12–1B)
       b. Measurements for an average adult range 22–26 inches.
   c. use a small piece of nonallergic tape to mark these two measurements.
10. Lubricate the tube's curved tip (and the guide if appropriate) with a small amount of water-soluble lubricant.
       10. Water-soluble lubrication decreases trauma and prevents oil aspiration if the tube enters the trachea. Be careful to avoid blocking the tube with lubricant.

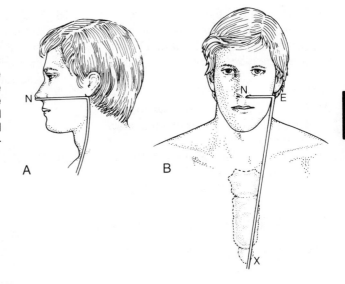

Figure 12–1. Nasogastric tube insertion procedures. *A,* Place the distal end of the tube at the tip of the patient's nose. Extend the tube to the earlobe. *B,* Extend the uncoiled portion from the earlobe to the xiphoid process.

A

B

UNIT 12

11. Establish a signal that the patient can use if a brief pause is needed during the procedure.

12. Position the emesis basin and tissues within easy reach.

   12. The patient can be asked to hold both.

SELECT NASAL ROUTE OR ORAL ROUTE*

Nasal Route

13. Assess nasal patency
    a. ask the patient to blow his or her nose gently to clear the nostrils
    b. use a penlight to inspect for a deviated septum
    c. ask the patient if he or she has a history of nose trauma
    d. occlude one nostril and ask the patient to breathe through the opposite nostril
    e. repeat a to d for the other nostril
    f. ask the patient which side he or she breathes easier.

   a. If both nostrils are not patent use the oral route.

   f. This side is the preferred nostril in which the tube will be inserted.

14. Position the patient with his or her head tilted back slightly.

15. Insert the lubricated tip of the tube.

16. Advance the tube along the nasal passage toward the ear on the same side.

   16. Avoid pressure on the turbinates.

17. Rotate the tube 180 degrees, as it passes the nasopharyngeal junction.

   17. This maneuver helps to prevent the tube from curving into the patient's mouth.

18. When you feel the tube begin to curve down the pharynx, have the patient tilt his head forward. *Do not force the tube.*

   18. You may wish to use a tongue blade and penlight to examine the mouth and throat, especially if the patient is unconscious. Tilting the patient's head forward helps to close the trachea and open the esophagus.

19. Unless contraindicated, have the patient sip some water through a straw or ask the patient to swallow.

20. Advance the tube as the patient swallows.

   20. Continue advancing the tube until the tape mark is reached.

---

*See Oral Route following step 20 of Nasal Route.

Oral Route

13. Remove any dentures.
14. Have the patient lower his or her chin and open his or her mouth if the patient is able to cooperate.
15. Place the tip of the tube at the back of the tongue.
16. If not contraindicated, ask the patient to sip water through a straw. Advance the tube as the patient swallows.
17. Continue advancing the tube until the tape mark reaches the lips.

18. If the patient is unable to swallow, you may need to use an insertion guide, to tilt his or her chin toward the chest, or both.

14. This maneuver closes the trachea.

16. Remind the patient not to clamp his or her teeth on the tube.

17. Stroke the patient's throat to facilitate passage of the tube down the esophagus.
18. Continue to stroke the patient's throat while advancing the tube between respirations.

Proper Tube Placement

Special Note. It is critical to carefully check for proper placement. However, be aware that misplaced, small-lumen tubes may not cause dramatic patient distress. If the tube enters the trachea, the patient may have difficulty breathing. If the patient is unable to speak, this sign may indicate that the tube is in the larynx.

1. Gently inject 10 cc of air through the tube as you auscultate the stomach for the rush of air.

2. If still unsure, try to *gently* aspirate gastric secretions.

3. If you cannot aspirate gastric contents, advance the tube slightly and repeat steps 1 and 2.

4. If you cannot aspirate gastric contents at this time, remove the tube and reinsert.

1. Place the stethoscope about 3 in below the xiphoid process. If the tube is in the stomach, you will hear a whooshing sound. If the tube is coiled in the esophagus, you will feel resistance.
2. Vigorous aspiration can result in tube collapse due to negative pressure. If you are able to aspirate gastric contents, placement is confirmed.
3. Never put the end of the tube into a container of water due to the risk of aspiration. Absence of bubbling does not confirm placement.

UNIT 12

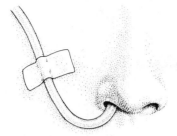

Figure 12–2. Tape the tube securely to the cheek or nose, avoiding excess pressure on the nostrils.

SECURING THE TUBE

1. Apply a small amount of tincture of benzoin to the skin area to be taped.

2. For a nasogastric tube
   a. tape the tube securely to the cheek or to the nose avoiding excess pressure on the nostrils (Fig. 12–2)
   b. to tape the tube to the nose, cut a 3 in long piece of 1 in-tape. Tear one end up the middle for about 1½ inches (Fig. 12–3A). Tape the untorn end to the nose and criss-cross the two free ends around the tube (Fig. 12–3B and 12–3C). Apply another piece of tape over the bridge of the nose for extra security.

3. For oral insertions, position the tube in the left buccal area between the cheek and teeth to reduce gagging. Tape the tube to the cheek (Fig. 12–4).

1. This will increase tape adherence and decrease skin irritation, particularly if the patient is diaphoretic.
2. There should be no distortion of the nostril's contour. Do not tape the tube to the patient's forehead.

   b. Prolonged nasogastric intubation can result in skin erosion at the the nostril. Careful taping and vigilant skin care avoids this problem.

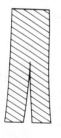
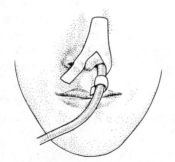
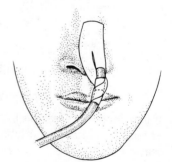

Figure 12–3. *A,* Cut a 3-in long piece of 1-in wide tape. Tear one end of the middle for about 1½ in. *B* and *C,* Tape the untorn end to the nose and crisscross the two free ends around the tube.

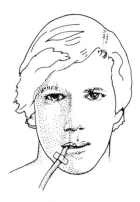

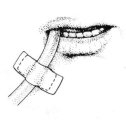

Figure 12–4. For oral insertions, position the tube in the left buccal area between the cheek and teeth to reduce gagging. Tape the tube to the cheek.

4. Use a rubber band to tie a slip knot around the tube. The rubber band can be secured with a safety pin to the clothing.

4. This additional method of securing the tube may prevent unnecessary pulling on the tube.

GENERAL CARE OF THE NOSE AND MOUTH

1. Plan for routine care of the nose.
   a. clean and lubricate both nostrils
   b. check carefully for any redness, bleeding, or numbness at the nostril.
2. Plan for routine care of the mouth.
   a. brush the teeth, gums, and tongue
   b. use mouthwash or salt solution
   c. moisten the lips with a lanolin-based cream.
3. Teach the patient/family care of the tube and skin.

1. Periodic removal of the tape is critical for complete skin assessment.

2. Mouth care is equally important for nasogastric insertions.

DOCUMENTATION

1. Record the date, time, type, and size of tube inserted. Include use of guide if appropriate.
2. Record the site of insertion (nasal/oral).
3. Document confirmation of proper tube placement.
4. Upon return visits record the condition of the skin.
5. Patient response to the procedure.
6. Patient/family teaching of tube and skin.

Nasogastric Tube Removal Procedure

PURPOSE

- To remove a nasogastric or feeding tube without injury and aspiration.

EQUIPMENT

- stethoscope
- 50 ml bulb or plunger syringe
- towel or absorbent pad
- adhesive remover
- mild soap and water
- tube clamp (optional)
- mouth care supplies

Special Note. Removal of feeding tubes weighted with mercury requires special handling for disposal. Radiopaque feeding tubes with tungsten do not require special handling.

Steps	Key Points
1. Explain the procedure to the patient/family.	1. Knowing what to expect increases patient compliance.
2. Provide privacy.	
3. Gather supplies.	
4. Wash hands	
5. If the tube's purpose was to remove gastric contents, check for bowel sounds prior to removing the tube.	
6. Place the patient in a high-Fowler position.	
7. Place the towel/absorbent pad over the patient's chest.	
8. Remove tape and/or any other devices securing the tube.	8. Do not allow the tube to move.
9. Flush the tube with 10 to 15 cc of air, then clamp or pinch the tube closed.	9. Clearing the tube of gastric contents decreases the risk of aspiration during removal.
10. Instruct the patient to hold his or her breath.	
11. Quickly but gently withdraw the tube (Fig. 12–5).	
12. Cover the tube with the towel/absorbent pad and remove it.	12. The tube's sight and odor may disturb the patient.

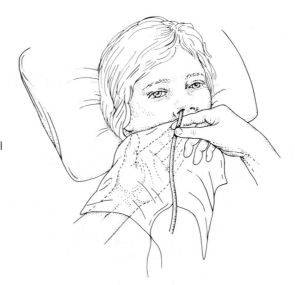

Figure 12–5. Nasogastric tube removal procedure. (See instructions in text.)

13. Assist the patient with oral hygiene as needed.
14. Clean the skin and remove any tape residue.
15. If the tube is to be reused, wash it with mild soap, rinse, and flush thoroughly with hot water.

13. A lubricant for nasal dryness may also be needed.

15. Check the tube carefully for any damage, hardening or cracks.

DOCUMENTATION

1. Describe, if appropriate, the color, consistency, and amount of gastric contents aspirated prior to removing the tube.

2. Record the date, time, size, and type of tube removed.

3. Describe the patient's tolerance of the procedure and the condition of the skin under the tape.

UNIT 12

Resources

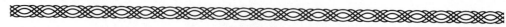

Gum Disease Warning Signs

1. Bleeding gums when teeth are brushed.
2. Bad breath.
3. Red, swollen, or tender gums.
4. Pus between teeth and gums when they are pressed.
5. Loose or separated permanent teeth.
6. Gums that have shrunk away from teeth.
7. A change in the way teeth come together when biting.
8. A change in the way dentures fit.

Bibliography

Bayer, L., Scholl, D., and Ford, E. Tube Feeding at Home. American Journal of Nursing, September 1983, pp. 1321–1325.

Given, B. A. and Simmons, S. J. Gastroenterology in Clinical Nursing, 4th ed. St. Louis: C. V. Mosby Co., 1983.

Gramse, C. A Review of Tube Feeding Techniques. Nursing 13(2): 1983, pp. 32B–32P.

Guenter, P. and Slocum, B. Hepatic Disease. Nutritional Implications. Nursing Clinics of North America, March 1983, pp. 71–80.

Harkaway, J. E. (ed.). Eating Disorders. Rockville, Maryland: Aspen Systems, 1987.

Home Tube Feeding Instructions. The Ross Medical Nutritional System, Columbus, Ohio: Ross Laboratories, 1982.

Konstantinides, N. and Shronts, E. Tube Feeding Managing the Basics. American Journal of Nursing, September 1983, pp. 1312–1320.

Larocca, F. E. (ed.). Eating Disorders. San Francisco: Jossey-Bass Inc., 1986.

Moghissi, K. and Boore, J. R. P. Parenteral and Enteral Nutrition for Nurses. Rockville, Maryland: Aspen Systems, 1983.

Moore, M. Do You Still Believe These Myths About Tube Feeding? RN, May 1987, pp. 51–54.

Sanger, E. and Cassino, T. Eating Disorders. Avoiding the Power Struggles. American Journal of Nursing, January 1984, pp. 31–35.

Hematology/Oncology Alterations

**UNIT
13**

Care Plans

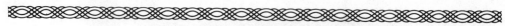

Chemotherapy Care Plan

CROSS REFERENCES

Constipation Care Plan
Depression Care Plan
Generic Cardiac Care Plan
Pain Care Plan
Spiritual Distress Care Plan

Home Safety Procedure
Home Health Aide Supervision Procedure
Indwelling Central Venous Catheter (Changing the Cap) Procedure
Indwelling Central Venous Catheter (Dressing Change) Procedure

Indwelling Central Venous Catheter (Heparinization) Procedure
Indwelling Central Venous Catheter (Withdrawing Blood) Procedure
Infection Control Procedure
Intravenous Therapy Procedure
Telephone Contact Procedure

Gum Disease (Warning Signs)

Mental Health Assessment/Intervention Guide

NURSING DIAGNOSES

1. Disturbance in self-concept related to
   a. alopecia
   b. weight loss/cachexia
   c. excessive fluid retention/weight gain
   d. changing/darkening skin pigmentation
   e. darkening/transverse ridging of nails
   f. premature menopause/amenorrhea
   g. decreased spermatogenesis
   h. ototoxic side effect
   i. dependence on others
   j. perceived sense of powerlessness
   k. other.
2. Alteration in nutrition (less than body requirements) related to
   a. nausea/vomiting
   b. anorexia
   c. dysphagia
   d. oral cavity tenderness/stomatitis
   e. diarrhea
   f. increased caloric needs
   g. depression
   h. distortion of taste and smell
   i. other.
3. Anxiety related to
   a. anticipation of side effects
   b. lack of understanding about side effects
   c. fatalistic misperceptions
   d. uncertainty about the future

    e. threat of long-term disability/life style changes
    f. change in urine color
    g. financial stress
    h. other.
 4. Potential for injury related to
    a. increased susceptibility to infection
    b. increased susceptibility to uncontrolled bleeding
    c. extravasation of vesicant/irritant drugs
    d. neurotoxic side effects
    e. ototoxic side effect
    f. other.
 5. Social isolation related to
    a. embarrassment regarding changed personal appearance
    b. weakness/decreased endurance
    c. fear of rejection by others
    d. depression
    e. fear of occurence of side effects in public
    f. other.
 6. Grieving related to loss of biopsychosocial well-being.
 7. Alteration in bowel elimination (constipation) related to
    a. neurotoxic side effects
    b. hypokalemia
    c. hypercalcemia
    d. other.
 8. Alteration in bowel elimination (diarrhea) related to
    a. gastrointestinal irritation
    b. anxiety
    c. fecal impaction
    d. other.
 9. Potential/actual fluid volume deficit related to
    a. diarrhea
    b. vomiting
    c. anorexia
    d. other.
10. Sexual dysfunction related to
    a. decreased vaginal lubrication
    b. ulceration of the genital tissues/organs
    c. other.
11. Alteration in patterns of urinary elimination related to genitourinary tract irritation.
12. Alteration in oral mucous membrane related to
    a. immunological deficit
    b. ineffective oral hygiene
    c. dehydration
    d. decreased/lack of salivation
    e. chemotherapeutic agent
    f. other.
13. Potential/actual impairment of skin integrity related to
    a. physical immobility
    b. skeletal prominence/emaciation
    c. altered metabolic state
    d. altered circulation
    e. altered sensation

UNIT 13

      f. immunological deficit

      g. contact with products of elimination

      h. extravasation of vesicant/irritant drug

      i. other.

14. Impaired physical mobility related to
   a. neurotoxic side effects
   b. altered metabolic state
   c. altered circulation
   d. other.

15. Self-care deficit (feeding, hygiene, grooming, toileting) related to
   a. decreased strength/endurance
   b. depression
   c. altered metabolic state
   d. neurotoxic side effects
   e. other.

16. Alteration in family process related to
   a. role modifications
   b. situational crisis of a chronically ill family member
   c. disruption of/change in usual pattern of family life
   d. other.

17. Ineffective family coping related to
   a. inadequate/incorrect understanding of chemotherapy by family members/significant others
   b. exhausted supportive capacity among family members
   c. ambivalent patient-family relationships
   d. resentment over forced reallocation of family resources/priorities
   e. financial stress
   f. sociocultural conflicts with treatment plan
   g. other.

18. Knowledge deficit (medication names; how chemotherapeutic agents work; side effects; early recognition of toxic effects; how to minimize, control, prevent side/toxic effects; purpose of chemotherapy; treatment plan; route of administration; signs and symptoms of anemia, bleeding, infection, altered metabolic states; methods of infection control; personal energy conservation methods; community resources; nutritional maintenance; oral and personal hygiene techniques) related to
   a. information misinterpretation
   b. cognitive limitation/impairment
   c. perplexity about treatment
   d. unfamiliarity with information resources
   e. patient/family request for no information
   f. denial/anxiety
   g. language barrier
   h. low readiness for acceptance of information
   i. sociocultural differences
   j. other.

PROCESS INDICATORS

1. The patient is protected against infection and injury.
Indicators
   a. patient's/family's recall of the signs and symptoms of infection

    b. patient's/family's recall of the signs and symptoms of bleeding
    c. patient's/family's recall of the signs and symptoms of neurotoxicity
    d. patient's/family's identification of how to control bleeding
    e. patient/family identifies household precautions/modifications to protect the patient
    f. patient/family states the situations necessitating contact with the nurse/physician.
2. The patient's physical health is maintained.

Indicators

    a. no signs and symptoms of infection
    b. no signs and symptoms of bleeding
    c. no signs and symptoms of altered metabolic states
    d. no skin irritation/breakdown
    e. intact oral mucosa
    f. patient is not dehydrated/overhydrated
    g. vital signs/laboratory values are within the patient's normal limits
    h. bowel and bladder patterns are regular/continent
    i. patient/family validates a balance between rest, nutrition, and exercise
    j. patient validation (verbally or nonverbally) that side effects are controlled/minimized.
3. The patient's psychosocial integrity is supported.

Indicators

    a. patient's performance of/participation in the activities of daily living are realistically commensurate with his or her capabilities
    b. patient maintains a satisfactory level of social/community interaction
    c. patient expresses satisfaction with his or her life experiences
    d. patient exhibits a reduction of anxiety-induced thoughts, feelings, and behaviors
    e. patient spontaneously shares his or her thoughts and feelings about his or her condition, changing life style, and so forth
    f. patient participates in a chemotherapy/cancer support group
    g. patient verbalizes acceptance of/comfort with his or her need to be dependent.
4. The family's psychosocial equilibrium is maintained.

Indicators

    a. familial feedback reflects an accurate understanding of cancer and chemotherapy
    b. familial feedback reflects that members are emotionally supportive of each other
    c. patient/family verbalizes acceptance of/comfort with role modifications
    d. patient's/sexual partner's feedback reflects satisfaction with sexual activity pattern
    e. each member's involvement in self-help groups/professional counselling
    f. patient/family appropriately utilizes community supports/resources
    g. family maintains its social/occupational responsibilities.

NURSING INTERVENTIONS

1. Assess the patient
    a. signs and symptoms of infection (fever, chills, aches, shortness of breath, dry hacking cough, dysuria, diarrhea, inflammation of skin/oral mucosa)
    b. signs and symptoms of bleeding (hemoptysis, petechiae, unexplained bruising, nosebleeds, bleeding gums, scleral hemorrhages, hematuria, irregular/excessive vaginal bleeding, abdominal pain, hypotension, tachycardia)
    c. signs and symptoms of anemia (pallor, weakness, fatigue, headache, tinnitus, palpitations, vertigo)
    d. signs and symptoms of neurotoxicity (tinnitus; abdominal cramping; imbalance; slapping gait; weakness, numbness, tingling of extremities; cranial nerve palsy; decreased/absent deep tendon reflexes)

UNIT
13

     e. cardiopulmonary status

     f. skin integrity

     g. signs and symptoms of overhydration/dehydration

     h. oral cavity status (dental caries, obvious peridontal disease, abscesses, mucosal ulceration)

     i. signs and symptoms of altered metabolic states (hypocalcemia/hypercalcemia, hypomagnesemia)

     j. presence/degree of chemotherapeutic-related side effects (alopecia, skin pigmentation/skin changes, nausea/vomiting, dermatitis, mood changes, sexual dysfunction)

     k. signs and symptoms of ototoxicity (hearing loss, tinnitus, vertigo)

     l. signs and symptoms of tissue necrosis (erythema, induration, tenderness)

     m. patterns of bowel/bladder elimination

     n. pattern of physical activity

     o. nutritional status/appetite

     p. psychological status

     q. cognitive ability

     r. readiness/motivation to learn.

2. Assess

     a. patient's/family's understanding of/perception of the chemotherapeutic treatment

     b. patient's/family's expectations of the chemotherapeutic treatment

     c. degree of difference/similarity between patient's/family's expections and health care team's expectations

     d. what meaning the patient/family attaches to the chemotherapeutic treatment

     e. patient's/family's sociocultural beliefs about the chemotherapeutic treatment

     f. changes in the family's routine attributed to the chemotherapeutic treatment

     g. interactions among the patient and family members

     h. extent of the patient's/family's socialization/social isolation

     i. cognitive abilities of the family members

     j. family's psychological status/strengths/weaknesses

     k. availability/reliability of support systems

     l. environmental hazards to the patient.

3. Provide instruction to the patient/family/home health aide about

     a. chemotherapy (medication name, side/toxic effects, route of administration, treatment plan, purpose, method of action)

     b. signs and symptoms of bleeding

     c. methods to minimize the risk of bleeding (avoid intramuscular injections when possible; avoid measuring temperature rectally; use electric razors; use soft-bristle toothbrushes; keep fingernails/toenails short and carefully trimmed; prevent constipation; routinely inspect mouth, skin, stool, and urine for signs of bleeding; avoid strenuous activity and activity that may cause trauma/injury; avoid use of aspirin-containing products; do not walk barefoot; do not use dental floss)

     d. signs and symptoms of infection

     e. how to minimize the risk of infection (frequent handwashing; good personal hygiene; well-ventilated rooms; little/no environmental clutter; avoid crowds and individuals with colds; avoid contact with animal/pet excreta; consult with physician about having a pet; avoid excessive exposure to the sun; do not squeeze/scratch pimples)

     f. environmental modifications for patient safety

     g. importance of maintaining an adequate fluid intake (at least 3000 ml daily if not contraindicated)

h. how to measure/monitor intake and output
i. importance of balancing rest, nutrition, and exercise
j. skin care
k. oral/personal hygiene
l. how to care for oral dryness/tenderness/stomatitis (rinse with saline, a 1:1 saline/hydrogen peroxide mixture, or a mixture of 1 teaspoon baking soda in 1 cup warm water at least every 2 hours; do not use commercial mouthwashes; avoid smoking and alcohol; avoid extremely hot foods and beverages; use soft foods with low-acid contents; avoid spices; use a soft-bristle toothbrush/toothette at least twice a day; use a topical anesthetic; suck on popsicles/hard candy; use lip balm/water-based lubricant; use artificial saliva)
m. techniques to stimulate appetite (eating at the table; food at room temperature or chilled; use of high calorie/protein supplements served over ice or with added flavors; eating at least a third of the day's total dietary requirements during breakfast; eating frequent small meals/snacks throughout the day)
n. personal energy conservation techniques
o. stress management/relaxation/imagery techniques
p. how some chemotherapeutic agents change urine/semen color/odor and that change is not a cause for alarm (provide information that is specifically related to the drug; doxorubicin and daunorubicin turn urine red; methotrexate turns urine bright yellow)
q. measures to minimize hair loss (cut hair in a short easy-to-manage style; use a mild shampoo; avoid excessive/overly brisk shampooing/brushing/combing; gently pat dry after rinsing; avoid use of electric hair dryers/curlers; air dry hair; avoid hair spray, hair dye, bobby pins, and hair clips; use a wide-tooth comb; use a satin pillow case)
r. how to cope with hair loss (use a wig/hair piece; wear hats/scarves/turbans; use a hairnet to minimize shedding; use an eyebrow pencil/false eyelashes)
s. how to cope with pruritus (use a water-based moisturizer; protect skin from temperature extremes; use cool/lukewarm water for showers and baths; add cornstarch, baking soda, oatmeal, or soybean powder to bath water; apply cool wet packs/ice bags to the skin; wear light weight/loose fitting/cotton clothes; control itching response; use a vibrator or finger/hand pressure on the itchy area; use distraction/imagery/relaxation techniques)
t. adjunct medications (purposes, side effects, administration).
4. Teach the patient/family how to avoid/cope with nausea and vomiting.
a. recall interventions/strategies that were successful during previous experiences with nausea/vomiting
b. avoid sights/sounds/odors that trigger the appetite response
c. avoid strong perfume, other individals who are vomiting, individuals with strong body odor, crowded places, and places with little ventilation
d. avoid eating heavy meals immediately before treatments
e. select/eat bland foods that are cold or at room temperature
f. eat crackers/toast/dry cereal
g. avoid foods that are fatty spicy/highly salted/fried/extremely sweet or rich
h. eat slowly and chew food well
i. drink clear fluids (apple juice, cranberry juice, lemonade, broth, ginger ale, cola, Gatorade, frozen fruit/ice popsicles, gelatins, weak tea)
j. eat/drink sour foods/beverages (lemons, pickles, hard candy, lemon water, lemon-lime drinks)
k. rest quietly after eating (do not lie flat for at least 2 hours after eating)

UNIT
13

    l. sleep if beginning to feel or anticipate being nauseated

    m. breathe slowly and deeply through mouth when feeling nauseated or during vomiting episodes

    n. experiment with eating/meal patterns

    o. seek/assure access to fresh air.

5. Teach the patient/family/home health aide to control bleeding by
   a. elevating the affected part, if possible
   b. applying cold compresses
   c. applying gentle pressure
   d. not moving the affected part after a clot has formed.

6. Teach the patient/family/home health aide to notify the nurse/physician if the patient experiences
   a. bleeding that is prolonged/does not stop
   b. signs and symptoms of infection
   c. shortness of breath
   d. palpitations
   e. extreme weakness/fatigue
   f. numbness/tingling of the extremities
   g. abrupt changes of personality/mental status
   h. urine or stool that contains blood
   i. urine that is cloudy, very dark, reddish, or brown.

7. Assist the patient/family in reorganizing daily patterns of living.

8. Confer and coordinate interventions with
   a. social worker
   b. physical therapist
   c. pharmacist
   d. pastoral care worker
   e. respite volunteer
   f. dentist.

9. Refer to the dietician and coordinate the patient's/family's utilization of the dietician's teaching to promote/maintain the patient's nutritional status.

10. Help the patient/family to identify and eliminate foods/habits that exacerbate diarrhea/constipation.

11. Create situations that facilitate the patient's independent action/decision-making.

12. Create situations that encourage the patient/family to express their thoughts and feelings about
    a. chemotherapeutic treatment plan
    b. side effects
    c. changes in life style
    d. unknown quality of their future.

13. Refer the patient/family to
    a. American Cancer Society
    b. Make Today Count
    c. National Cancer Institute
    d. self-help support groups.

14. Request and obtain orders/prescriptions, as necessary, from the attending physician.

15. Monitor and evaluate
    a. fluid and electrolyte balance
    b. urine pH
    c. white blood cell count
    d. platelet count

e. red blood cell count
f. serum levels (calcium, glucose, uric acid, potassium, magnesium)
g. urine levels (glucose, uric acid).
16. Send progress notes and a discharge summary to the attending physician.

THERAPEUTIC ACHIEVEMENT

- The patient/family adapts to the life style changes induced by the side effects of chemotherapy.
- The patient's self-esteem and sense of identity are maintained.
- The family unit is preserved.

RELATED PATIENT INSTRUCTIONS

A Daily Food Guide—Four Basic Food Groups
Antibiotic Medications
Anticonvulsant Medications
Comfort Measures for Dehydration
Constipation
General Comfort Measures
Guidelines for Describing Seizure Activity
Hair Loss
Healthy Heart
Heart Medications
Heparin Lock

Indwelling Central Venous Catheter
Infection Control for the Home
Intramuscular Injections
Intravenous Therapy
Making the Home Environment Safe
Management of Seizure Activity
Medication Compliance
Pain Medications
Reality Orientation
Seizure Precautions
Skin Care
When to Call for Help

**UNIT
13**

Leukemia Care Plan

CROSS REFERENCES

Bereavement Care Plan
Chemotherapy Care Plan
Constipation Care Plan
Generic Cardiac Care Plan
Pain Care Plan

Home Health Aid Supervision Procedure
Home Safety Procedure
Infection Control Procedure
Oxygen Therapy Procedure
Range of Motion Procedure

Medication Compliance Management Guidelines

NURSING DIAGNOSIS

1. Alteration in nutrition (less than body requirements) related to
   a. anorexia
   b. nausea/vomiting
   c. depression
   d. dysphagia
   e. oral lesions/tenderness
   f. increased metabolic rate
   g. other.
2. Potential/actual fluid volume deficit related to
   a. increased metabolic rate
   b. vomiting
   c. diarrhea
   d. anorexia
   e. other.
3. Potential/actual impairment of skin integrity related to
   a. inadequate hygiene/skin care
   b. decreased mobility/immobility
   c. emaciation/skeletal prominence
   d. radiation
   e. other.
4. Activity intolerance related to
   a. imbalance between oxygen supply and demand
   b. disease progression
   c. cardiopulmonary insufficiency
   d. other.
5. Alteration in comfort (pain) related to
   a. side effects of chemotherapy/radiation therapy
   b. hyperuricemia
   c. enlarged lymph nodes/body organs
   d. accumulation of white blood cells in bone marrow
   e. other.
6. Anxiety/fear related to
   a. increased susceptibility to infection
   b. increased susceptibility to uncontrolled bleeding

    c. uncertainty about the future
    d. financial stress
    e. knowledge deficits
    f. other.
7. Potential for injury related to
    a. increased susceptibility to infection
    b. increased susceptibility to uncontrolled bleeding
    c. orthostatic hypotension
    d. environmental safety hazards
    e. other.
8. Grieving related to chronic, potentially fatal disease.
9. Impaired physical mobility related to
    a. decreased strength/endurance
    b. pain/discomfort
    c. depression/anxiety
    d. fear of injury/trauma
    e. dizziness
    f. chronic fatigue
    g. other.
10. Ineffective breathing pattern related to
    a. pain/discomfort
    b. anxiety
    c. decreased oxygen-carrying capacity of blood
    d. fluid retention/cardiopulmonary edema
    e. other.
11. Social isolation related to
    a. change in physical appearance
    b. fear of exposure to infection
    c. fear of injury/trauma
    d. depression
    e. weakness/fatigue
    f. other.
12. Alteration in family process related to
    a. situational crisis of a chronically/fatally ill family member
    b. disruption of usual pattern of family life
    c. lack of support among/from significant others
    d. resentment over forced reallocation of family resources/priorities
    e. financial stress
    f. role modifications
    g. other.
13. Sleep pattern disturbance related to
    a. fear/anxiety
    b. pain/discomfort
    c. other.
14. Self-care deficit (feeding, bathing/hygiene, dressing/grooming, toileting) related to
    a. decreased strength/endurance
    b. chronic fatigue
    c. pain/discomfort
    d. depression
    e. other.
15. Knowledge deficit (pathophysiology and progression of leukemia; treatments/therapies; medications; signs and symptoms of anemia, bleeding and increased intracranial

UNIT 13

pressure; methods of infection control; personal energy conservation techniques; skin care/hygiene techniques; community resources; temperature taking; nutritional maintenance; methods to promote sleep/rest; signs and symptoms of infection) related to

a. information misinterpretation
b. cognitive limitation
c. perplexity about treatment
d. denial
e. other.

PROCESS INDICATORS

1. The patient is protected against infection and injury.
Indicators
    a. patient/family recall of the signs and symptoms of infection
    b. patient/family recall of the signs and symptoms of bleeding
    c. patient/family identification of how to control bleeding
    d. patient/family identifies the adoption of household precautions/modifications to protect the patient
    e. patient/family recall of the purpose and administration of prescribed antibiotics
    f. patient/family state the situations that necessitate contact with the nurse/physician.

2. The patient's biopsychosocial integrity is maintained.
Indicators
    a. no signs and symptoms of infection
    b. no signs and symptoms of bleeding
    c. no signs and symptoms of hyperuricemia
    d. no skin irritation/breakdown
    e. intact oral mucosa
    f. patient is not dehydrated/overhydrated
    g. patient's performance of/participation in the activities of daily living are realistically commensurate with his or her capabilities
    h. patient maintains a satisfactory level of social/community interaction
    i. patient/family validates a balance between rest, nutrition, and exercise
    j. patient verbalizes acceptance of/comfort with his or her need to be dependent
    k. vital signs/laboratory values are within the patient's normal limits
    l. patient demonstrates/verbalizes increased tolerance for exercise/activity
    m. patient validates (verbally/nonverbally) that pain/discomfort are controlled/minimized.

3. The family's psychosocial integrity is maintained.
Indicators
    a. familial feedback reflects an understanding of leukemia and its resultant disabilities
    b. patient/family verbalizes acceptance of/comfort with role modifications
    c. patient/family utilizes community resources
    d. each family member participates in the patient's care
    e. familial feedback reflects that members are emotionally supportive of each other.

NURSING INTERVENTIONS

1. Assess the patient
    a. signs and symptoms of bleeding (hemoptysis, petechiae, unexplained bruising,

nosebleeds, bleeding gums, scleral hemorrhages, hematuria, irregular vaginal bleeding, abdominal pain, hypotension, tachycardia)
   b. signs and symptoms of increased intracranial pressure (headache, papilledema, double vision, blurred vision, cranial nerve palsies, change in level of consciousness, impaired verbal communication)
   c. cardiopulmonary status
   d. signs and symptoms of hyperuricemia (lethargy, nausea, vomiting, hematuria, renal/kidney area pain, oliguria or anuria, joint/back pain, joint swelling/redness)
   e. signs and symptoms of infection
   f. skin integrity
   g. nutritional status/appetite
   h. signs and symptoms of dehydration
   i. signs and symptoms of anemia (pallor, weakness, fatigue, headache, tinnitus, palpitations, vertigo)
   j. patterns of bowel/bladder elimination
   k. presence/degree of pain/discomfort
   l. pattern of physical activity
   m. psychological status
   n. cognitive ability.
2. Assess
   a. environmental hazards to the patient
   b. availability/reliability of support systems
   c. interactions among the patient and family members
   d. changes in the family's routine
   e. what the diagnosis of leukemia means to the patient/family
   f. cognitive abilities of the family members.
3. Provide instruction to the patient/family/home health aide about
   a. pathophysiology and course of leukemia
   b. signs and symptoms of bleeding
   c. methods to minimize the risk of bleeding (avoid intramuscular injections when possible; use electric razors; use soft-bristle toothbrushes; keep fingernails and toenails short and carefully trimmed; avoid measuring temperature rectally; prevent constipation; routinely inspect mouth, skin, stool, and urine for signs or bleeding; avoid aspirin and products containing aspirin or ibuprofen; avoid strenuous activity and activity that may cause trauma/injury)
   d. signs and symptoms of infection
   e. how to minimize the risk of infection (frequent handwashing; avoid crowds/individuals with colds; practice good personal hygiene)
   f. importance of administering antibiotics on the prescribed schedule to maintain therapeutic blood levels
   g. importance of maintaining an adequate daily fluid intake (at least 3000 ml if not contraindicated)
   h. how to measure/monitor intake and output
   i. importance of getting weighed daily (on the same scale)
   j. importance of avoiding foods high in purine (nuts, wine/alcohol, fried foods, dried beans and peas, tea, asparagus, avocados, sardines, liver, kidney, tripe)
   k. skin care
   l. oral hygiene
   m. techniques to conserve personal energy
   n. methods to induce sleep
   o. oxygen therapy

UNIT 13

      p. medications (purpose, side effects, administration)
      q. environmental modifications for patient safety
      r. importance of graded/progressive exercise
      s. value of wearing an emergency medical identification tag/bracelet
      t. techniques of pain management.

4. Teach the patient/family home health aide to control bleeding by
      a. elevating the affected part if possible
      b. applying cold compresses
      c. applying gentle pressure
      d. not moving the affected part after a clot has formed.

5. Teach the patient/family/home health aide to immediately notify the nurse/physician if the patient experiences
      a. bleeding that is prolonged/does not stop
      b. signs and symptoms of infection
      c. persistent progressively worse headache.

6. Request/obtain orders, as necessary, for medications, laboratory tests, oxygen, and so forth from the attending physician.

7. Monitor
      a. fluid and electrolyte balance
      b. platelet count
      c. white blood cell count
      d. serum uric acid level
      e. blood, sputum, urine, wound cultures.

8. Refer to and coordinate nutrition-based interventions with the dietician.

9. Coordinate referrals to/interventions with
      a. social worker
      b. physical therapist
      c. occupational therapist
      d. durable medical equipment suppliers
      e. pastoral care
      f. hospice workers
      g. respite volunteers.

10. Refer to
      a. American Cancer Society
      b. Leukemia Society of America
      c. Make Today Count
      d. self-help support groups.

11. Assist the patient/family to
      a. reorganize daily patterns of living
      b. develop safe travel plans.

12. Provide opportunities that facilitate the patient's independent action and/or decision making.

13. Create situations that encourage the patient/family to express their thoughts and feelings.

14. Send progress notes and a discharge summary to the attending physician.

THERAPEUTIC ACHIEVEMENT

- The patient/family adapts to the life style changes induced as a result of leukemia.
- The family unit is preserved.

RELATED PATIENT INSTRUCTIONS

A Daily Food Guide–Four Basic Food Groups
Antibiotic Medications
Comfort Measures for Dehydration
Constipation
General Comfort Measures
Healthy Heart
Infection Control for the Home
Making the Home Environment Safe

Measuring Liquid Intake and Output
Mouth Care
Oxygen Therapy
Pain Medications
Range of Motion Exercises
Skin Care
Ways to Save Your Energy

Lung Cancer Care Plan

CROSS REFERENCES

Bereavement Care Plan
Chemotherapy Care Plan
Generic Cardiac Care Plan
Pain Care Plan
Terminal Illness Care Plan

Indwelling Central Venous Catheter (Changing the Cap) Procedure
Indwelling Central Venous Catheter (Dressing Change)
Indwelling Central Venous Catheter (Heparinization) Procedure

Indwelling Central Venous Catheter (Withdrawing Blood) Procedure
Infection Control Procedure
Oxygen Therapy Procedure
Suctioning (Oronasopharyngeal) Procedure
Telephone Contact with Patient/Family Procedure

Medication Compliance Management Guidelines
Mental Health Assessment/Intervention Guide
Suction Catheter Sizes

NURSING DIAGNOSES

1. Ineffective airway clearance related to
   a. thick/tenacious/copious secretions
   b. nonproductive/minimally productive cough
   c. obstructing tumor
   d. other.
2. Ineffective breathing patterns related to
   a. obstructing tumor pressure
   b. decreased energy/fatigue
   c. decreased lung expansion
   d. other.
3. Impaired verbal communication related to obstructing tumor pressure.
4. Alteration in nutrition (less than body requirements) related to
   a. depression
   b. anxiety
   c. dysphagia
   d. side effects of chemotherapy/radiation therapy
   e. other.
5. Potential/actual impairment of skin integrity related to
   a. radiation therapy
   b. decreased mobility/immobility
   c. emaciation/skeletal prominence
   d. other.
6. Potential for injury related to
   a. necrotic cell buildup (infection)
   b. erosion of blood vessels (hemorrhage)
   c. other.
7. Anxiety/fear related to
   a. being dependent on others for care
   b. potential/actual metastatic disease
   c. dyspnea
   d. lack of control over disease progression

    e. financial stress
    f. perceived/actual inability to communicate
    g. uncertainty about the future
    h. other.

8. Alteration in comfort (pain) related to
    a. obstructing tumor pressure
    b. metastatic disease
    c. side effects of chemotherapy/radiation therapy
    d. other.

9. Sleep pattern disturbance related to
    a. orthopnea
    b. coughing
    c. fear/anxiety
    d. other.

10. Activity intolerance related to
    a. inadequate nutritional status
    b. imbalance between oxygen supply and demand
    c. fatigue/decreased energy
    d. metastatic disease
    e. other.

11. Self-care deficit (feeding, hygiene, grooming, toileting) related to
    a. decreased strength/endurance
    b. dyspnea
    c. depression
    d. disease progression
    e. other.

12. Knowledge deficit (pathohysiology, progression, and etiology of lung cancer; treatments/therapies; medications; personal energy conservation methods; signs and symptoms of infection; community resources; pulmonary toilet; nutritional maintenance; methods to promote sleep/rest) related to
    a. information misinterpretation
    b. cognitive limitation
    c. perplexity about treatment
    d. denial
    e. low readiness for acceptance of information
    f. patient's/family's request for no information
    g. other.

13. Alteration in thought process related to
    a. metastatic disease
    b. hypercalcemia
    c. other.

14. Impaired physical mobility related to incision pain/discomfort.

PROCESS INDICATORS

1. The patient's physical integrity is maintained.
Indicators
    a. no signs and symptoms of infection
    b. decreased amount/loose tracheobronchial secretions
    c. patient decreases/stops smoking

UNIT 13

    d. no cyanosis
    e. rearrangement of the home environment to eliminate known safety hazards
    f. weight gained/maintained
    g. patient demonstrates recommended methods to prevent/relieve breathlessness
    h. patient/family demonstrates measures that improve bronchial hygiene
    i. patient/family verbalizes an understanding of how to minimize/prevent pulmonary irritation
    j. patient/family recalls signs and symptoms of respiratory infection/deterioration
    k. patient validation (verbally or nonverbally) that pain/discomfort are minimized/controlled
    l. patient/family recalls the purpose, side effects, and precautions associated with prescribed medications, treatments, therapies
    m. patient/family validates a balance between rest, nutrition, exercise.

2. The patient participates in the activities of life to the extent of his or her capabilities.

Indicators

    a. patient realistically identifies his or her physical limitations
    b. patient demonstrates personal energy conservation methods
    c. patient revises his or her daily pattern of interaction with others to incorporate the limitations imposed by lung cancer and its treatment
    d. patient maintains his or her social/occupational responsibilities
    e. patient verbalizes his or her acceptance of/comfort with his or her need to be dependent
    f. patient can/does communicate.

3. The family's psychosocial integrity is maintained.

Indicators

    a. familial feedback indicates an understanding of lung cancer and its resultant disabilities
    b. familial feedback reflects an understanding of the typical behavior patterns of chronically ill respiratory patients
    c. familial feedback reflects acceptance of/comfort with role modifications
    d. patient's/family's appropriate utilization of community resources
    e. each member verbalizes thoughts and feelings about lung cancer and its associated changes.

NURSING INTERVENTIONS

1. Assess the patient
    a. cardiopulmonary status
    b. signs and symptoms of respiratory infection
    c. signs and symptoms of obstructing tumor pressure (facial flushing; edema of face, arms, neck; nosebleeds; chest, shoulder, arm, back pain)
    d. signs and symptoms of hypercalcemia (anorexia, lethargy, cardiac arrhythmia, confusion)
    e. signs and symptoms of brain metastases (change in mental status, personality changes, loss of memory, blurred vision, headaches, seizures)
    f. presence/degree of pain/discomfort
    g. pattern of physical activity
    h. pattern of sleep/rest
    i. nutritional status/appetite
    j. patterns of bowel/bladder elimination

    k. signs/symptoms of dehydration/electrolyte imbalance

    l. psychological status (depression, anger, anxiety)

    m. psychological strengths and weaknesses

    n. cognitive ability

    o. what meaning he or she assigns to the lung cancer

    p. method/quality of communication

    q. smoking habits

    r. pattern of oxygen use.

2. Assess

    a. environmental hazards to the patient

    b. what meaning the family attaches to the lung cancer

    c. method/quality of the family's communication with the patient

    d. each family member's willingness to participate in the patient's care

    e. availability/reliability of support systems

    f. changes in the family's routine

    g. cognitive abilities of the family members.

3. Provide instruction to the patient/family/home health aide about

    a. pathophysiology, etiology, and course of lung cancer

    b. signs and symptoms of respiratory infection

    c. how to minimize the risk of infection (handwashing, good personal hygiene, avoid crowds/individuals with colds)

    d. benefits of not smoking (less coughing, reduced sputum production, increased resistance to respiratory infections)

    e. how to avoid/reduce bronchopulmonary irritation (check air pollution levels daily and avoid outdoor activity when levels are high; use radiant heat/air conditioning when feasible; keep home temperatures about 70° F during the day and 65° F at night; change/clean air filters in forced air-conditioning systems; do not use fireplaces or coal/wood-burning stoves; use exhaust fan in kitchen/bathroom; avoid using substances containing ammonia/chlorine bleach; frequently dust/damp mop)

    f. identification and avoidance of bronchopulmonary irritants (dust, fumes, smoke, chemicals with strong odors, powders, paint, smog, particulates, dogs, cats, pigeons, farm animals)

    g. personal energy conservation techniques (pacing activities; sitting instead of standing; moving slowly; including "fatigue time" when scheduling the day's activities; avoiding straining, bending, squatting; loose/light weight clothing; slip-on shoes)

    h. measures to improve bronchial hygiene (postural drainage with percussion/vibration; adequate fluid intake; slow, deep breathing with prolonged expiratory phase; pursed-lip breathing)

    i. positions to relieve dyspnea (sit in a firm chair, rest forearms on thighs; sit in a firm chair, lean forward, rest forearms on table)

    j. the importance of balancing rest, nutrition, exercise

    k. setting a regular schedule for activities of life and daily care

    l. recognizing abrupt changes in the patient's mental status

    m. methods to induce sleep

    n. use/cleaning/maintenance of respiratory equipment

    o. techniques of pain management

    p. skin care/personal hygiene

    q. importance of not washing off the guiding red marks for radiation therapy from the patient's skin

UNIT 13

    r. importance of adequate oral/dental hygiene

    s. stress management/relaxation techniques

    t. verbal/nonverbal communication techniques.

4. Teach the patient/family/home health aide about oxygen therapy
   a. need for low flow rate
   b. use of oxygen at mealtimes, when febrile, and during exercise/strenuous activity
   c. need to regard oxygen as medication
   d. importance of not increasing the flow rate without a physician/nurse so advising
   e. not using oxygen near an open flame.

5. Teach the family/home health aide guidelines for effective communication with the patient by
   a. responding to the patient, no matter how awkward or minimal his or her speech efforts are
   b. avoiding pressuring the patient into conversation
   c. asking questions so that yes-or-no answers suffice
   d. not yelling when speaking to the patient
   e. not answering questions or giving responses for the patient
   f. encouraging the patient's self-expression through any available means (hand signals, magic-erase slate, flash cards, writing, lip reading, art, music).

6. Refer to and coordinate nutrition-based interventions with the dietician.

7. Coordinate referrals to/interventions with
   a. social worker
   b. physical therapist
   c. speech therapist
   d. pastoral care worker
   e. hospice workers
   f. respite volunteers
   g. durable medical equipment suppliers.

8. Refer to
   a. American Cancer Society
   a. Make Today Count
   b. self-help support groups.

9. Request/obtain orders, as necessary, for medications, laboratory tests, oxygen, and so forth from the attending physician.

10. Provide opportunities that facilitate the patient's independent action and/or decision making.

11. Create situations that encourage the patient/family to express their thoughts and feelings.

12. Send progress notes and a discharge summary to the attending physician.

THERAPEUTIC ACHIEVEMENT

- The patient/family adapts to the life style changes induced as a result of the lung cancer.
- The family unit is preserved.

RELATED PATIENT INSTRUCTIONS

A Daily Food Guide—Four Basic Food Groups
Bronchopulmonary Health
General Comfort Measures
Healthy Heart
Heparin Lock
Indwelling Central Venous Catheter
Infection Control for the Home
Medication Compliance

Mouth Care
Oral Suctioning
Oxygen Therapy
Pain Medications
Skin Care
Ways to Save Your Energy
When to Call for Help

Mastectomy Care Plan

CROSS REFERENCES

Bereavement Care Plan
Chemotherapy Care Plan
Pain Care Plan

Breast Self-Examination Procedure

Infection Control Procedure

Mental Health Assessment/Intervention Guide
Post Mastectomy Exercises

NURSING DIAGNOSES

1. Anxiety/fear related to
   a. response of husband/sexual partner to mastectomy
   b. being dependent on others for care
   c. potential/actual metastases
   d. potential of recurrence
   e. vulnerability to lymphedema
   f. other.
2. Sleep pattern disturbance related to
   a. anxiety
   b. depression
   c. incisional discomfort
   d. other.
3. Impaired physical mobility related to
   a. pain
   b. muscle stiffness
   c. lymphedema
   d. other.
4. Disturbance in self-concept (body image) related to
   a. phantom breast symptoms
   b. loss of breast
   c. use of breast prosthesis
   d. perceived loss of a sense of femininity
   e. other.
5. Sexual dysfunction related to
   a. response of husband/sexual partner to mastectomy
   b. embarrassment
   c. pain/discomfort
   d. other.
6. Self-care deficit (feeding, bathing/hygiene, dressing/grooming) related to
   a. decreased strength/endurance
   b. pain/discomfort
   c. depression/anxiety
   d. lymphedema
   e. muscle stiffness
   f. other.

7. Activity tolerance related to generalized weakness.
8. Knowledge deficit (arm care, incision care, dressing change, community resources, breast self-examination, frequency of health follow-up, mammography, prosthesis, lymphedema, prevention of secondary lymphedema, prevention of infection) related to
   a. information misinterpretation
   b. cognitive limitation
   c. perplexity about treatment
   d. denial
   e. other.
9. Grieving related to
   a. loss of breast
   b. perceived loss of a sense of femininity
   c. other.
10. Alteration in comfort (pain) related to
    a. side effects of chemotherapy/radiation therapy
    b. incisional healing
    c. surgical manipulation
    d. other.

PROCESS INDICATORS

1. The patient's physical health is maintained.
Indicators
   a. no signs and symptoms of incisional infection/inflammation
   b. patient validation (verbally or nonverbally) that pain/discomfort are controlled/minimized
   c. patient identification of how to protect the arm on the operative side from infection and injury
   d. no lymphedema of the arm on the operative side
   e. patient demonstration of preoperative level of function/range of motion of the arm on the operative side
   f. patient demonstration of breast and mastectomy site self-examination
   g. patient demonstration of appropriate techniques of incision/mastectomy site care
   h. patient/family validates a balance between rest, nutrition, exercise.
2. The patient participates in the activities of life to the extent of her capabilities.
Indicators
   a. patient realistically identifies her physical limitations
   b. patient demonstration of personal energy conservation methods
   c. patient maintains her social/occupational responsibilities
   d. patient/family realistically identifies the amount/type of activity the patient can undertake
   e. patient verbalizes/demonstrates increased tolerance for exercise/activity.
3. The patient's/family's psychosocial integrity is maintained.
Indicators
   a. patient/family feedback reflects an accurate understanding of the mastectomy
   b. patient and sexual partner state a return to their previous pattern of sexual activity
   c. patient identifies the normalcy of the phantom breast phenomenon
   d. patient demonstration/explanation of proper prosthesis use
   e. patient and sexual partner verbalize acceptance of/comfort with sexual behavior modifications
   f. patient/family utilization of community resources/self-help groups.

UNIT
13

NURSING INTERVENTIONS

1. Assess the patient
   a. signs and symptoms of incisional infection
   b. signs and symptoms of lymphedema
   c. presence and degree of pain/discomfort
   d. pattern of physical activity
   e. pattern of rest/sleep
   f. psychological strengths/weaknesses
   g. psychological status (anger, depression, anxiety)
   h. current stresses/life changes being experienced (negative changes related to self/sexual identity, such as menopause, weight gain, and muscle tone loss, tend to increase the negative impact of the mastectomy on the patient's life)
   i. what meaning the patient assigns to the mastectomy
   j. presence/frequency of the phantom breast phenomenon
   k. ability to do/learn techniques of breast/mastectomy site care/health follow-up.
2. Assess the sexual partner/family
   a. availability/reliability as a support system
   b. changes attributed to the mastectomy
   c. sexual partner's/family's understanding of the mastectomy
   d. what meaning the sexual partner/family assigns to the mastectomy
   e. interactions among the patient/sexual partner/family members
   f. cognitive abilities.
3. Provide instruction to the patient/family/home health aide about
   a. signs and symptoms of infection (tenderness, redness, swelling, purulent drainage at surgical site; fever; malaise)
   b. most frequent sources of infection (burns, cuts, abrasions, inflammation around fingernails) and importance of preventing their occurrence
   c. measures to prevent injury to the arm of the operative side (no blood work/blood pressure testing/injections on/in this arm; no jewelry/watch on this arm; use of a gradient elastic sleeve; avoid reaching into a hot oven with the hand on operative side; wear loose rubber gloves when washing dishes/using harsh detergents)
   d. dressing change
   e. importance of regular exercise to prevent lymphedema and to increase upper limb mobility
   f. vulnerability to secondary lymphedema in the arm on the operative side for the rest of the patient's life
   g. how to incorporate arm exercises into activities of daily living/personal hygiene
   h. how to do post-mastectomy exercises/range of motion exercises
   i. importance of contacting the nurse/physician if the arm on the operative side becomes red, warm, swollen, or unusually hard
   j. physiology of mastectomy
   k. value of wearing a medical emergency identification tag or bracelet
   l. how to examine the mastectomy site (palpate the incision site and axilla; inspect the skin for changes)
   m. how to do breast self-examination
   n. personal energy conservation methods
   o. mammography (women 40 to 49 years of age should have one done every 1 to 2 years; women over 50, yearly; women with related personal/family histories, as recommended by personal physicians; 45 to 60 minutes usually required to complete the procedure; some minor discomfort associated with the procedure)

    p. medications (side effects, purpose, administration)
    q. need to balance rest, nutrition, exercise
    r. major emotional distress, such as grief reactions, associated with mastectomy that are relatively short-term for many women (astute nursing judgment and acute sensitivity are necessary when broaching this intervention)
    s. how the redness and swelling of the mastectomy site fade with time
    t. mastectomy site care after the incision heals (massage the area with cocoa butter or cold cream to keep skin soft; use cornstarch or plain talcum powder to reduce itching/irritation of the area)
    u. purchasing a breast prosthesis (do not purchase a permanent prosthesis until the incision is fully healed; prostheses are expensive; clothing styles are easily adapted to the prosthesis; where prostheses can be obtained)
    v. types of breast prostheses (foam rubber, air-filled, fluid-filled)
    w. importance of diligent health care follow-up
    x. normal frequency of health care follow-up (initially every 3 to 4 months, then every 6 to 12 months)
    y. breast reconstruction (best results are obtained 3 to 6 months post-mastectomy; health insurance may not cover the cost; contraindicated with local disease present and with inflammatory breast cancer)
    z. pain management techniques.

4. Teach the patient and partner how to adapt their sexual activities to the mastectomy
    a. use a position that is comfortable and easy to assume
    b. emphasize enjoyment over performance
    c. temporary options for decreasing anxiety (undress in the dark; wear a bra at night)
    d. teach the sexual partner to massage the mastectomy site with lotion/change the dressing
    e. change positions so the sexual partner caresses the unaffected side (particularly helpful when the affected side is still painful/tender)
    f. importance of continuing their usual pattern of communicating affection/love
    g. select a time for sexual intercourse that allows for experimentation/sharing/resting.

5. Confer and coordinate interventions with
    a. physical therapist
    b. occupational therapist
    c. social worker
    d. hospice worker
    e. pastoral care worker.

6. Refer the patient/family to
    a. American Cancer Society (Reach to Recovery)
    b. self-help and living-with-cancer groups
    c. prosthesis shops.

7. Provide opportunities that facilitate the patient's independent action and/or decision making.

8. Create opportunities that encourage the patient/family to express
    a. feelings about the mastectomy
    b. uncertainty about the future
    c. fears and concerns
    d. grief.

9. Request/obtain orders/prescriptions as necessary from the attending physician.

10. Provide progress notes and a discharge summary to the primary physician.

UNIT 13

THERAPEUTIC ACHIEVEMENT

- The patient adapts to the life style changes induced as a result of the mastectomy.

RELATED PATIENT INSTRUCTIONS

A Daily Food Guide—Four Basic Food Groups
Antibiotic Medications
Breast Self-Examination
Changing Dressings
General Comfort Measures

Infection Control for the Home
Pain Medications
Post-Mastectomy Exercises
Skin Care

Procedures

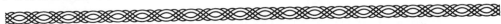

Breast Self-Examination Procedure

PURPOSE

- To detect changes in the breast tissue and axillary nodes.
- To reinforce the importance of breast self-examination (BSE).
- To teach the procedure of BSE.
- To familiarize the patient with the way her breasts look/feel normally.

EQUIPMENT

- pillow or folded towel
- mirror
- breast self-examination (described in *Patient and Family Instructions*)

Steps	Key Points

1. Assess for
  a. family history of breast cancer, fibroids, mother's use of diethylstilbestrol (DES)
  b. personal history of obesity, diabetes, hypertension, use of estrogens, high dietary intake of animal fats, smoking, exposure to carcinogens, cancer, fibrocystic disease, chronic stress, early menarche or late menopause, surgical procedures
  c. recent changes in breast tissue (lumps, pain, discharge, dimpling, contour, appearance).
	1. A graph that notes the areas of lumps/thickened tissue is a helpful baseline comparison for a woman with fibrocystic disease.

2. Have patient disrobe to the waist in front of a mirror.	
3. Tell the patient to relax her arms in her lap.	

4. Inspect the breasts for
  a. changes in contour
  b. swelling
  c. dimpling of skin
  d. changes in the nipple
  e. diffuse blue casts
  f. peau d'orange (large-pored, edematous skin).
	4. Breasts normally deviate slightly in symmetry and size.

UNIT 13

5. Instruct the patient to raise her arms over her head and inspect the breasts.

6. Instruct the patient to rest her palms on her hips, press down firmly, and visually inspect her breasts (front, left side, right side).

7. Palpate the breasts and axillae.
   a. sweep the breasts bilaterally with the palm and the pads of the fingers from the clavicles to the nipple
   b. grasp the tissue of the axillae and gently squeeze in a rolling motion
   c. instruct the patient that this segment of BSE is easier if done in the shower.

7. Malignancies most often occur in the upper outer quadrants. Determine the mobility, consistency, and boundary discreteness of any mass.

8. Have the patient lie down, put the pillow or folded towel under the right shoulder, and have her place her right hand behind her head.

8. This position evenly distributes the breast tissue over the chest wall.

9. Palpate the right breast, with the finger pads of the left hand, in concentric circles starting at 12 o'clock and proceeding to 1 o'clock, 2 o'clock and so forth.

9. The procedure can be made easier if the patient liberally applies lotion to the fingertips/pads.

10. Inch the fingers toward the nipple and repeat the concentric circle. Continue this until the entire breast has been examined.

10. A ridge of firm tissue at the lower curve of the breast is normal. Tenderness is an abnormality.

11. Squeeze the nipple gently between the thumb and index finger to assess for discharge. Then depress the nipple with the index and middle fingers to palpate the area beneath the nipple.

11. Any discharge from a nonlactating breast is significant. If present, note the color, amount, odor, and consistency.

12. Have the patient put the pillow under her left shoulder, place her left hand behind her head and repeat the procedure with the nurse watching.

13. Instruct the patient
   a. to do BSE monthly (1 week after menses or once each month on the same date, e.g., the seventeenth, if menopausal)
   b. to contact the attending physician immediately if a lump, discharge, or dimple is discovered
   c. to speak with the attending physician about mammography.

13. Breast cancers that are found easily and treated promptly have the best chances for cure. The American Cancer Society recommends that mammography be done once between ages 35 and 40 for a baseline, every two years from ages 40 to 49, and once a year after age 50.

14. Discuss with the patient
    a. her feelings about BSE
    b. her feelings about seeking follow-up for abnormalities.
15. Contact the attending physician if any abnormalities are discovered in order to obtain an early appointment for evaluation.
16. Examination of the male breast follows the same procedure.

14. The discovery of an abnormality can produce paralyzing anxiety in the patient.

DOCUMENTATION

1. The procedure, teaching, and quality of the return demonstration.

2. The findings. If lumps are found, describe their location, size in centimeters, consistency shape, tenderness, and mobility. If discharge is present, describe its color, consistency, odor, amount, and circumstances of its appearance (e.g., "Discharge apparent only when nipple squeezed").

3. The patient's response to the procedure.

4. Interactions with the attending physician (date, time, person spoken with, substance of conversation).

5. The need for follow-up (instruction, physician appointment, psychotherapeutic intervention for anxiety).

UNIT 13

Chemotherapy Administration Procedure

PURPOSE

- To ensure safe administration of antineoplastic agents.

EQUIPMENT

- plastic-backed absorbent pad
- long-sleeve disposable gown
- disposable gloves
- goggles/protective glasses
- intravenous fluid (amount and type per physician's order)
- intravenous tubing
- intravenous pole or substitute
- prescribed antineoplastic agents
- emergency box (contents per agency policy)
- container for disposal of used equipment
- items for initiation of infusion site (see Heparin Lock Wing-tipped Needle Insertion Procedure)

Steps

1. Explain the procedure to the patient/family.
2. Assess the patient's laboratory test values.

3. Wash your hands.
4. Assess the patient's vital signs.

5. Select a work area.

6. Place the plastic-backed absorbent pad on the work area.
7. Put on the gown, gloves, and goggles.
8. Prepare the intravenous solution and antineoplastic agents over the work area.

Key Points

1. Knowing what to expect increases patient/family compliance.
2. Notify the atteding physician of
   a. increased blood urea nitrogen level
   b. increased serum creatinine level
   c. abnormal liver function studies
   d. decreased white blood cell count
   e. decreased hematocrit value
   f. decreased platelet count.

4. Notify the attending physician if the patient's temperature is above 101°F.
5. Kitchen and bathroom counters are easily cleaned and often convenient heights.

8. Refer to the Intravenous Therapy Procedure.

Special Note. If an antineoplastic agent is accidentally spilled, wipe it up with paper towels. Thoroughly rinse the area with water.

9. Verify the prepared intravenous solution and antineoplastic agents with the physician's order.
10. Attach the intravenous tubing to the patient's venous access device/site.
11. Infuse the intravenous solution and antineoplastic agents.

11. If giving the antineoplastic agents via the IV push method, give the drugs slowly. Flush the intravenous line with 10 to 15 ml of solution between each drug.

12. Ask the patient to alert you to sensations felt during the infusion.

12. Observe the insertion site for swelling, redness, or hives.

Special Note. If *extravasation* of a vesicant agent occurs or is suspected (1) stop the infusion; (2) aspirate the residual solution and blood from the tubing, needle and site; (3) instill an intravenous antidote (per agency policy); (4) remove the intravenous needle (if in a peripheral site); (5) inject a subcutaneous antidote (per agency policy); (6) apply a topical ointment (per agency policy) and cover with a sterile occlusive dressing; (7) apply hot or cold compresses (per agency policy); and (8) notify the attending physician of the extravasation and subsequent interventions.

If the patient exhibits the signs and symptoms of an *anaphylactic reaction* (1) stop the infusion, (2) maintain the intravenous line with normal saline, (3) put the patient into a supine position, (4) monitor the patient's vital signs, (5) maintain a patent airway, (6) notify the attending physician, and (7) administer antihistamine per physician's orders.

13. After the intravenous solution and antineoplastic agents have been infused, dispose of used equipment and supplies (according to agency policy) in a leak-proof, puncture-proof container labeled "Hazardous Waste."
14. Wash your hands.
15. Instruct the patient/family about
    a. specific patient care details relative to the chemotherapeutic regimen
    b. signs and symptoms to report to the nurse/physician (bleeding that is prolonged/does not stop, elevated temperature, chills, shortness of breath, palpitations, extreme weakness/fatigue, numbness/tingling of the extremities, abrupt changes of personality/mental status, blood in urine or stool, urine that is cloudy/very dark/reddish or brown, vomiting that continues more than 24 hours after the infusion).

13. If the container is to be collected later by the vendor, store it in an area where the patient, family and pets are least likely to disturb it.

a. Refer to the Chemotherapy Care Plan.

UNIT
13

DOCUMENTATION

1. The date and time of the procedure.
2. The administered solution and antineoplastic agents.
3. The venous access site/device used.
4. The patient's/family's response to the procedure.
5. The teaching done.
6. Plan for follow-up.

Resources

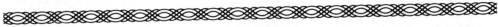

Cancer Warning Signs

1. Change in bowel or bladder habits.
2. A sore that does not heal.
3. Unusual bleeding or discharge.
4. Thickening or lump in the breast or elsewhere.
5. Persistent indigestion or loss of appetite.
6. Obvious change in a wart or mole.
7. Nagging cough or hoarseness.

Post-Mastectomy Exercises

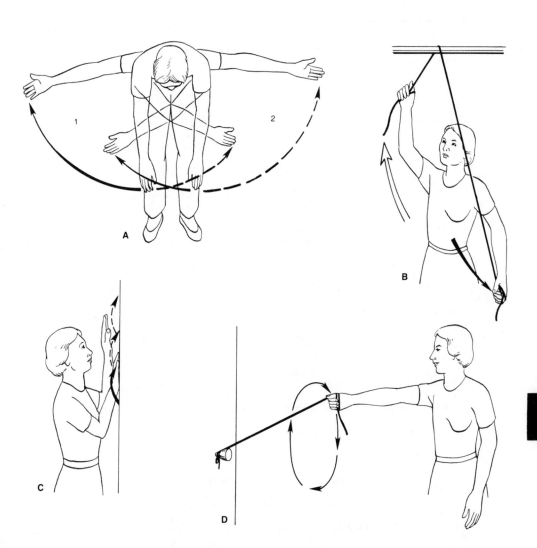

UNIT
13

Postmastectomy exercises. *A, Arm swings.* Stand with feet 8 inches apart. Bend forward from waist, allowing arms to hang toward floor. Swing both arms up to sides to reach shoulder level. Swing back to center, then cross arms at center. Do not bend elbows. If possible, do this and other exercises in front of mirror to ensure even posture and correct motion. *B. Pulley motion.* Using operated arm, toss 6-foot rope over a shower curtain rod (or over top of a door that has a nail in the top to hold the rope in place for the exercise). Grasp one end of rope in each hand. Slowly raise operated arm as far as comfortable by pulling down on the rope on opposite side. Keep raised arm close to your head. Reverse to raise unoperated arm by lowering the operated arm. Repeat. *C, Hand wall climbing.* Stand facing wall with toes 6 to 12 inches from wall. Bend elbows and place palms against wall at shoulder level. Gradually move both hands up the wall parallel to each other until incisional pulling or pain occurs. (Mark that spot on wall to measure progress.) Work hands down to shoulder level. Move closer to wall as height of reach improves. *D, Rope turning.* Tie rope to door handle. Hold rope in hand of operated side. Back away from door until arm is extended away from body, parallel to floor. Swing rope in as wide a circle as possible. Increase size of the circle as mobility returns. (Reproduced with permission from Luckmann, J. and Sorensen, K. C. Medical-Surgical Nursing, A Psychophysiologic Approach, 3rd ed. Philadelphia: W. B. Saunders Co., 1987, pp. 1823.)

Bibliography

Ahanna, D. and Kunishi, M. Cancer Care Protocols for Hospital and Home Care Use. New York: Springer Publishing Company, 1986.

Anderson, J. and Brown, M. The Cancer Patient in the Community: A Nursing Challenge. Nursing Clinics of North America, 15(2): 1980, pp. 373–388.

Bouchard-Kurtz, R. and Speese-Owens, N. Nursing Care of the Cancer Patient, 4th ed. St. Louis: C. V. Mosby Co., 1981.

Burns, N. Nursing and Cancer. Philadelphia: W. B. Saunders Co., 1982.

Donovan, M. and Girton, S. Cancer Care Nursing. Norwalk, Connecticut: Appleton-Century-Crofts, 1984.

Dwyer, J. and Held, D. Home Management of the Adult Patient with Leukemia. Nursing Clinics of North America, 17(4): 1982, pp. 665–675.

Fergusson, J. and Hobbie, W. Home Visits for the Child with Cancer. Nursing Clinics of North America, 20(1): 1985, pp. 109–116.

Gallagher M. and Wyland, N. Leukemia: When White Cells Run Wild. RN, November 1986, pp. 33–37.

Gibbons, M. and Boren, H. Stress Reduction: A Spectrum of Strategies in Pediatric Oncology Nursing. Nursing Clinics of North America, 20(1): 1985, pp. 83–103.

Gregory-Addesa, G. Helping Your Patient When Nausea Goes With the Treatment. RN, April 1986, pp. 43–44.

Herbeth, L. and Gosnell, D. Nursing Diagnoses for Oncology Nursing Practice. Cancer Nursing, 10(1); 1987, pp. 41–51.

Huldij, A., et al. Alterations in Taste Appreciation in Cancer Patients During Treatment. Cancer Nursing, 9(1): 1986, pp. 38–42.

Koocher, G. Psychosocial Care of the Child Cured of Cancer. Pediatric Nursing, 11(2): 1985, pp. 91–93.

Knox, L. S. Nutrition and Cancer. Nursing Clinics of North America, March, 18(1): 1983, pp. 97–109.

Kramer, R. and Perin, G. Patient Education and Pediatric Oncology. Nursing Clinics of North America, 20(1): 1985, pp. 31–48.

McCormick, R. Infections in Patients with Solid Tumors. Nursing Clinics of North America, 20(1): 1985, pp. 199–206.

Mosely, J. Alterations in Comfort. Nursing Clinics of North America, 20(2): 1985, pp. 427–438.

Newman, K. The Leukemias. Nursing Clinics of North America, 20(1): 1985, pp. 227–234.

Reheis, C. Neutropenia: Causes, Complications, Treatment, and Resulting Nursing Care. Nursing Clinics of North America, 20(1): 1985, 219–226.

Ristuccia, A. Hematologic Effects of Cancer Therapy. Nursing Clinics of North America, 20(1): 1985, pp. 235–240.

Ross, D. and Ross, S. Stress Reduction Procedures for the School-Age Hospitalized Leukemia Child. Pediatric Nursing, 10(6): 1984, pp. 393–395.

Schaffner, A. Safety Precautions in Home Chemotherapy. American Journal of Nursing, 84(3): 1984, pp. 346–347.

Walter, J. Care of the Patient Receiving Antineoplastic Drugs. Nursing Clinics of North America, 17(4): 1982, pp. 607–629.

Wesseer, R. Care of the Hospitalized Adult Patient with Leukemia. Nursing Clinics of North America, 17(4): 1982, pp. 649–663.

Yasko, J. and Greene, P. Coping with Problems Related to Cancer and Cancer Treatment. CA-A Cancer Journal for Clinicians, 37(2): 1987, pp. 106–125.

Intravenous Therapy

Procedures

UNIT
14

Procedures

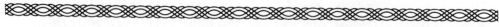

Heparin Lock
(Administration of Fluids/
Medications) Procedure

PURPOSE

- To ensure patency of the heparin lock when administering intermittent intravenous fluids or medications.

EQUIPMENT

- intravenous fluid or medication (per physician's prescription)
- intravenous tubing and attached 25-gauge needle (if intravenous fluids are being administered or if the medication is diluted in a bag/bottle of intravenous fluid)
- sterile syringe with 4 ml of sterile normal saline and an attached 25-gauge needle
- sterile syringe with heparinized solution (per physician's prescription) and attached 25-gauge needle
- alcohol swabs

Steps	Key Points
1. Explain the procedure to the patient.	1. Knowing what to expect increases patient compliance.
2. Determine the most comfortable place for the patient during fluid/medication administration and help the patient into a semi-Fowler position.	
3. Organize equipment within reach and prepare it for use.	3. If intravenous fluids are being administered or if the medication is diluted in a bag/bottle of intravenous fluids, spike the fluid container with the intravenous tubing and prime the tubing and attached needle.
4. Wipe the injection port with an alcohol swab.	
5. Insert the needle of the syringe containing sterile normal saline, aspirate a blood return to ensure position of the heparin lock, and inject 2 ml of saline.	5. This step flushes heparin from the catheter. Do not force injection if resistance is met.
6. Remove the needle and syringe and recap the needle.	
7. Insert the intravenous fluid or medication needle.	

8. Inject the medication slowly or infuse the intravenous fluid at the prescribed rate.
9. Observe the patient for side effects of the medication.
10. Remove the needle when the medication or fluid has been infused.
11. Insert the needle of the syringe containing sterile normal saline and inject the remaining 2 ml of saline.
12. Remove the needle and syringe.
13. Insert the needle of the syringe containing the heparinized solution and inject the solution.
14. Remove the needle and syringe.
15. Clean the injection port with an alcohol swab.
16. Dispose of equipment.

8. Medications diluted in intravenous fluids should be infused at the rate recommended on the package insert.

10. Remember to clamp intravenous tubing before removal.

13. The heparinized solution fills the lock and helps ensure future patency.

DOCUMENTATION

1. The date and time of administration.
2. The intravenous fluids, medications, dilutants (specify amount), and rates of infusion.
3. The administration of sterile normal saline (specify amount) and heparinized solution (specify amount).
4. Patient's response to the procedure.

UNIT 14

Heparin Lock (Wing-tipped Needle Insertion) Procedure

PURPOSE

- To provide an available site for short-term intermittent intravenous therapy or medication administration.

EQUIPMENT

- wing-tipped heparin lock needle
- alcohol swabs
- sterile 4×4 gauze pads
- tourniquet
- povidone-iodine ointment
- air occlusive tape
- polyurethane film dressing (optional)

CONTRAINDICATIONS

Venipuncture is contraindicted in veins with hematomas. Do not place in the arm on the operative side of a postmastectomy patient. Arteriovenous shunts should also be left undisturbed, utilizing the patient's opposite arm.

Special Note. Assess that the patient and family are willing and able to assume the activities related to management of the heparin lock. Evaluate the sanitary practices in the home, as this is a sterile procedure and care of the heparin lock must be done under aseptic technique.

Steps	Key Points
1. Explain the procedure to the patient/family.	1. Knowing what to expect increases patient/family compliance.
2. Help the patient into a comfortable semi-Fowler or supine position, with arms extended.	
3. Organize the equipment within reach.	
4. Inspect the patient's arms for a straight prominent vein that is not swollen, inflamed, or irritated.	4. Pulsating vessels are arteries and should be avoided.
5. Select a venipuncture site.	5. Begin selection of venipuncture site at the distal end of the veins. Avoid joints as needles are easily dislodged at these sites by patient movement.

6. Apply the tourniquet 2 to 6 in above the selected site and tell the patient to clench his or her fist.
7. Palpate the selected vein.

6. The tourniquet should not occlude the distal arterial pulse.

7. The vein should rebound on palpation. A vein that rolls and/or is rigid is difficult to puncture.

Special Note. If the vein cannot be easily palpated remove the tourniquet and apply warm compresses over the selected site for 10 to 20 minutes.

8. Cleanse the selected site with an alcohol swab moving in a circular motion out from the site about 2 in.
9. Remove the cover from the needle.
10. Place the thumb of your nondominant hand slightly below the selected site and pull the skin taut.
11. Pinch the plastic flaps together; hold the needle with the bevel up at a 30- to 45-degree angle from the selected site.
12. Tell the patient that he or she will feel a stick and then pierce the skin.
13. Carefully insert the needle into the vein, decreasing the angle of the needle to 15 degrees.

8. Allow the alcohol to dry before inserting the needle.

10. This step helps stabilize the vein.

13. Slow introduction of the needle prevents puncture on the opposite side of the vein.

Special Note. Blood should begin flowing into the tubing.

14. Advance the needle and continue to decrease the angle until the needle is lying flat on the patient's arm.
15. Release the tourniquet and tell the patient to open his or her fist.
16. Secure the needle and tubing with air occlusive tape.
17. Apply povidone-iodine ointment to the venipuncture site.
18. Dress the site with either sterile 4 × 4 gauze pads and an occlusive dressing or with a polyurethane film dressing.
19. Write the date, time, type and size of needle, and your name on the dressing.
20. Swab the injection port with an alcohol wipe.
21. Insert the syringe with heparinized solution, inject the solution, and remove the syringe.
22. Swab the injection port with an alcohol wipe.

14. If the venipuncture is unsuccessful, try again with another sterile needle at a proximal site.

18. Keep the heparin lock's injection port exposed for access.

21. Be careful not to pierce the catheter tubing with the needle.

UNIT 14

23. Help the patient to a more comfortable position.
24. Dispose of equipment.
25. Instruct the patient and at least one other responsible family member regarding
    a. changing the dressing if it is soiled, wet, or opened
    b. signs and symptoms of infection (swelling, redness, tenderness)
    c. the importance of checking the site at regular intervals

    a. Stress the importance of aseptic technique.

    c. Visual inspection of the site is not necessary if the patient has no fever and feels no discomfort when the site is gently palpated through the dressing.

    d. covering the site with a plastic bag or plastic wrap when bathing
    e. steps to take if the needle becomes dislodged (remove the dressing and needle, apply pressure at the site for at least 5 minutes or until bleeding stops, cover the site with a Band-Aid, notify the nurse).
26. Plan to rotate the site every 72 hours, if possible and necessary.

    26. The rate of infection increases significantly after 72 hours.

27. Schedule visits so that the administration of intravenous fluids and medications is coordinated to enhance maintenance of the heparin lock's patency.

DOCUMENTATION

1. The date and time of the procedure.
2. The location of the heparin lock.
3. The type and size of the needle inserted.
4. The administration of heparinized solution (specify amount).
5. The patient's/family's response to the procedure.
6. The teaching done (names and relationships of persons taught other than the patient).
7. Plans for follow-up.

Implanted Venous Portal System (Accessing) Procedure

PURPOSE

- To establish entry into the implanted venous portal system.

EQUIPMENT

- povidone-iodine swabs
- sterile 4 × 4 gauze
- sterile gloves
- sterile drape
- Huber needle (20 or 22 gauge; straight or 90-degree angle)
- extension tubing with stopcock (must be compatible with implanted system)
- 10 ml syringe filled with normal saline

Steps

1. Explain the procedure to the patient/ family.
2. Wash your hands.
3. Locate the portal system.

4. Inspect the portal site and gently palpate the port between your fingers.
5. Locate the portal septum (rubber top of the port) with your fingers.
6. Clean the portal site with povidone-iodine.
7. Repeat step 6.
8. Wipe the excess povidone-iodine off the skin with a sterile 4 × 4 gauze.
9. Place the sterile drape on the patient near the portal site.
10. Open the sterile equipment (Huber needle, extension tubing) onto a sterile field.
11. Put on sterile gloves.
12. Attach the extension tubing to the filled 10-ml syringe.
13. Attach the extension tubing to the Huber needle.

Key Points

1. Knowing what to expect increases patient compliance.

3. A small bump in the middle to upper chest area may be seen and/or felt.
4. Notify the physician of signs and symptoms of inflammation (redness, tenderness, pain, swelling).

6. Start cleaning at the portal septum and move outward about 3 in, in a circular motion.

UNIT 14

14. Prime the extension tubing and Huber needle with 5 ml of normal saline.
15. Close the stopcock on the extension tubing.
16. Place the syringe and the extension tubing on the sterile drape while continuing to hold the Huber needle.
17. Locate the portal septum by palpation.
18. Push the Huber needle firmly through the skin and portal septum.

19. Open the stopcock and check for a blood return by aspirating the syringe.

14. Do not disconnect the syringe from the tubing.

18. Push until the needle hits the bottom of the portal chamber. Avoid tilting or rocking the Huber needle.
19. If blood does not return
    a. reposition the needle (do not remove it) and aspirate the syringe again
    b. change the patient's position and aspirate the syringe again
    c. flush with 5 ml of saline and aspirate the syringe again (do not flush if resistance is met)
    d. discontinue the procedure and notify the physician.

20. Inject the remaining 5 ml of normal saline.
21. Close the stopcock.

21. Always close the extension tubing when the Huber needle is in the portal chamber to prevent the introduction of air into the system.

22. Proceed with the
    a. heparinization
    b. withdrawing of blood.

DOCUMENTATION

1. The date and time of the procedure.
2. Size of the Huber needle.
3. Difficulties encountered and corrective actions.
4. Patient teaching done.
5. Patient's response to the procedure.

Implanted Venous Portal System (Heparinization) Procedure

PURPOSE

- To maintain patency of the implanted system.

EQUIPMENT

- 5-ml syringe filled with heparinized solution
- Band-aid

Special Note. Heparinization of the implanted system is done upon completion of a particular therapy (e.g., withdrawing blood) and at least once every 4 weeks when the system is not in use.

Steps

1. Follow steps 1 to 21 in the Implanted Venous Portal System (Accessing) Procedure.
2. Remove the empty syringe.
3. Attach the 5-ml syringe filled with heparinized solution.
4. Open the stopcock.
5. Slowly inject the heparinized solution.
6. While injecting the last 1 ml of heparinized solution, bend the extension tubing with your fingers until resistance is met.
7. Keeping the tubing bent, press down on the port with two fingers, and remove the Huber needle.
8. Apply a Band-aid to the site.

Key Points

6. This step will produce a heparin lock and prevent reflux when withdrawing the needle from the port.

DOCUMENTATION

1. The date and time of the procedure.
2. Amount of heparinized solution used.
3. Difficulties encountered and corrective actions.
4. Condition of the portal site.
5. Patient's response to the procedure.
6. Patient teaching done.

UNIT 14

Implanted Venous Portal System (Withdrawing Blood) Procedure

PURPOSE

- To draw blood for sampling purposes.

EQUIPMENT

- Vacu-tainer tube adapter
- laboratory tubes
- 5-ml syringe filled with heparinized solution

Steps	Key Points
1. Follow steps 1 to 21 in the Implanted Venous Portal System (Accessing) Procedure.	
2. Label one laboratory tube "discard."	
3. Remove the empty syringe.	
4. Connect the Vacu-tainer tube adapter.	
5. Insert the adapter needle into the laboratory tube labeled "discard" and open the stopcock.	5. This fluid will be discarded later.
6. Fill the tube, close the stopcock, and remove the tube.	6. Difficulty in withdrawing blood is usually due to the patient's position. Ask the patient to a. change position b. take a deep breath c. lift one or both arms.
7. Fill the other laboratory tubes following steps 5 and 6.	
8. Attach the 5-ml syringe filled with heparinized solution.	
9. Open the stopcock.	
10. Inject the heparinized solution slowly.	
11. While injecting the last 1 ml of heparinized solution, bend the extension tubing with your fingers until resistance is met.	11. This step will produce a heparin lock and prevent reflux when withdrawing the needle from the port.
12. Keeping the tubing bent, press down on the port with two fingers, and remove the Huber needle.	
13. Apply a Band-Aid to the site.	
14. Properly label all the laboratory tubes with the date, time, and patient's name.	

DOCUMENTATION

1. The date and time of the procedure.
2. Laboratory tests for which the blood was drawn.
3. Difficulties encountered and corrective actions.
4. Patient's response to the procedure.
5. Disposition of the laboratory tubes.

Indwelling Central Venous Catheter (Changing the Cap) Procedure

PURPOSE

- To maintain an adequate barrier between the patient's vascular system and the environment.
- To teach/demonstrate routine care of an indwelling central venous catheter to the patient/family.

EQUIPMENT

- sterile catheter cap
- cannula clamp/toothless hemostat/rubber-tipped hemostat
- alcohol wipes
- receptacle for used disposable supplies

Steps	*Key Points*
1. Review the procedure with the patient.	1. Knowing what to expect increases patient compliance.
2. Have the patient wash his or her hands.	2. Good handwashing is an essential component of clean technique.
3. Help the patient organize the supplies within his or her reach.	
4. Instruct the patient to clamp the catheter near the cap, over the taped portion of the catheter.	4. If the patient is using a rubber-tipped hemostat, he or she does not need to clamp over the tape.
5. Have the patient unscrew and discard the old cap.	
6. Have the patient wipe the end of the catheter with an alcohol wipe.	6. Remind the patient that this precaution is taken to reduce the chance of infection.
7. Instruct the patient to screw on the new cap.	7. Remind the patient to make sure the cap is screwed on tightly.
8. Have the patient unclamp the catheter.	

9. Instruct the patient
  a. about the critical need to keep the catheter clamped when changing the cap
  b. about the importance of using only a toothless hemostat, rubber-tipped hemostat, or cannula clamp
	
	  a. Air embolus is a potential complication if the catheter is not clamped.
	  b. Instruments with teeth can damage the catheter.

c. about the importance of clamping over tape if using a toothless hemostat or a cannula clamp

d. to change the cap at least once a week.

10. Teach the patient what to do if air enters the catheter.

a. clamp the catheter
b. telephone the doctor
c. lie down on his or her left side with his or her head lower than the body
d. follow the doctor's further instructions.

11. Have the patient demonstrate the procedure without nursing assistance.

12. Teach the procedure to at least one other responsible family member.

c. Clamping over the tape reduces the risk of damage to the catheter.

10. The patient should follow steps 10.a to 10.d if he or she experiences chest pain, cyanosis, dyspnea, or confusion.

11. Repeat this step on future visits to assess whether the patient has correctly learned and is compliant with the procedure.

12. It is important for another family member to know the procedure in the event the patient is unable to change the catheter cap.

DOCUMENTATION

1. The teaching, procedure, quality of the return demonstration, and name plus relationship of the person taught, if other than the patient.
2. The patient's/family's response to the procedure.
3. Plans for follow-up.

Indwelling Central Venous Catheter (Dressing Change) Procedure

PURPOSE

- To observe the exit site.
- To prevent infection at the exit site.
- To teach/demonstrate routine care of an indwelling central venous catheter to the patient/family.

EQUIPMENT

- hydrogen peroxide
- sterile swabs
- povidone-iodine ointment/swabs
- alcohol swabs
- sterile 2×2 gauze (precut)
- sterile 4×4 gauze
- paper tape
- paper bag to dispose of used supplies

Special Note. Never use acetone on the catheter, as it will cause the silicone to deteriorate.

Steps	*Key Points*
1. Review the procedure with the patient.	1. Knowing what to expect increases patient compliance.
2. Have the patient wash his or her hands.	2. Good handwashing is an essential component of clean technique.
3. Help the patient organize the supplies within his or her reach.	
4. Instruct the patient to remove the old dressing.	4. Discard the old dressing into the paper bag.
5. Have the patient inspect the exit site for any signs of infection (redness, swelling, tenderness, drainage).	5. Remind the patient to notify the nurse/physician if these signs are present.
6. Have the patient clean the exit site with hydrogen peroxide, using the sterile swabs.	6. Remind the patient to start cleaning at the exit site and move outward, about 3 in, in a circular motion.
7. Instruct the patient to remove old tape and clean the catheter from the exit site to the distal catheter end with an alcohol swab.	7. Remind the patient not to tug or pull on the catheter.
8. Have the patient apply povidone-iodine ointment to the exit site.	8. Be sure the patient includes the inferior side by gently lifting the catheter up from his or her chest wall.

9. Instruct the patient to apply a precut sterile 2×2 gauze to the exit site and to secure it with paper tape.
10. Have the patient wrap the catheter with tape about 3 in from its distal end. Show the patient how to fold the tape ends to make tabs for easy removal.
11. Have the patient loop the catheter on the dressing with the cap pointing upward.
12. Have the patient cover the looped catheter with a sterile 4×4 gauze and tape it occlusively in place.
13. Instruct the patient
    a. to change the dressing every other day or when it becomes wet, soiled, or opened
    b. about the signs and symptoms of infection (redness, swelling, tenderness, fatigue, fever, anorexia)
    c. about the importance of good handwashing.
14. Have the patient demonstrate the procedure without nursing assistance.

15. Teach the procedure to at least one other responsible family member.

9. Remind the patient to never use scissors near the line.

10. If the patient's standard supplies include a rubber-tipped hemostat, the tape is unnecessary.

11. Remind the patient to make sure there are no kinks in the line.

12. Remind the patient that the catheter cap should extend beyond the 4×4 gauze.

14. Repeat this step on future visits to assess whether the patient has correctly learned and is compliant with the procedure.

15. It is important for another family member to know the procedure in the event that the patient is unable to change the dressing.

DOCUMENTATION

1. The teaching, procedure, quality of the return demonstration, and name plus relationship of the person taught, if other than the patient.
2. The appearance of the exit site.
3. The patient's/family's response to the procedure.
4. Plans for follow-up.

Indwelling Central Venous Catheter (Heparinization) Procedure

PURPOSE

- To maintain patency of the catheter when it is not in use, i.e., not connected to an infusing solution.
- To teach/demonstrate routine care of an indwelling central venous catheter to the patient/family.

EQUIPMENT

- heparinized solution (amount/strength prescribed by the patient's physician)
- alcohol wipes
- sterile syringe with 25-gauge needle
- cannula clamp/toothless hemostat/rubber-tipped hemostat

Steps	Key Points
1. Review the procedure with the patient.	1. Knowing what to expect increases patient compliance.
2. Have the patient wash his or her hands.	2. Good handwashing is an essential component of clean technique.
3. Help the patient organize the supplies within his or her reach.	
4. Have the patient wipe the top of the heparinized solution bottle with an alcohol swab.	
5. Instruct the patient to inject an amount of air equal to the amount of solution to be withdrawn into the heparinized solution vial.	
6. Have the patient turn the vial upside down and withdraw the desired amount of heparinized solution.	6. Remind the patient to make sure there are no air bubbles in the syringe.

Special Note. If the patient contaminates the equipment he or she should begin the procedure again with fresh sterile supplies.

7. Have the patient wipe the catheter cap with an alcohol swab.	7. Remind the patient to let the catheter cap air dry.
8. Instruct the patient to inject all but the last 0.5 ml of heparinized solution into the center of the cap.	8. Remind the patient to be very careful not to pierce the catheter with the needle.

Special Note. If any resistance is felt when injecting the heparinized solution, the patient should stop the procedure and notify the nurse/physician.

9. Instruct the patient to clamp the catheter.

10. Have the patient inject the last 0.5 ml of solution.

11. Have the patient remove the needle and syringe, wipe the catheter cap with an alcohol wipe, and unclamp the catheter.

12. Instruct the patient to flush the catheter with heparinized solution once a day.

13. Have the patient demonstrate the procedure without nursing assistance.

14. Teach the procedure to at least one other responsible family member.

9. If using a toothless hemostat or a cannula clamp, clamp over the taped portion of the catheter.

10. This step creates positive pressure in the catheter, thus preventing back-flow and clotting of blood.

12. More frequent flushing may be necessary if the patient is receiving intravenous fluids on an intermittent basis.

13. Repeat this step on future visits to assess whether the patient has correctly learned and is compliant with the procedure.

14. It is important for another family member to know the procedure in the event the patient is unable to heparinize the catheter.

DOCUMENTATION

1. The teaching, procedure, difficulties encountered, corrective actions, quality of the return demonstration, and name plus relationship of the person taught, if other than the patient.

2. The patient's/family's response to the procedure.

3. Plans for follow-up.

UNIT 14

Indwelling Central Venous Catheter (Withdrawing Blood) Procedure

PURPOSE

- To draw blood for sampling purposes.

EQUIPMENT

- 10-ml syringe with an attached needle
- syringe for drawing blood samples (syringe size determined by amount of blood needed for laboratory tests)
- laboratory tubes
- 10-ml syringe filled with heparinized solution
- cannula clamp/toothless hemostat/rubber-tipped hemostat
- sterile 25-gauge, 1-in needle

Steps	*Key Points*
1. Explain the procedure to the patient.	1. Knowing what to expect reduces patient anxiety.
2. Wash your hands.	
3. Clamp the catheter.	3. If using a toothless hemostat or a cannula clamp, clamp over the taped portion of the catheter.
4. Remove the catheter cap.	4. Remove the needle from the empty 10-ml syringe and attach it to the catheter.
5. Securely connect the empty 10-ml syringe to the catheter.	
6. Remove the clamp.	
7. Withdraw 6 ml of fluid.	7. This fluid may be discarded later.
8. Reclamp the catheter and disconnect the syringe.	
9. Securely connect the sampling syringe.	
10. Unclamp the catheter and withdraw the amount of blood necessary for the laboratory tests.	10. Difficulty in withdrawing blood is usually due to the patient's position. Ask the patient to a. change position b. take a deep breath c. lift one or both arms. If difficulty persists, do not use force in withdrawal attempts. Notify the attending physician.

11. Reclamp the catheter and remove the sampling syringe.
12. Securely connect the 6-ml syringe with the heparinized solution.
13. Unclamp the catheter and inject all but 0.5 ml of the solution.
14. Reclamp the catheter and inject the remining solution.

15. Remove the syringe and replace the catheter cap.
16. Unclamp the catheter.
17. Transfer the blood from the sampling syringe to the laboratory tube.

11. Attach the sampling syringe to the sterile 25-gauge needle.

14. This step creates positive pressure in the line, thus clearing the catheter of blood and preventing its backflow into the catheter.
15. Remember to detach the cap from the needle.

17. Properly label all the laboratory tubes with the time, date, and patient's name.

DOCUMENTATION

1. The procedure, difficulties encountered, actions taken, and laboratory tests for which the blood was drawn.
2. The patient's/family's response to the procedure.
3. Disposition of the laboratory tubes.

UNIT 14

Intravenous Therapy Procedure

PURPOSE

- To provide a peripheral site for short-term administration of intravenous fluids.

EQUIPMENT

- over-the-needle catheter ("Angiocath")
- alcohol swabs
- sterile 4×4 gauze pads
- povidone-iodine ointment
- air occlusive tape
- polyurethane film dressing (optional)
- intravenous fluid (amount and type per physician's prescription)
- intravenous tubing
- intravenous pole or substitute
- tourniquet

CONTRAINDICATIONS

Venipuncture is contraindicated in veins with hematomas. Do not place in the arm on the operative side of a post-mastectomy patient. Arteriovenous shunts should also be left undisturbed, utilizing the patient's opposite arm.

Special Note. Assess that the patient and family are willing and able to assume the activities related to management of intravenous therapy. Evaluate the sanitary practices in the home, as this is a sterile procedure and care of the peripheral line must be done under aseptic technique.

Steps	Key Points
1. Explain the procedure to the patient/family.	1. Knowing what to expect increases patient/family compliance.
2. Determine the most comfortable place for the patient during intravenous therapy and help the patient into a semi-Fowler position.	
3. Organize equipment within reach.	
4. Spike the fluid container with the intravenous tubing, prime the tubing, and clamp it.	4. Label the tubing with date and time.
5. Inspect the patient's arms for a straight prominent vein that is not swollen, inflamed, or irritated.	5. Pulsating vessels are arteries and should be avoided.

6. Select a venipuncture site.

6. Begin selection of the venipuncture site at the distal end of the veins. Avoid joints as needles are easily dislodged at these sites by the patient's movements.

7. Apply the tourniquet 2 to 6 in above the selected site and tell the patient to clench his or her fist.

7. The tourniquet should not occlude the distal arterial pulse.

8. Palpate the selected vein.

8. The vein should rebound on palpation. A vein that rolls and/or is rigid is difficult to puncture.

Special Note. If the vein cannot be easily palpated, remove the tourniquet and apply warm compresses over the selected site for 10 to 20 minutes.

9. Cleanse the selected site with an alcohol swab, moving in a circular motion out from the site about 2 in.

9. Allow the alcohol to dry before inserting the needle.

10. Place the thumb of your nondominant hand slightly below the selected site and pull the skin taut.

10. This step helps stabilize the vein.

11. Hold the angiocath with the bevel up at a 30- to 45-degree angle from the selected site.

12. Tell the patient that he or she will feel a stick and then pierce the skin.

13. Carefully insert the needle into the vein, decreasing the angle of the needle to 15 degrees.

13. Slow introduction of the needle prevents puncture on the opposite side of the vein.

Special Note. Blood should begin flowing into the plastic hub of the needle.

14. Advance the catheter into the vein until its hub rests at the venipuncture site.

14. Secure the needle hub with one hand to prevent its advancement. Do not remove the needle.

15. Release the tourniquet and tell the patient to open his or her fist.

16. Withdraw the needle from the catheter and attach the primed intravenous tubing.

16. Prompt connection of the intravenous tubing prevents uncontrollable blood return.

17. Open the roller clamp slowly and observe the venipuncture site.

18. Secure the catheter and tubing with air occlusive tape.

19. Apply povidone-iodine ointment to the venipuncture site.

20. Dress the venipuncture site with either sterile 4 × 4 gauze pads and an occlusive dressing or a polyurethane film dressing.
21. Write the time, date, type and size catheter, and your name on the dressing.
22. Adjust the infusion rate per the physician's prescription.
23. Dispose of equipment.
24. Instruct the patient and at least one other responsible family member regarding
    a. changing the dressing if it is wet, soiled, or opened
    b. keeping the drip chamber at least half full but not completely full
    c. how to monitor the drip rate
    d. how to change fluid containers when necessary
    e. importance of not using fluids that are cloudy or have particulate matter
    f. importance of checking the site at regular intervals

    g. signs and symptoms of infection/infiltration (redness, swelling, tenderness)

    h. steps to take if the catheter becomes dislodged (remove the catheter and dressing, apply pressure at the site for at least 5 minutes or until the bleeding stops, cover site with a Band-Aid, notify the nurse)
    i. covering the site with a plastic bag or plastic wrap when bathing
    j. wearing clothes with large sleeves to facilitate changing.

20. If necessary, immobilize the extremity with an arm board or splint.

    a. Stress the importance of aseptic technique.

    d. When 10 ml is remaining in the fluid container, a new container should be placed near the patient for easy accessibility.

    f. Visual inspection of the site is not necessary if the patient has no fever and feels no discomfort when the site is gently palpated through the dressing.
    g. Stress the importance of notifying the nurse immediately if the patient experiences pain at the venipuncture site, increased skin temperature at the site, or erythema along the vein of the venipuncture.
    h. Be sure the patient/family has a telephone number that gives them 24-hour access to a professional nurse.

25. Plan to
    a. rotate the venipuncture site every 72 hours, if possible and necessary
    b. change the intravenous tubing every 48 hours
    c. change the fluid container every 24 hours (if more frequent changes are not dictated by infusion rate)
    d. assess the patient for changes in fluid and electrolyte status and signs and symptoms of infiltration, infection, and phlebitis.
26. Discontinue the intravenous therapy when the prescribed course of treatment is completed.

a. The rate of infection increases significantly after 72 hours.

DOCUMENTATION

1. The date and time of the procedure.
2. The location and status of the intravenous venipuncture site.
3. The type and size of the catheter inserted.
4. The prescribed/administered fluid, infusion rate, and time begun.
5. The patient's/family's response to the procedure.
6. The teaching done (names and relationships of persons taught other than the patient).
7. Plan for follow-up.

UNIT
14

Venipuncture Procedure

PURPOSE

- To obtain blood samples for analysis.

EQUIPMENT

- alcohol swabs
- sterile 2×2 gauze
- rubber tourniquet
- Band-Aid
- Vacu-tainer with needle holder
- sterile double-ended needle (20- to 21-gauge for adults; 23- to 25-gauge for children)
- appropriate blood tubes
- laboratory requisitions

CONTRAINDICATIONS

Venipuncture is contraindicated in veins with hematomas or near intravenous infusion sites. Do not place in the arm on the operative side of a post-mastectomy patient. Arteriovenous shunts should also be left undisturbed, utilizing the patient's opposite arm.

Steps	Key Points
1. Explain the procedure to the patient/family.	1. Knowing what to expect increases patient/family compliance.
2. Assess that the patient has been NPO (nothing by mouth), if necessary.	
3. Assess the patient's ability to cooperate during the procedure.	3. Ask family members to restrain and/or hold a confused/restless patient or child.
4. Help patient into a comfortable semi-Fowler or supine position, with arms extended.	
5. Inspect the patient's arms for a straight prominent vein that is not swollen, inflamed, or irritated.	5. Pulsating vessels are arteries and should be avoided.
6. Select a venipuncture site (for adults, the antecubital fossa site is most often used; for children, veins on the dorsal aspect of the foot are used).	
7. Apply the tourniquet 2 to 6 in above the selected site.	7. The tourniquet should not occlude the distal arterial pulse.

8. Palpate the selected vein.

8. The vein should rebound on palpation. A vein that rolls and/or is rigid is difficult to puncture.

Special Note. If the vein cannot be easily palpated, remove the tourniquet and apply warm compresses over the selected site for 10 to 20 minutes.

9. Cleanse the venipuncture site with an alcohol wipe, moving in a circular motion out from the site about 2 in.

9. Allow the alcohol to dry before inserting the needle.

10. Screw the double-ended needle into the Vacu-tainer

11. Place a blood tube in the Vacu-tainer, resting the rubber stopper against the shorter needle end.

11. Do not puncture the blood tube's rubber top.

12. Remove the needle cover.

13. Place the thumb of your nondominant hand about 1 in below the selected venipuncture site and pull the skin taut.

13. This step helps stabilize the vein.

14. Hold the Vacu-tainer at a 15- to 30-degree angle from the patient's arm with the bevel up.

15. Tell the patient that he or she will feel a stick and then pierce the skin.

16. Carefully insert the needle into the vein.

16. Slow introduction of the needle prevents puncture on the opposite side of the vein.

17. Hold the Vacu-tainer firmly and advance the blood tube against the needle.

17. Take care not to further advance the needle into the patient's arm.

Special Note. Blood should immediately begin flowing into the tube. If it does not, either the vacuum in the tube has been lost or the needle is not in the vein.

19. Once the blood tube is filled, remove it. Insert and fill additional tubes as needed.

19. Be careful with each removal and insertion to firmly hold the Vacu-tainer and not to dislodge the needle.

20. Place a sterile 2 × 2 gauze pad over the puncture site.

20. Do not apply pressure.

21. Withdraw the needle from the vein and immediately apply pressure to the site.

21. Maintain pressure for 1 to 3 min or until the bleeding stops.

Special Note. Patients receiving anticoagulants may require pressure over the site for at least 5 minutes.

22. Apply the Band-Aid to the puncture site.

UNIT 14

23. Gently rotate all blood tubes containing additives. Do not shake.

23. Do not shake the tubes as shaking can cause hemolysis of the red blood cells (RBCs) and inaccurate test results.

24. Help the patient to a more comfortable position.
25. Securely attach identification label and requisition forms to the blood tubes per agency procedure.

25. Transfer blood samples to laboratory per agency procedure.

26. Dispose of equipment.
27. Wash your hands.

DOCUMENTATION

1. The date and time of the procedure.
2. The patient's response to the procedure.
3. The blood specimens taken (specify tests).
4. The location and condition of the venipuncture site after the specimen collection.

Bibliography

Birdsall, C. What are Dos and Don'ts for Hickman/Broviac Catheters. American Journal of Nursing, 86(4): 1986, pp. 385.

Cozad, J. Indwelling Central Venous Catheters. Point of View, 22(3): 1985, pp. 14–15.

Hower, D. Using Special I.V. Lines at Home. Nursing 17(7): 1987, pp. 56–58.

Klass, K. Trouble-shooting Central Line Complications. Nursing, 11:1987, pp. 58–61.

Moore C. L. et al. Nursing Care and Management of Venous Access Ports. Oncology Nursing Forum, 13(3): 1987, pp. 35–39.

Schakenbach, L. and Dennis, M. And Now, a Quad-lumen I.V. Catheter. Nursing, 15(11): 50 November, 1985.

Wainstock, J. Make a Choice: The Venous Access Method You Prefer. Oncology Nursing Forum, 14(1): 1987, pp. 79–82.

APPENDICES

Appendix A

General Bibliography

Bates, B. A Guide to Physical Examination, 3rd ed. Philadelphia: J. B. Lippincott Co., 1983.

Borden, J. W. Nurses as Health Teachers: A Practical Guide. Philadelphia: W. B. Saunders Co., 1987.

Brunner, L. and Suddarth, D. The Lippincott Manual of Nursing Practice, 5th ed. Philadelphia: J. B. Lippincott Co., 1987.

Govoni, L. E. and Hayes, J. E. Drugs and Nursing Implications, 5th ed. Norwalk, Connecticut: Appleton-Century-Crofts, 1985.

Griffith, H. W. Instructions for Patients, 3rd ed. Philadelphia: W. B. Saunders Co., 1982.

Kim, M., McFarland, J. A., and McLane, A. (eds.). Pocket Guide to Nursing Diagnoses. St. Louis: C. V. Mosby Co., 1984.

Lederer, J. et al. Care Planning Pocket Guide: A Nursing Diagnoses Approach. Menlo Park, California: Addison-Wesley Publishing Co., 1986.

Luckmann, J. and Sorensen, K. Medical-Surgical Nursing: A Psychophysiologic Approach. Philadelphia: W. B. Saunders Co., 1987.

Metheny, N. M. Fluid and Electrolyte Balance: Nursing Consideration. Philadelphia: J. B. Lippincott Co., 1987.

National Association of Orthopaedic Nurses. Core Curriculum for Orthopaedic Nurses. Pitman, New Jersey, 1986.

Redman, B. K. The Process of Patient Education, 5th ed. St. Louis: C. V. Mosby Co., 1984.

Smith, C. E. (ed.). Patient Education: Nurses in Partnership with Other Health Professionals. Orlando, Florida: Grune & Stratton, 1987.

Ulrich, S. P., Canale, S. W., and Wendell, S. A. Nursing Care Planning Guides. Philadelphia: W. B. Saunders Co., 1986.

Whitman, N. I. et al. Teaching in Nursing Practice: A Professional Model. Norwalk, Connecticut: Appleton-Century-Crofts, 1986.

Appendix B

Conversion Tables

Celsius	Fahrenheit	Celsius	Fahrenheit
34.0	93.2	38.6	101.5
34.2	93.6	38.8	101.8
34.4	93.9	39.0	102.2
34.6	94.3	39.2	102.6
34.8	94.6	39.4	102.9
35.0	95.0	39.6	103.3
35.2	95.4	39.8	103.6
35.4	95.7	40.0	104.0
35.6	96.1	40.2	104.4
35.8	96.4	40.4	104.7
36.0	96.8	40.6	105.2
36.2	97.2	40.8	105.4
36.4	97.5	41.0	105.9
36.6	97.9	41.2	106.1
36.8	98.2	41.4	106.5
37.0	98.6	41.6	106.8
37.2	99.0	41.8	107.2
37.4	99.3	42.0	107.6
37.6	99.7	42.2	108.0
37.8	100.0	42.4	108.3
38.0	100.4	42.6	108.7
38.2	100.8	42.8	109.0
38.4	101.1	43.0	109.4

$$(°C \times \tfrac{9}{5}) + 32 = °F \qquad (°F - 32) \times \tfrac{5}{9} = °C$$

°C = temperature in Celsius (centigrade) degrees
°F = temperature in Fahrenheit degrees

Weights and Measures

1 Tsp = 5 gm	2 Cups	= 16 oz
5 cc*	(approx)	1 lb
3 Tsp = 1 Tbsp		1 pt
1 Tbsp = 15 gm		480 gm
15 cc	4 Cups	= 1 quart
½ oz		2 pt
2 Tbsp = 1 oz		960 cc
= ⅛ cup	1 Pint	= 480 cc
30 cc		16 oz
30 gm		2 cups
4 Tbsp = 2 oz	1 Quart	= 960 cc
¼ cup		32 oz
8 Tbsp = 4 oz	4 Quarts	= 1 gallon
½ cup	1 Liter	= 1 kilogram
16 Tbsp = 8 oz		1000 cc
1 cup		2.2 lb
½ lb	1 oz Dry	= 28.35 gm
240 gm	1 oz Liquid	= 30 gm
1 Cup = ½ pt		2 Tbsp
8 oz		30cc
240 cc	1 Lb	= 480 gm
½ lb		0.45 kilogram

*The cubic centimeter (cc) is considered equivalent to 1 gram (1 cc = 1 gm). One ounce equals 28.35 gm. For computing purposes, 30 gm or 30 cc is considered equivalent to 1 oz.

Conversion Factors for Weight, Volume, and Length

Weight

Ounces	× 30*	= grams
Pounds	× 0.45	= kilograms
Grams	× 0.035	= ounces
Kilograms	× 2.2	= pounds

Volume

Tsp	× 5	= milliliters
Tbsp	× 15	= milliliters
Fl Ounce	× 30	= milliliters
Cups	× 0.24	= liters
Pints	× 0.47	= liters
Quarts	× 0.95	= liters
Gallons	× 3.8	= liters
Milliliters	× 0.03	= fluid ounces
Liters	× 2.1	= pints
Liters	× 1.06	= quarts
Liters	× 0.26	= gallons

Length

Inches	× 2.5	= centimeters
Feet	× 30	= centimeters
Yards	× 0.9	= meters
Millimeters	× 0.04	= inches
Centimeters	× 0.4	= inches
Meters	× 3.3	= feet
Meters	× 1.1	= yards

*The actual figure is 28.25.

Appendix C

This community resource list includes associations, foundations, and self-help groups you might wish to contact for additional information. The address of the national office is listed beneath the name of each organization. Use the space provided next to each name to fill in the local addresses and phone numbers of organizations you contact frequently.

NATIONAL OFFICE	LOCAL ADDRESS AND PHONE NUMBER

Alcoholics Anonymous
Box 459
Grand Central Station
New York, NY 10163

Alzheimer's Disease and Related Disorders
   Association, Inc.
70 East Lake Street
Suite 600
Chicago, IL 60601

American Allergy Association
Box 7273
Menlo Park, CA 94026

American Anorexia and Bulimia Association, Inc.
133 Cedar Lane
Teaneck, NJ 07666

American Cancer Society, Inc.
National Office
777 Third Avenue
New York, NY 10017

American Council for Healthful Living
439 Main Street
Orange, NJ 07050

American Diabetes Association
P. O. Box 25757
1660 Duke Street
Alexandria, VA 22313

American Foundation for the Blind
1800 Johnson Street
Baltimore, MD 21230

American Heart Association
7320 Greenville Avenue
Dallas, TX 75231

American Kidney Fund
7315 Wisconsin Avenue
Bethesda, MD 20814

American Liver Foundation
998 Pompton Avenue
Cedar Grove, NJ 07009

American Lung Association
1740 Broadway
New York, NY 10019

American Parkinson's Disease
  Association, Inc.
116 John Street
New York, NY 10038

American Occupational Therapy
  Association, Inc.
1383 Piccard Drive
P.O. Box 1725
Rockville, MD 20850-4375

American Physical Therapy Association
1156 15th Street, NW
Washington, DC 20005

American Social Health Association
P.O. Box 100
Palo Alto, CA 94302

American Speech and Hearing Association
1081 Rockville Pike
Rockville, MD 20852

Amyotrophic Lateral Sclerosis Society
  of America
15300 Ventura Boulevard
Suite 315
Sherman Oaks, CA 91413

Anorexia Nervosa and Associated
  Disorders, Inc. (ANAD)
P.O. Box 271
Highland Park, IL 60035

Arthritis Foundation
1314 Spring Street, NW
Atlanta, GA 30309

Autism Helpline and Information
  Clearinghouse
123 Franklin Corner Road
Suite 215
Lawrenceville, NJ 08648

Cancer Information Service
(800)4-CANCER

Cystic Fibrosis Foundation
6931 Arlington Road
Bethesda, MD 20814

Division for the for the Blind and Physically
  Handicapped
Library of Congress
Washington, DC 20542

Epilepsy Foundation of America
4351 Garden City Drive
Landover, MD 20785

Herpes Resource Center
P.O. Box 13827
Research Triangle Park, NC 27709

International Association of
  Laryngectomees
c/o American Cancer Society
90 Park Avenue
New York, NY 10016

Leukemia Society of America
733 Third Avenue
New York, NY 10017

Make Today Count
514 Tama Building
Box 303
Burlington, Iowa 52601

Muscular Dystrophy Association of
  America, Inc.
810 Seventh Avenue
New York, NY 10019

National Alliance for the Mentally Ill
1901 North Fort Meyer Drive
Suite 500
Arlington, VA 22209

National Anorexic Aid Society, Inc.
5796 Karl Road
Columbus, Ohio 43229

National Cancer Institute
Bethesda, MD 20205

Narcotics Anonymous
P.O. Box 9999
Van Nuys, CA 92409

National Kidney Foundation
116 E. 27th Street
New York, NY 10016

National Multiple Sclerosis Society
205 East 42nd Street
New York, NY 10017

National Self Help Clearinghouse
City University of New York
Graduate Center
Room 1206A
New York, NY 10036

National Sudden Infant Death
   Syndrome Foundation
8200 Professional Place
Suite 104
Landover, MD 20785

Self Help for Hard of Hearing People, Inc.
7800 Wisconsin Avenue
Bethesda, MD 20814

Society for the Right to Die
250 West 57th Street
New York, NY 10107

United Cerebral Palsy Association, Inc.
66 East 34th Street
New York, NY 10016

United Ostomy Association
2001 West Beverly Boulevard
Los Angeles, CA 90057-2491

Index